Eat to Beat Illness

80 Simple, Delicious Recipes Inspired by
the Science of Food as Medicine

DR. RUPY AUJLA

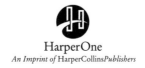

HarperOne
An Imprint of HarperCollins*Publishers*

HarperOne

EAT TO BEAT ILLNESS © 2019 by Rupy Aujla. All rights reserved. Printed in Canada.
No part of this book may be used or reproduced in any manner whatsoever without written permission except in the case of brief quotations embodied in critical articles and reviews. For information, address HarperCollins Publishers, 195 Broadway, New York, NY 10007.

HarperCollins books may be purchased for educational, business, or sales promotional use. For information, please email the Special Markets Department at SPsales@harpercollins.com.

Originally published as *The Doctor's Kitchen: Eat to Beat Illness* in the United Kingdom in 2019 by Thorsons, an imprint of HarperCollins UK.

FIRST US EDITION

Photography © Faith Mason 2019
Food stylist: Marina Filippelli
Prop stylist: Sarah Birks

Library of Congress Cataloging in Publication Data is available upon request.

ISBN 978-0-06-291628-0

19 20 21 22 23 TC 10 9 8 7 6 5 4 3 2 1

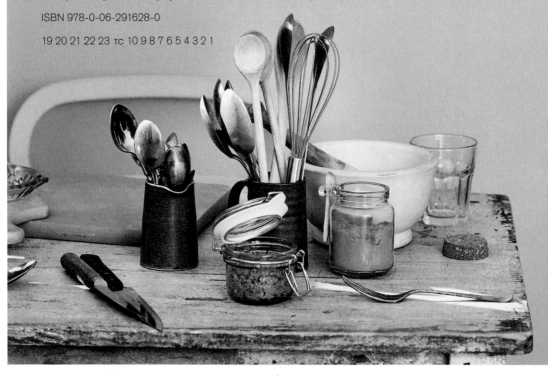

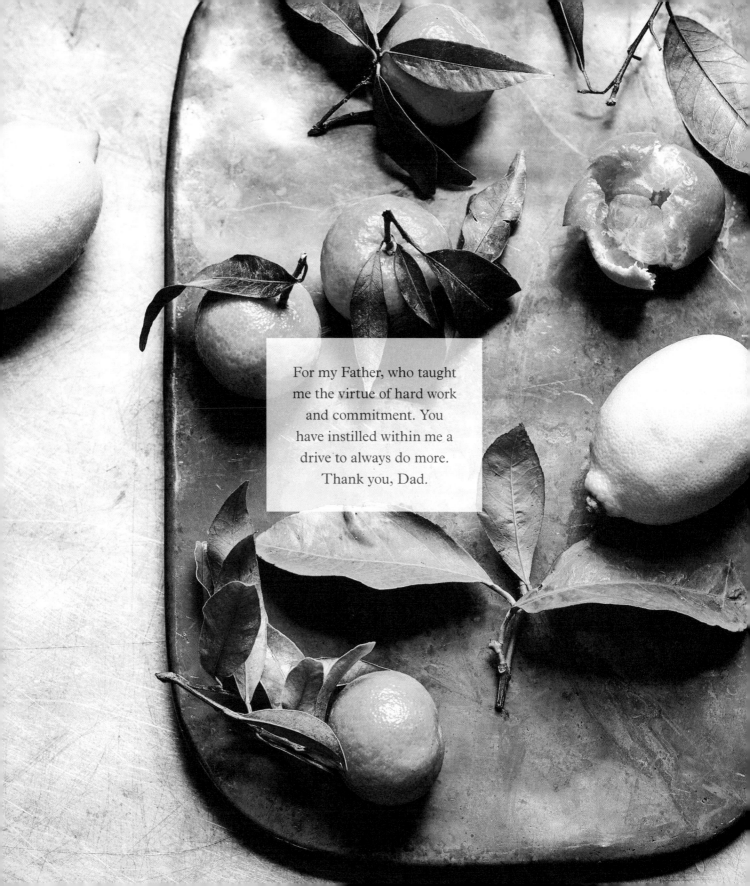

For my Father, who taught
me the virtue of hard work
and commitment. You
have instilled within me a
drive to always do more.
Thank you, Dad.

CONTENTS

Introduction 6

Eat for Your Brain 12

Eat for Your Heart 22

Eat for Inflammation 34

Eat for Immunity 48

Eat to Beat Cancer 62

Eat for Your Mood 74

Eat for Your Skin 86

Eat for Your Eyes 98

Eating and Living for
Ultimate Health 108

Recipes

Breakfast

Cajun Sweet Potato Hash 116
One-Pan Greek Breakfast 119
One-Pan Cajun Scramble 119
One-Pan Spicy Bean and Mushroom
   Breakfast 120
Watercress, Walnut, and Crayfish 121
Pimenton Oats with Poached Salmon 122
Wild Mushroom and Herb Frittata 124
Oats and Butter Bean Breakfast 125
My Best Breakfast Bowl 127

Small plates

Greek Skewers with Tzatziki 130
Spring Asparagus, Peas, and Scallops with
   Tarragon Butter 133
Sage Eggplant and Broccoli 134
Sri Lankan–Style Oats 135
Speedy Gazpacho 137
Lemon, Thyme, and Hazelnut Roast
   Vegetables 138
Cajun Corn Bites 141
Citrus and Pineapple Asian Salad 142
Herby Cauliflower Steaks 145
Fennel and Carrots with Star Anise 146
Almond and Hazelnut Lentils with Capers 147
Radicchio, Peach, and Fennel Salad
   with Balsamic Croutons 148
Baked Rainbow Chard with Apricot
   and Walnuts 151
Fennel, Cumin, and Mackerel Salad 152
Polenta and Greens 153
Greek-Style Giant Beans 154

Rapid meals

Carrot and Zucchini Laksa 158
Spinach and Sorrel Borscht 161
Rendang Stir-Fry 162
Harissa Beans and Greens 164
Butter Beans, Butternut Squash, and
   Spicy Couscous 165
Creole Couscous with White Beans
   and Parsley 166
Black Bean Goulash 167
Pea Orecchiette with Purple Sprouting
   Broccoli and Hazelnuts 169
Spanish Chickpea Stew with Roasted Peppers 170

Spicy Peanut and Lime Stir-Fry	172
Sunflower Sprouts with Caraway and Porcini Mushrooms	173
5-Spice Sticky Eggplant Bake	175
Cod Bites with Lemon and Seaweed	176
Sweet Cajun Salmon	179
Fennel Sardines with Pine Nuts	180
Chili and Lime Fish Skewers with Mint and Red Cabbage Salad	181
Heirloom Tomatoes, Horta, and Mackerel	182

Main meals

Seasonal Soup with Red Pesto	186
Roast Walnut and Squash Medley with Persillade	188
Chicken Thighs with Red Onion, Apple, and Chestnuts	190
Glazed Asian Vegetable Rice Bowls	193
Crispy Mushroom Bowl	194
Herby Walnut and Cashew Roast	195
Eggplant and Walnut Ragu	197
Aromatic Vietnamese Pho	199
Okra and Lentil Curry with Buckwheat Uttapam	200
Sri Lankan Cashew Curry	203
Jambalaya	204
Thyme and Ginger Comfort Soup	207
Parsnip and Butternut Squash with Flatbreads	208
Umami Mushroom Tacos	210
Poke Bowl	211
Ethiopian Berbere Curry	213
Asian-Style Lettuce Wraps with Mint and Thai Basil	214
Roast Squash Curry with Cashew Sauce	216
Herbes de Provence Chicken Skewers	217
Coconut Chicken with Spicy Peas and Potato	219
Mussels in Parsley and Lemon Dressing with Rye Croutons	220
Spinach and Vegetable Lasagne	222
Split Green Pea and Pearl Barley Pan	223
Vibrant Malay Salad	225
Thai-Style Salmon Burgers	226
Bengali-Style Cod	228
Celeriac and Broad Bean Rendang Curry	229

Desserts

Coconut Bananas with Maple Cream	232
Candied Almonds with Spiced Strawberries	234
Roasted Apricots with Cardamom and Lime	235
Orange-Zest Chocolate Bark with Berries	237
Banana Berry Scoops	238
Glazed Peaches with Thyme	241

Pastes, spices, and teas

Creole Spice Blend	245
Rupy's Ras El Hanout	245
Malaysian Laksa Paste	246
Rendang Curry Paste	246
Chili Melon Relish	249
Roasted Red Pepper Salsa	249
Aromatic Citrus-ade	250
Fresh Tea Blends	253

Notes	255
Index	264
Acknowledgments	271

Introduction

My name is Rupy. I'm a National Health Service medical doctor, I founded the non-profit Culinary Medicine UK, and I'm passionate about teaching everybody how to use food and lifestyle as medicine. I firmly believe the key to a happy, healthy life starts in our kitchen. *Eat to Beat Illness* is a blueprint that demonstrates the intersection of diet and lifestyle factors across multiple medical specialties and shows you how you can improve your ultimate level of well-being today.

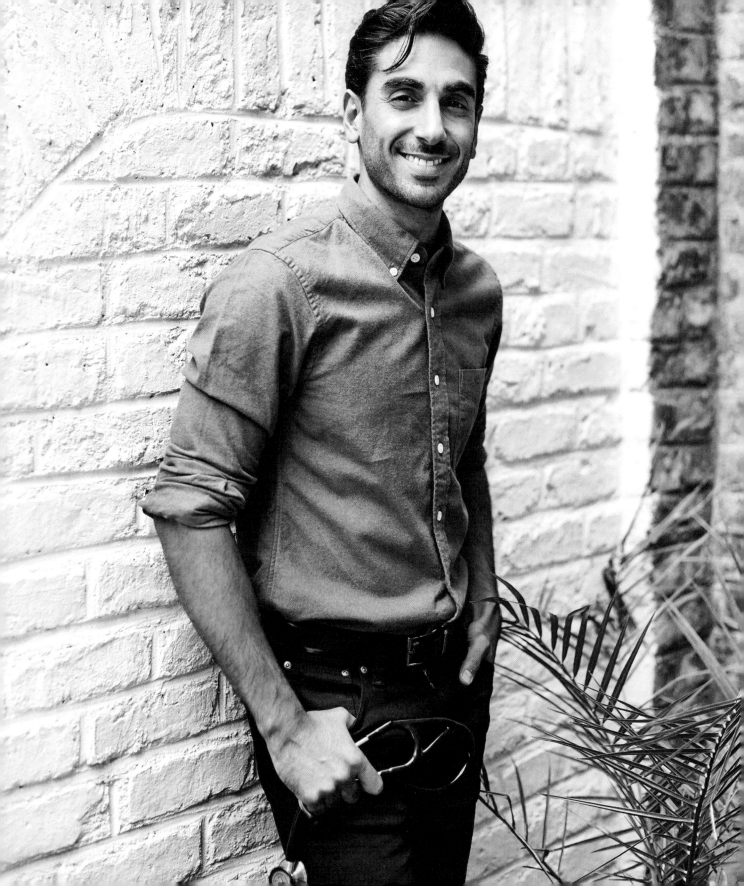

8   As a doctor, it's my responsibility to deliver credible, evidence-based information, which is why I'm very comfortable talking about the medicinal effects of eating well. Research is clearly demonstrating that improving our diet and lifestyle can enhance our health, and the traditional skepticism surrounding this topic is changing. More doctors are taking an active interest in this area either because of personal experience or anecdotes from their patients or simply because people are starting to demand more from their doctors than purely pharmaceutical fixes that are unsustainable.

    The decision about which topics to discuss in this new cookbook has been heavily influenced by my experience as a doctor. Patients often tell me that they didn't realize how food can impact a variety of conditions beyond heart disease and sugar control. Whether it's their bones, arthritis, skin, or even sleep and mood, I always have a chat with my patients about food and discuss the relevance of nutrition and lifestyle to their overall health. There is an incredible amount of research looking at the impact of diet, and it is the vital first step in the resolution of many problems. Every patient deserves this information, and this new book will give you an insight into why I'm so vocal about the subject.

    The principles of a healthy diet are simple: eat whole, colorful, mostly plant-based

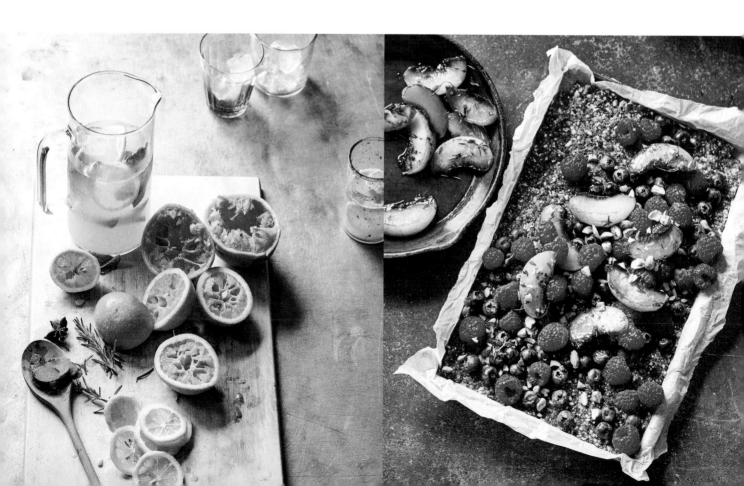

foods, including quality fats and plenty of fiber, and treat meat and fish as luxury items
rather than staples. You'll see this theme is woven throughout this book, and I'll also be
dissecting exactly why these principles are so important by showing how this way of eating
affects different conditions and parts of our body. Using the lens of science, the hundreds
of research papers I've read, and a good dose of common sense, I aim to demonstrate
exactly why our food can be so impactful on healthcare today.

Although I touched on the clear link between food and overall health in my first book,
The Doctor's Kitchen, here I examine in more depth how food affects our mental health,
making us think more clearly as well as protecting us from disease. I discuss the impact
of nutrition on skin quality and even how our eyes are affected by diet. It's a fascinating
and overwhelming field, but after reading these chapters you're going to be even more
motivated to eat well for life, and the simple recipes to complement the science will ease
you into a deliciously healthy lifestyle.

On this journey we're going to be talking about how simple changes to what you eat can
protect and amplify your body's own defenses against ill health. Your immune system can
be thought of as a complex network of specialized proteins, specific parts of the body, and
the population of microbes concentrated in your gut. I'll walk you through how nourishing
our bodies with incredible, accessible ingredients can ensure the correct functioning of our
immune systems. What's more exciting, however, is that the food choices I encourage you to
make are culturally diverse and vibrant. The complex flavors found in widely available spices,
for example, not only deliver exceptional taste, but have clear benefits to our health.

Most healthy-eating books concentrate on heart health and weight, but it's not
commonly recognized that lifestyle and nutrition can impact the most important organ in your
body—the brain. I'll be introducing you to a way of eating that embraces quality fats plus a
variety of colorful and exciting ingredients that have scientifically recognized benefits for the
brain. Eating a diet according to these principles helps protect you from one of the worst
diagnoses we as doctors have to deliver—dementia—while helping you achieve a sharper,
clearer mind.

I'll also talk through the concepts of inflammation and oxidative stress, and tackle the
uncomfortable subject of cancer. By covering all these topics, I hope to convince you that
your diet is not simply something to manipulate to improve your aesthetic appearance or
weight. We can certainly achieve those results with our lifestyle, but it is so much more
important than just this. It is the very foundation for a happy life and for improving every
aspect of your body's function.

I have high aspirations to create a movement that considers food as medicine. I mean
this in the most literal sense. I am not a naturopath or an alternative care practitioner. I'm

an NHS GP with an interest in emergency medicine. But I recognize that there is a lot that conventional physicians can learn from the lifestyle principles of ancient medicine. By approaching disease with a holistic perspective, of which food is a vital part, we can tackle the root causes of disease and help our patients truly live well. Our plates are more powerful than pills, and it is a key starting point for lifestyle changes that can protect against disease and boost our health.

Medicine is changing. Our global healthcare systems are struggling under the weight of treating lifestyle-related disease; without a lifestyle-related solution we must really address how we tackle this uncertain landscape. Now that we understand the molecular mechanisms by which dietary and lifestyle factors can affect chronic inflammation, mental health, and the immune system, we can confidently encourage nutrition as a health strategy. Judging from the medical conferences I attend globally, there has never been more interest in nutritional science, and I'm hopeful that the future of modern healthcare has an immense focus on this subject.

Since I wrote my last book, Culinary Medicine UK has taken shape, and a few medical schools are pioneering this method of teaching their students the foundations of clinical nutrition, as well as how to cook. Governments across the world are seriously considering nutrition training as part of public schooling, and cooking classes for patients could become part of treatment within the healthcare system. This is the future of medicine, and I'm glad to see it unfold in small steps, but we need to accelerate its adoption. By purchasing this book, reading it, and applying it to your own life, you are now part of this conversation and contributing to the mission.

I believe my role as a health professional is to increase your awareness of the choices that will benefit your health. What you'll find in this book is a diverse selection of recipes bursting with flavor, which will help empower you to make healthy meal choices that are easy to put into practice and infinitely beneficial to your well-being. They will focus on speed, simplicity of ingredients, incredible flavor, and high nutritional value. This combination of information and recipes will keep you in flourishing health, and I'm certain that you will find this way of life fulfilling and achievable.

As well as showing you the benefits of food, I've highlighted "**Lifestyle 360**" changes that are relevant to each subject discussed in the chapters. I'll be talking through the evidence behind deep breathing exercises, meditation practices, and the importance of sleep and exercise through the lens of different conditions. It's essential that everybody reading this understands the overall value of all these lifestyle factors and their impact on health. By utilizing all these factors in unison, we can deliver a package that has great synergy and is, in essence, medicinal.

"By approaching disease with a holistic perspective, of which food is a vital part, we can tackle the root causes of disease and help our patients truly live well."

Although exercise and rest are critical to our health, eating is a particularly special feature of our lifestyle that naturally has greater importance to our well-being. Food is a universal language. Some of our strongest memories and emotions are linked to meals and, luckily for most of you reading this, it's not purely to nourish. We celebrate with food, break barriers, solidify relationships over shared plates, and communicate across cultures through the enjoyment of each other's recipes. For this reason, although this is a "health" book, my recipes will travel through different cuisines to reflect my belief that food the world over can be healthy and incredibly tasty.

Health starts on our plates. My promise to you is that although my recipes are influenced by the thousands of research studies I've read on nutrition and medicine, they are far from boring. My motto in the kitchen is **Flavor as well as Function,** and you'll learn how a delicious diet can create a more resilient body and mind. Step away from the scale and calorie counters and open yourself up to the wonderful world of eating to benefit your body and beat illness.

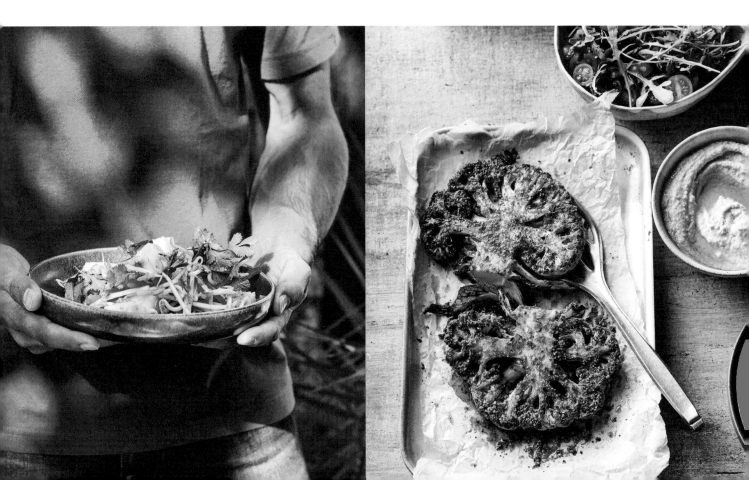

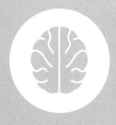

Eat for Your Brain

To kick off the "eating to beat illness" discussion, there is simply nowhere more fascinating to start than with the brain. Our most prized possession, it controls the centers for movement, thought, emotion, and all the automatic processes such as breathing and heart rate that we do not have to consciously concern ourselves with. Quite literally, it is the most advanced machine ever known to us and, unlike the latest computer or most sought-after gadget, we all have one.

Our skull houses trillions of neural synapses (the junctions between nerve cells); these carry information across different brain centers that have specific functional roles for the body. The beautiful coordination of these electrical signals determines our actions and thoughts, which are generated in these centers.

Of late, however, our brains are under fire. As a medical doctor, I witness the aftermath of conditions such as dementia and strokes all too often, and the prevalence of these is increasing.[1] These conditions reveal the vulnerability of the brain and body once these centers become affected and a culmination of insults have taken place.

Dementia is now the leading cause of death in the UK, and cases are rising.[2] Before you assume it is a natural part of aging and a consequence of our population living for longer, there is clear evidence to suggest the contrary. Our lifestyles drastically impact the health of our brain, and this chapter will help you understand why and how we can protect ourselves and optimize our brain power.[3]

Loss of emotional intelligence, inhibition of thoughts, motor-control deficits, memory impairment, and many more signs illustrate exactly why diseases of the brain are so life-changing. It's the experiences of these patients that push me to highlight the impact of diet and lifestyle and how we use the tools within our control. And it starts with our plates. I haven't written these symptoms to scare you, but rather to highlight how beautifully coordinated our brains are and the consequences of poor lifestyle choices that are preventable.[4] We tend only to value the importance of such organs when we have lost control of their precious functions and, while you may consider these conditions to only be relevant in later age, I'm here to inform you that looking after your brain is a lifelong process.[5] The acceptance that you "naturally" lose brain function as you age is a myth[6], and I want to show you that looking after your brain can be enjoyable and delicious!

NEUROPLASTICITY

The ability of our brain to harness new neural connections, create new brain cells, and positively adapt its function in response to stimuli from our environment is a concept known as "neuroplasticity." It is one of the most fascinating and promising topics I have come across in recent years, and one where food and lifestyle play a pivotal role.[7] Previously, it was not commonly believed that cells of the nervous system could regenerate or improve their function. It was conventional thinking that after childhood development, our brains were relatively "static."[8] However, research is demonstrating that not only can we change the synapses to improve our memory and the general functioning of our brain, but it could be a useful tool in the management of conditions such as neurodegenerative disease, like dementia.[9] As you read, you will understand how diet and lifestyle are involved in this neuroplastic process in a way that can positively impact our brain health.

BRAIN INFLAMMATION

By changing the internal environment of the body, we can create the perfect setting for the cells of our nervous system to function optimally.[7] Oxidative stress is a topic we will visit later on (pages 34–47), but our brains are particularly susceptible to an imbalance in inflammatory proteins. It has been demonstrated in many studies that an "inflammatory western diet" (high in sugar, refined carbohydrates, processed foods, and salt) is disastrous for brain health.[10, 11] In addition to putting people at risk of heart disease and stroke, which all raise the risk of neurological disorders, this western-style diet promotes inflammation that could disrupt the blood-brain barrier—a protective layer that surrounds the central nervous system and is integral to the health of your brain.[10]

In contrast, diets high in polyphenols (the types of plant chemicals that we find in colorful fruits and vegetables) are shown to reduce oxidative stress, which may explain their benefits to brain health.[12] The Mediterranean diet contains an abundance of different polyphenols and has long been recognized as one of the healthiest diets for most people to follow.[13] In general, it consists predominantly of plant-based proteins, plenty of pulses, quality fats from nuts and seeds, as well as colorful vegetables and oily fish. The diet has been shown to reduce the incidence of vascular disease that can contribute to poor brain health, and protects against diabetes, which we know is related to declining mental ability.[14] Oxidative stress and inflammation are generally reduced in those adhering to a Mediterranean style of eating, which is in part explained by the sheer number of antioxidants found in the fruits and vegetables consumed.[15]

MIND DIETS

As well as the potential of diet and lifestyle to reduce the incidence of neurodegenerative conditions, I think it's also important to bring attention to some of my patients' anecdotes following improvements to their diet and lifestyle. I regularly hear comments such as, "I feel clearer in my head," "My mood has improved," or even, "I have so much more energy these days." I recognize that these are soft and subjective statements but—despite no concrete, clinically validated method of measuring these outcomes—it gives me further hope that positive diet and lifestyle changes could improve the lives of everyone and not just those labeled with a condition. The improvements in mental clarity and mood could potentially be explained by reducing inflammation in the brain and oxidative stress, but there's a lot more to learn in this field.[16]

A specific diet, appropriately called the MIND diet, was born out of some of the research looking at the correlation of high vegetable intakes and lower rates of dementia.[17] This study, plus many others, have highlighted certain ingredients as beneficial to the resilience of our brains, and I'd like to bring attention to them. The following is by no means a definitive list of ingredients you "must have" to protect your brain, nor is it a suggestion that we can radically renew our brain cells using these foods. However, it is an introduction into how incredible and impactful our diet can be to the function of our brain.[3] Hopefully this will prompt you towards a healthier perspective that could potentially offer protection to this vital organ.

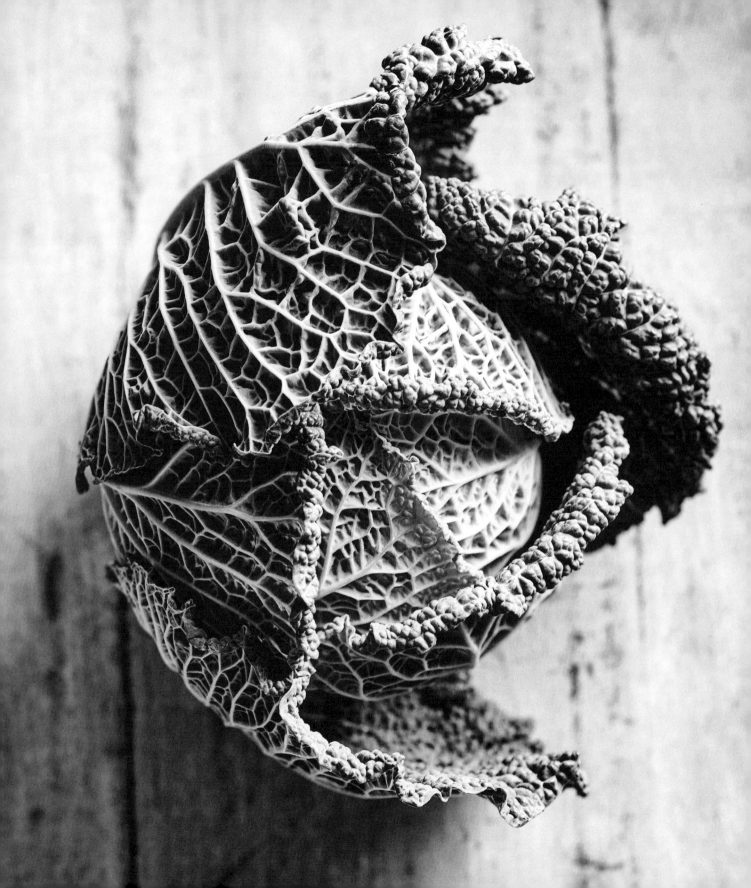

+ Greens These can impact multiple systems of the body, including the brain, and are one of the most important parts of a healthy diet. Ingredients such as cavolo nero, spinach, arugula, and sprouts contain high amounts of phytonutrients that drastically reduce inflammation in the body.[18] Inflammation is a key component of why brain processes can become disrupted, leading to symptoms of fatigue and sometimes low mood.[19] Dark leafy greens are also a source of fiber that could benefit the gut bacterial population found in the digestive tract, which is also involved in the regulation of inflammation in the body.[20] Try the Harissa Beans and Greens (see page 164) for a spicy and delicious way of including more greens.

+ Omega-3-rich fats These are found in oily fish, nuts and seeds, plus extra-virgin olive oil. The long-chain Omega-3 fatty acids are of particular interest, as they have been shown to promote the growth of brain cells, which can help maintain the adaptability of the brain.[21] These sorts of fats are potentially key components of the brain's neuroplastic ability. Another benefit of nuts, seeds, and oily fish in the diet is the quality protein they provide. These ingredients are broken down into amino acids (the building blocks of protein), which are used for the production of neurotransmitters, the chemical messengers of the brain that are created every time your brain centers need to send signals.[22] Adequate stores of good-quality protein ensure the

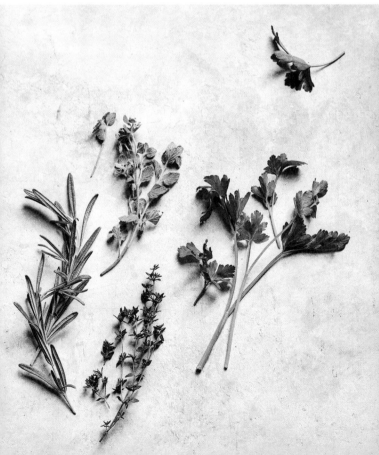
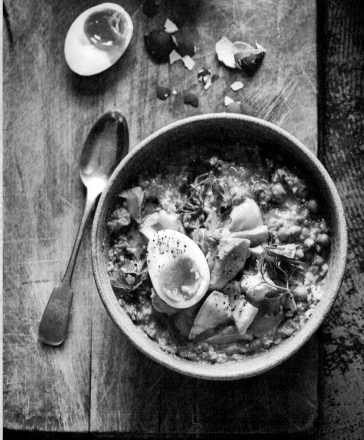

availability of these nutrients for the production of these essential chemicals. Try the Almond and Hazelnut Lentils with Capers (see page 147) to get nuts into recipes.

+ **Berries** These have received a lot of attention for being brain protective, with good reason. They are rich sources of polyphenols, including anti-inflammatory resveratrol and quercetin, but they may also be involved in the production of brain-derived neurotrophic factor (BDNF).[23] BDNF is involved in the maintenance and survival of nerve cells and could be a critical component of protecting the brain against disease but also enhancing cognitive ability. I always have a mixture of berries in my freezer at home for convenience because they are as nutrient-dense as fresh and much less expensive.

+ **Whole grains** Examples of these, including red rice, rolled oats, and quinoa, are great sources of antioxidants, fiber, and B vitamins, which are essential for brain health.[3] The brain is a sugar-dependent organ, but excessive sugar that disrupts the normal mechanisms governing the control of glucose in the bloodstream has been shown to negatively impact brain cells.[11, 24, 25]

This is why whole grains with the fiber attached are so important from the perspective of sugar control. Rather than blindly counting carbohydrates and removing anything labeled a "carb," I urge patients to consider the quality of ingredients. Barley, corn, and millet are nutritionally very different from breads, pasta, and cakes, yet they are all lumped together under the same banner of "carbohydrate." Whole grains are what we should be eating as they release sugar into the blood gradually and have not had the important nutrients stripped away from them. My Sri Lankan–Style Oats (see page 135) are a great way of using whole grains in an unusual dish.

+ **Water** Perhaps the easiest to access and the most commonly forgotten ingredient of all is simply water. All too often I ask patients about their drinking habits only to discover a shockingly low amount of hydration! Discounting certain medical conditions that would contradict 8½ cups of plain water a day, and excluding tea and coffee (which can actually dehydrate us), this is how much we should be aiming for. It is essential for nutrient transfer across brain cells, delivering oxygen as well as maintaining the integrity of cell structures. The simple act of hydration has been demonstrated in clinical studies to improve cognitive performance, and there's no reason why we shouldn't all be drinking adequate amounts.[26] Drink for your mind.

+ **Herbs and spices** Most of these contain key antioxidants and phytochemicals (chemicals produced by plants) that can reduce oxidative stress.[27] As a general rule of thumb, using simple kitchen herbs like rosemary, basil, oregano, and mint in your cooking is a great way to reduce inflammation and improve the enjoyment of food. Certain chemicals labeled "adaptogens" or nutraceuticals, including ashwagandha, curcumin, and gingko (to name just a few), have been given a lot of attention in the press over recent years, claiming to boost brain health with regular consumption. While I welcome greater research into compounds that are safe and well tolerated, the biggest impact on brain health is not going to come from a nutraceutical pill. I wouldn't like anyone to believe that simply taking supplements in isolation is the best way to protect your brain. It's going to be your plate and lifestyle that have the biggest impact.

LIFESTYLE 360

I could talk extensively about micronutrients, including vitamins E and D, or the power of individual phytochemicals, but this would neglect the importance of "food synergy." We don't eat nutrients in isolation, and I'm a firm believer of an integrated dietary approach. By overanalyzing single elements of our diet, we miss the wider picture about the combinations of food we consume and how difficult it is to tease out what's having an impact. We need to experiment with new and delicious ingredients, but in addition, the synergistic effect of lifestyle alongside diet is a powerful combination to be reckoned with.

+ **Mental training and stimulation** These have been observed to increase a type of material in the brain called "grey matter" that makes up parts of the brain involved in emotion, coordination, and perception.[28] You don't have to just do sudoku or mathematical exercises—meditation and mindfulness regimens have also been shown to demonstrate increases in grey matter.[29] Playing a musical instrument, singing, and any activity that focuses attention may lead to benefits and are worth the time investment to keep your brain healthy.

+ **Chronic stress** It has been shown that a high level of stress induces structural changes in the brain, which suggests our emotions are potent modulators of our brain's anatomy.[30, 31] In clinic, I emphasize the need for simple stress-relieving strategies, such as yoga, deep breathing, and meditation, that heighten neural activity in the brain's pleasure centers and improve our tolerance to stress.[32] These powerful tools are accessible to everybody and, if taught appropriately, research shows can be very effective.

+ **Exercise** High-intensity interval training (HIIT) and endurance exercises reduce the incidence of cardiovascular disease, which would ultimately reduce the likelihood of cognitive decline. But exercise itself also induces the production of "neurotrophic" factors that enhance nerve cell generation and protect against shrinkage of the brain that occurs as we age.[33] Our bodies are designed to move constantly, but I find that many patients are confined to their desks in their working environments. Whether it's a case of getting a standing desk or taking the stairs, I advise to try to move as much as possible throughout the day—exercise is not confined to the gym. Your brain will thank you for it.

+ Sleep Sleeping to both protect and greatly enhance brain function is the lowest hanging fruit, yet few of us practice good sleep hygiene. The constant stimulation from TV platforms and mobile electronic devices creates an environment associated with disrupted sleep. During sleep your brain's lymphatic system (the system that removes toxins and waste products as a result of normal cellular processes) gets to work to clear debris that can impact the functioning of your nerve cells.[34] There is a clear link between poor sleep and a higher likelihood of cognitive decline, and on the other side of the spectrum, boosted cognitive performance when you are well rested. Getting a good quality 8–9 hours of rest per 24 hours is one of the simplest ways to boost brain health. Make yourself a promise: try it for 7 days and monitor how you feel. It will revolutionize what you prioritize.

By employing all these tactics we can positively impact our brain on multiple levels. We have the power with our diet to reduce inflammation, stimulate brain growth factors, promote neuronal cell production, reduce oxidative stress, and improve many other processes that we have yet to discover. As well as all these dietary and lifestyle changes being protective, the aforementioned activities are also being considered in management to improve outcomes or prevent further decline in patients to good effect. This is where we need to invest more of our time and resources, but I'm making this vital information accessible to you right here. Don't wait for the prescription pad. Take advantage of these points and start looking after your brain health right now. As you'll discover in all the other chapters in this introduction, eating and living well doesn't solely affect your brain health, but rather your entire ecosystem.

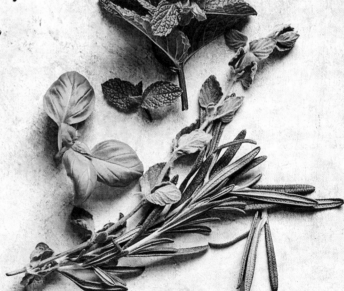

Whole Grains
red rice, rolled oats, quinoa

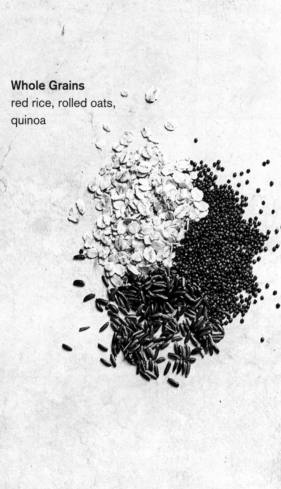

Berries
blackberries, blueberries, raspberries

Water

Herbs
rosemary, basil, oregano, mint

Food for Your Brain

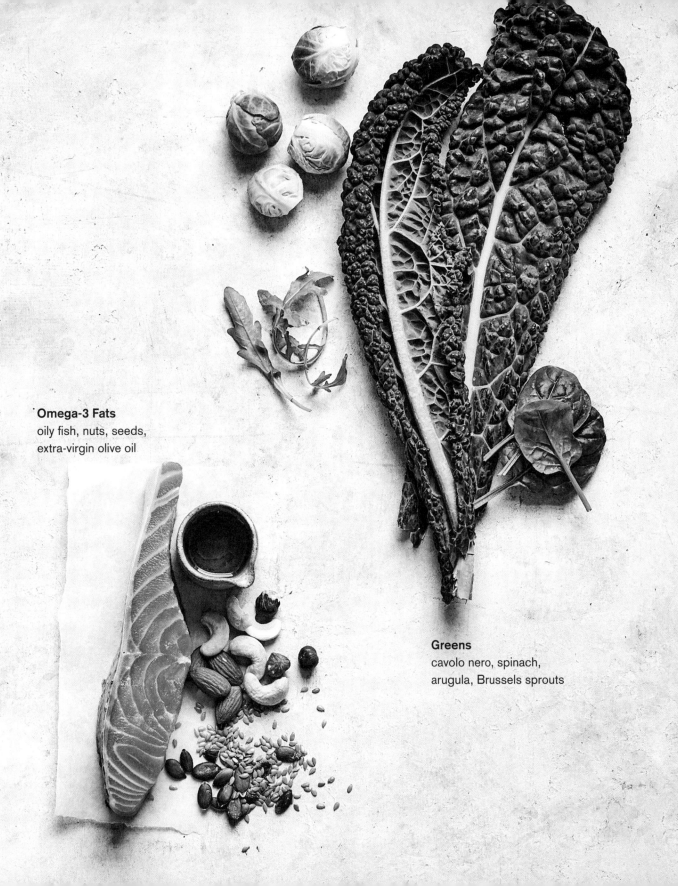

Omega-3 Fats
oily fish, nuts, seeds,
extra-virgin olive oil

Greens
cavolo nero, spinach,
arugula, Brussels sprouts

Eat for Your Heart

If you're tempted to skip over this chapter because you're in your mid-twenties or early thirties and you believe heart disease is only something of concern in later life, think carefully about flicking past these pages. Heart disease isn't something that suddenly becomes relevant as soon as we reach a certain age threshold. We build the foundations for a healthy or unhealthy heart in our childhood, and we are starting to see the early signs of atherosclerosis (narrowed, inflamed arteries) in those as young as teenagers.[35] But rather than scaring you into booking a CT angiogram to determine the state of your vital organ, I want to show you how much control you have using your fork.

Our heart is a complex machine that generates electrical energy to synchronously contract its muscles, pumping blood around our network of vessels. The blood contains vital oxygen molecules, as well as nutrients to feed every cell in our body, but the heart itself is desperately reliant on the same nutritional need. Micronutrients like potassium, magnesium, and calcium are essential to ensure the contractility of this muscular organ that, hopefully, will never stop throughout our entire existence.

If you hit the gym harder than usual and you're dehydrated, or perhaps you haven't had adequate nutrition prior to your workout, your muscles will feel stiff and generally fatigued. Feed yourself the right fuel, however, and you're less likely to feel the negative effects of training. Our heart muscles are categorically different from the skeletal muscles in our limbs, but the general principles of feeding our muscle tissue still apply. It's vital to ensure your heart is adequately nourished to perform its function throughout its lifetime and make lifestyle choices that nurture this beautiful, industrious machine. Thankfully, this isn't hard, and the food you can enjoy is still incredibly delicious and exciting.

It's important to remember that the heart (like most organs) is incredibly resilient. As demonstrated by some impressive studies, reversal of atherosclerosis can be achieved with a lifestyle that encourages your body to look after itself.[36] A number of cardiologists have demonstrated, using both blood tests and imaging to look at the vasculature of the heart, that a healthy lifestyle can reduce blockages of the arteries.[37, 38] This is absolutely groundbreaking and something not thought possible up until a few years ago. In fact, some lifestyle medicine programs have become so effective at reversing cardiovascular disease that they're now covered by American health insurers.[39, 40]

But rather than trying to just reverse heart disease, I want to focus on the habits that will prevent the life-changing event of a heart attack that happens to over 700,000 American citizens per year. Yes, there is evidence to suggest that we can drastically improve post–heart attack symptoms with intense lifestyle changes, but the better and more effective aspiration is to prevent that stage in the first place.

THE MEDITERRANEAN WAY

The Mediterranean diet has been heralded as the most heart-healthy diet, and evidence supports this. When we look at large population studies, it's clear that a Mediterranean way of eating, which includes plenty of fruits, vegetables, good-quality oils, and healthy fats, significantly reduces the likelihood of high blood pressure, strokes, and heart disease.[41, 42] A representative dish of how to eat with this focus in mind is my Roast Walnut and Squash Medley with Persillade (see page 188) or the Eggplant and Walnut Ragu (see page 197).

We can analyze why this may be the case by examining the components of a

Mediterranean way of eating. The focus is on colorful vegetables such as tomatoes, squash, lentils, and dark leafy greens, which are fantastic sources of the micronutrients necessary for optimum cardiac muscle function.[43, 44] The most extensively studied of these micronutrients include potassium, calcium, magnesium, and co-enzyme Q10,[45] but there are a huge number of other plant chemicals found in the same foods that we still haven't fully investigated the effects of.[46]

There are now over 30 years of data, including the results of the Lyon Heart Study, PREDIMED studies, and other large research projects that all point towards Mediterranean-style diets and lifestyle modifications as being significantly more effective at prevention of cardiovascular disease than drugs combined.[41] To put this another way, if you change your lifestyle and eating habits, it has a more powerful effect on your health than any number of medication combinations I can prescribe. This is simply not common knowledge among our population, nor medical professionals, and quite frankly, it should be printed on the front door of every cardiac unit and family physicians office in the country. Considering the exorbitant cost of medications and interventions directed at preventing cardiovascular events that our healthcare system invests in,[47] there is simply no excuse for why diet education should not play a central role in healthcare. We do ourselves a disservice by not engaging in this conversation, and it is where we need to direct our resources.

NUTRIGENETICS

If you happen to have a family history of heart disease, you may be thinking to yourself that your genes are your destiny and there isn't much you can do about your "dirty DNA." On the contrary: studies have shown that we are more in control of our heart disease risk than previously thought. Our genetic blueprint is inherited from our parents; this information is stored in every cell of your body and it is unchangeable. However, we can change the *output* of our genes by changing what we put *in* to our system.[48] The ability to change the expression of our genes is a concept I introduced in my first book. Nutrigenetics, nutrigenomics, and epigenetics are among a few novel science disciplines that focus their attention on the role of nutrients and bioactive food compounds in gene expression.[49] When I personally learned more about this field, it revolutionized my perspective on just how important food and our lifestyle are.

Once we begin to understand and believe in the power of environmental influences on the very foundations of our existence, it becomes clear why diet is one of the most technologically advanced treatments we have in our armory against disease. When you consume food, it "speaks" to your DNA, and this communication can either lead to an overall positive or negative outcome. By introducing colorful foods, nutrient-dense ingredients, and good-quality fats (which all the recipes in this book contain), we not only provide micronutrients and proteins for heart function, but we are also changing the messages transmitted via our DNA.[50] Cardiologists are now warming to the idea that nutrigenomics has a role in their specialty, and I see more specialists attending lectures in nutrition, engaging with me on social media and at talks, wanting to learn more. This area of research gives us further mechanistic information about why particular diets like the Mediterranean diet are so cardio protective,[50] and I'm sure biomedical informatics will help tackle the complexity of this field.

What we can be certain of is that the root cause of—and solution to—the clear majority of cardiovascular diseases that I see in the emergency department and primary care is manageable with lifestyle. This fact alone should give us a clue as to where we should be concentrating our attention and resources.

STOP THE STRESS

Beyond the nutrients necessary for contracting the muscular walls of our heart, this organ is vulnerable to "oxidative stress," a topic we discuss in the chapter exploring inflammation (pages 34–47). High levels of inflammation have been shown in many animal and human models to be detrimental to the walls of arteries.[51] Oxidative stress can be created by

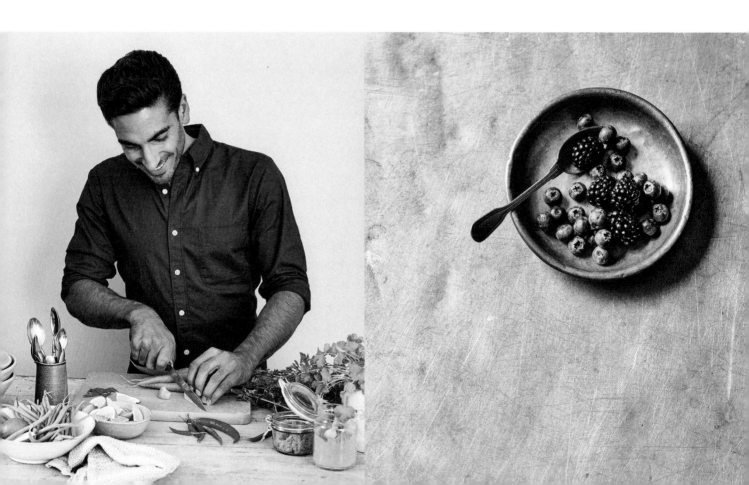

high blood pressure, smoking, as well as high-sugar diets that can lead to the creation of "advanced glycemic end products" (AGEs). These products concentrate in parts of the heart vessels, creating inflammation that can lead to plaque formation.[52] By ensuring your lifestyle reduces inflammation, limits foods high in sugar and refined carbohydrates (like white rice, bread, pasta, cookies, and cakes), you can prevent unnecessary oxidative stress and fuel your body's natural inflammation-balancing mechanisms.

A Mediterranean-style diet has been shown to reduce oxidative stress, lower blood pressure, and improve the health of blood vessels.[41] In addition, a diet high in green vegetables such as broccoli, parsley, and sprouts not only contains oxidant scavengers like vitamin C and heart-stabilizing minerals like magnesium,[53] but phytochemicals including sulfurophane, indole-3-carbinol, and quercetin that are known to be potent anti-inflammatory ingredients.[54]

BALANCED FATS

Despite years of being told fat should be stripped out of our diets, sources of good-quality fat such as nuts, seeds, and extra-virgin olive oil feature heavily in Mediterranean diets, which are heart healthy. The detrimental low-fat message needs to be addressed. It's been heavily over-simplified, and it's a confusing topic for many patients who still believe all sources of fat are harmful. To put it simply, whole sources of fat such as pecans, walnuts, sunflower seeds, and minimally processed extra-virgin olive oil are fantastic additions to your diet from a heart-health perspective. Not only do they contain key minerals like selenium and magnesium but they provide antioxidants such as vitamin E, which can protect the heart from oxidative stress.[55] Algae oil and wild oily fish also contain long-chain Omega-3 fatty acids that have been shown to be anti-inflammatory[56] and vital additions to a heart-healthy diet.

Two types of fatty acids, Omega-3 and Omega-6, have been given a lot more attention in studies trying to explain the rise of heart disease in western countries. Omega-6 is found in cereals, wheat, and animal products but also within vegetable oils, nuts, and seeds. Omega-6 is generally thought to be pro-inflammatory, but as we will learn in the inflammation chapter (pages 34–47), the process of inflammation is essential for our body, and this is why we need some sources of Omega-6 in our diet. The issue appears to arise where the ratio of Omega-6 to Omega-3 in our body falls out of balance. Throughout our evolution we would have had equal amounts of 3 and 6 or a ratio between 1:1 to 1:4.[57] However, western diets high in poor-quality industrial corn and soy oils, refined cereals, wheat, and animal products tip the balance to one that has a much higher ratio of Omega-6 than is sensible for human health.

"Whole sources of fat such as pecans, walnuts, sunflower seeds, and minimally processed extra-virgin olive oil are fantastic additions to your diet from a heart-health perspective."

The mechanism by which different fats impact our health is more complicated than simply turning inflammation on and off. Fatty acids modify the blood's ability to clot and even influence gene expression of cells in our vessels.[58] To put it simply, it's all about ratio, but rather than suggesting we all diligently calculate our Omega-3 to Omega-6 percentages, my advice would be to concentrate your fat sources on whole foods such as nuts and seeds. Use minimally processed oils like extra-virgin olive oil, and limit your intake of cookies, fried foods, and refined snacks like chips. Follow these principles, and your ratios are likely to be optimal for general as well as heart health without having to obsess about the numbers.

Our plates are a gateway to using the thousands of compounds that assist our body's inherent ability to look after itself. Recipes such as my Eggplant and Walnut Ragu (see page 197) or the Jambalaya (see page 204) are great examples of the types of food we need to concentrate our diet around. These include vegetables, fruits, spices, and specific fats that help reduce our risk of heart disease through a multitude of cellular processes. Here are some of the foods I regularly recommend to patients interested in heart-healthy meals:

+ **A rainbow of colors** There is a significant body of clinical data and large studies to demonstrate that antioxidant-rich diets reduce blood pressure and cardiovascular risk,[59] and as a general rule of thumb, colors mean antioxidants. Look for a rainbow of colors in your diet, and you're likely to be including a plethora of micronutrients that will positively impact your heart. Of particular note, I like to include red and purple foods such as berries, beets, red cabbage, and grapes. These contain phytochemicals such as the betalains and anthocyanins that have been shown to relax blood vessels and lower high blood pressure.[60, 61, 62]

+ **Calcium and potassium** These minerals are essential for vascular health. You'll find calcium in ingredients such as chickpeas, puy lentils, and sesame seeds, and both potassium and magnesium are abundant in dark greens such as cavolo nero, spring greens, and Swiss chard. The heart is an energy-generating organ that relies on these minerals to appropriately conduct electricity through its tissue fibers. By eating these types of foods, you ensure the availability of these essential nutrients to safeguard optimal heart function.

+ **Fiber** As well as the minerals contained within beans, legumes, and pulses, these foods offer a variety of fiber sources. As with most aspects of health, your gut microbes have a significant role in cardiovascular disease, and there is a clear "gut-heart" connection.[63] Inflammation is an important contributor to the mechanism of cardiovascular disease, and nurturing a robust gut population with plenty of fiber sources reduces inflammation and can prevent damage to arteries that can cause heart attacks and strokes. In addition to pulses and legumes, chicory, garlic, onion, and leeks are fantastic fiber sources that will encourage a healthy microbiota.

+ **Good-quality fats** These have been shown to have positive effects on the expression of your genes, which create a more favorable cholesterol profile and improve fat distribution around your body.[49] The fats to focus on are those from whole plant sources: concentrate on the least refined types. These include walnuts, pistachios, almonds, oily fish, cold-pressed virgin oils (like avocado, rapeseed, and olive), and seeds. These tend to have higher amounts of unsaturated versus saturated fats, but I'd rather you pay attention to foods rather than the biochemical profiles of ingredients. I've found in clinical practice that it's a waste of mental energy to try and entertain the different arguments for and against certain fats. The reality is, all fats contain both unsaturated and saturated categories in varying proportions and subtypes. It doesn't make any sense to suggest we should remove all saturated fats from your diet when every fat you can think of will contain some amount of saturated fat. Trust me on this one: your heart will thank you for focusing on plentiful whole, largely plant-based fats and enjoying fats from animal products like meat and dairy on occasion.

LIFESTYLE 360

Diet is just one of the many strategies to positively impact metabolism, genetic expression, body-fat distribution, and many more processes that benefit your heart.[64] Now consider the extra medicinal benefit of complementing delicious food with lifestyle modifications. As a starting point, the recommendations of smoking cessation, alcohol moderation, and exercise are essential, but this is not where lifestyle advice stops. Over and above these well-known factors are other extensively studied recommendations that I've outlined below.

+ **Sleep** If there was one thing I could change about my patients' habits, from the perspective of improving heart function, it would be to get more sleep. Sleep deprivation is correlated with higher blood pressure, higher measures of inflammation, and worsening cholesterol profiles, all of which contribute to heart disease.[65] Findings from multiple studies demonstrate that a lack of sleep causes raised stress hormone levels and activation of your "fight or flight" system, which leads to changes in your mental ability as well as causing strain on your heart. In addition to the direct impact, after a poor night's sleep your brain sends signals to make you hungrier, making you more likely to crave that

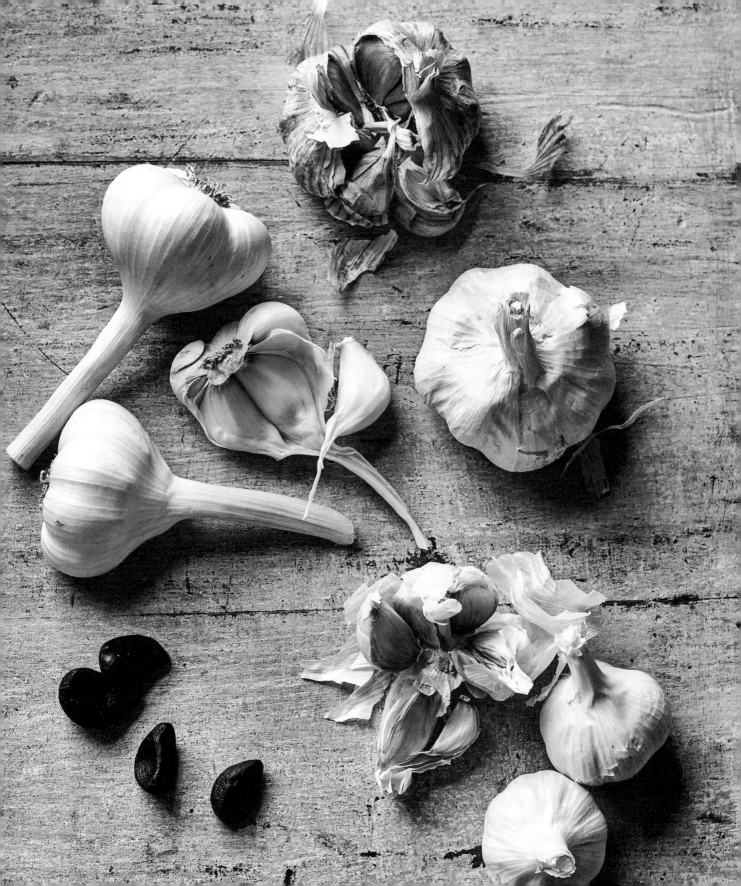

sugary croissant or salty fried snack, which will compound the detrimental impact.[66] As with most things in medicine, it's not about quantity but quality. Seven to nine hours a night is a general rule of thumb, but try measuring how long you sleep on the weekend without an alarm waking you the next day and being aware of how refreshed you feel. This will give you a personal indication of generally how much sleep you should be aiming for during the working week, too.

+ Stress-relieving techniques As an adjunct to improving stress hormone levels and reducing inflammation, stress-relieving techniques and mind–body interventions including deep breathing exercises, meditation, and yoga can have positive effects on heart health. It may seem slightly left-field for a conventionally trained doctor to be recommending this, but actually mental stress has been shown in many studies to be a significant contributing factor to heart disease.[67, 68] Stress activates the immune system to create an inflammatory environment as it perceives the body is "under attack," and this can lead to oxidative stress that damages and weakens blood vessels. These same stress hormones can increase sugars in your bloodstream, which can impact fat production by the liver as well as cholesterol ratios. There are robust clinical reasons behind why one of the most effective lifestyle programs for heart disease, the Dr. Ornish Program for Reversing Heart Disease, has an intense focus on stress-relieving techniques. We would all benefit from one of these in our daily routine, and you can check the website www.thedoctorskitchen.com.

+ When we eat The timing of when we eat has been shown to have a significant impact on our blood sugar, cholesterol ratios, and the overall impact on our heart health.[69] It is an unfortunate and well-recognized fact that shift workers who experience regular disruption to their circadian rhythm (the rough 24-hour cycle that all our cells are aligned to) have a greater risk of heart disease, obesity, and dementia and generally live shorter lives.[70] However, there are certain practices that even shift workers can employ to mitigate the effect of cycle interference. Studying this population of workers has led to some interesting recommendations that even those who are lucky enough not to have to do odd working patterns can employ. As a guide, it has been suggested that night-shift workers should eat at the start of their shift (dinner) and at the end (breakfast) to minimize the negative impact of eating when their bodies should be asleep. This practice of "defining periods of eating" to a rough 10- to 12-hour window (during hours that you are awake) has also been shown to have favorable effects on markers of disease risk.[71–73] As a general rule of thumb, this practice allows cells of your liver, pancreas, and gut to better tolerate the food you ingest so that it is less likely to cause blood sugar spikes and cholesterol imbalances that can affect your heart. It's a simple guide that not only gives your gut a rest (allowing it to perform the numerous other functions it needs to do) and minimizes disturbance to your important rhythms, but it also discourages the mindless snacking in the late evenings that most of us do out of boredom.

These simple diet and lifestyle practices are incredibly powerful and accessible to the entire population. Combining these with the other chapters that demonstrate how to improve your immune system, balance inflammation, and relieve stress produces a collective medicinal package that is so powerful in the fight against the biggest killer in the US today. Our food and lifestyle are powerful tools that I encourage you to use, whatever your age, for the optimal functioning of this principal organ.

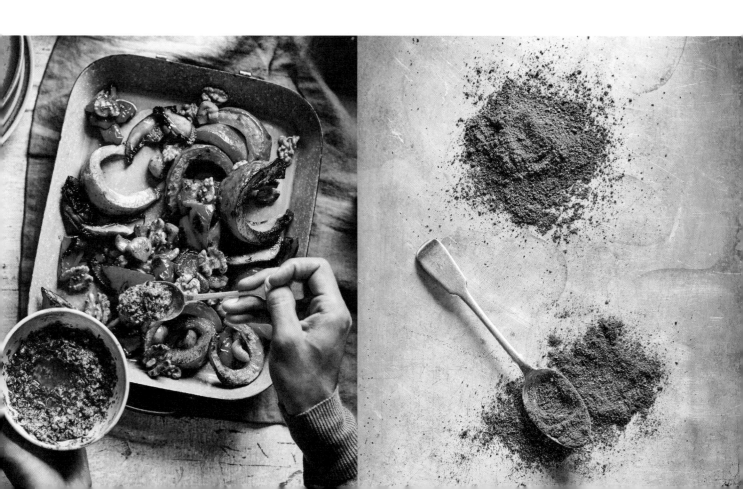

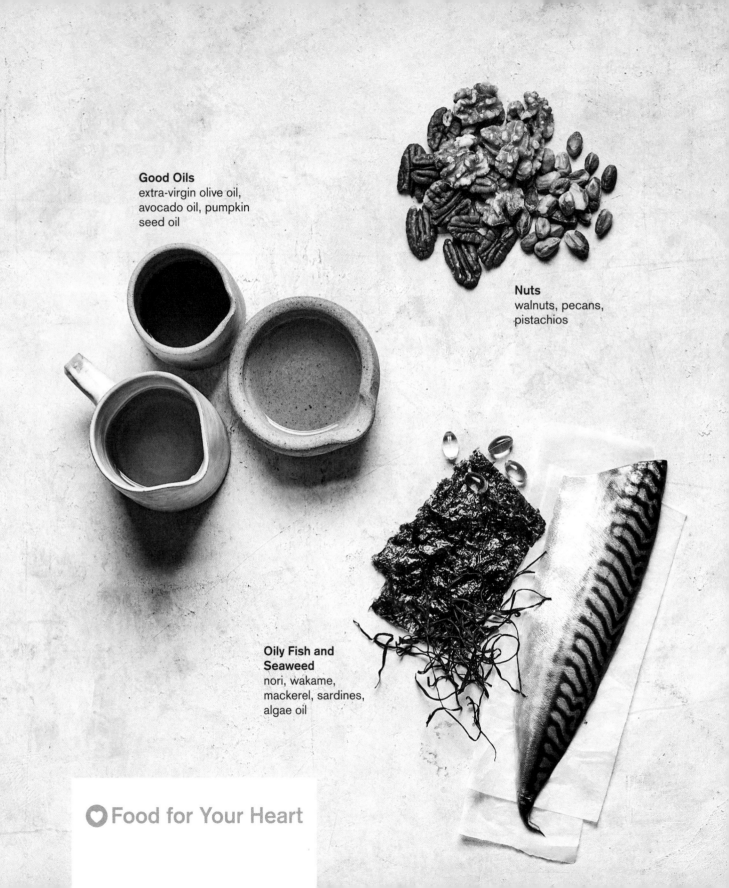

Good Oils
extra-virgin olive oil,
avocado oil, pumpkin
seed oil

Nuts
walnuts, pecans,
pistachios

**Oily Fish and
Seaweed**
nori, wakame,
mackerel, sardines,
algae oil

Food for Your Heart

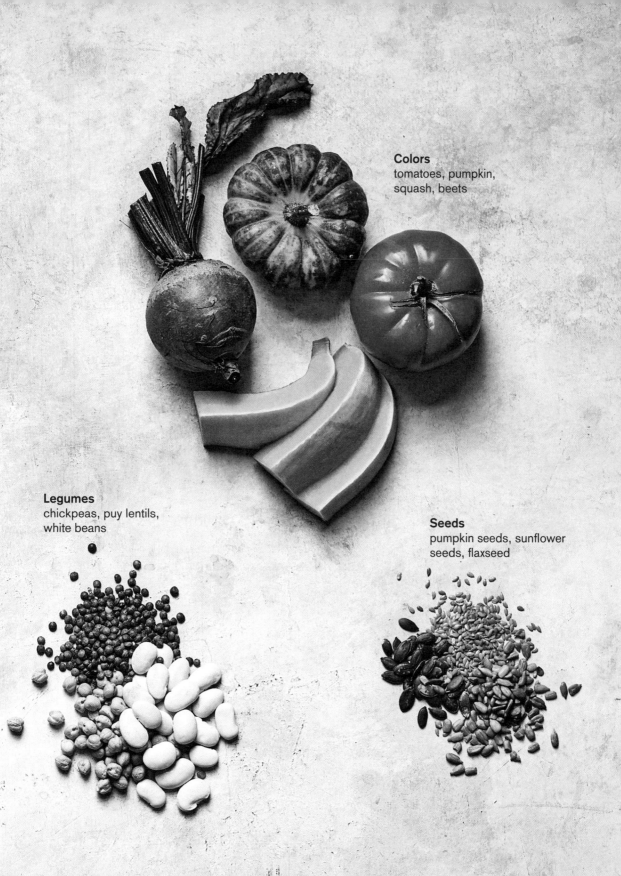

Colors
tomatoes, pumpkin,
squash, beets

Legumes
chickpeas, puy lentils,
white beans

Seeds
pumpkin seeds, sunflower
seeds, flaxseed

Eat for Inflammation

It's amazing how many times I see "inflammation" as a concept coming up in different medical specialties as one of the potential causes of disease. It has almost become a unifying theory that links conditions of the modern world to our lifestyles. You might think I'm talking just about the swollen ankle that happens after an injury, or the redness that surrounds a cut on the skin, but high blood pressure, heart disease, dementia, diabetes, and mental health problems all have links to an imbalance of inflammation in the body at a cellular level.[75]

I see many products being labeled as "anti-inflammatory," and I think there is a lot of misunderstanding about what inflammation really is. This chapter will give you more of a tangible idea about the role of inflammation in our health as well as how to tackle the problems related to an imbalance of this essential system.

Inflammation is your body's normal response to events that cause damage to cells, like an injury or infection. The process involves proteins being released in response to the damage, and these proteins send signals to the cells of the immune system to come and help. This is usually a short-lived, adaptive response that involves coordination of many complex signals and organs.[74]

The inflammation process is very important: without it our cells would not be aware of bacteria causing something like a simple skin infection, and leaving the bacteria undetected in our body could lead to an uncontrolled severe infection with significant consequences. Inflammation is critical for infection prevention and to keep the body alert. We have, in essence, evolved to be able to fight infections, and a host of other stressors to the human body, effectively and swiftly using inflammation as an important tool.[76]

However, inflammation is meant to be a temporary, protective response. Whether that's a reaction to a knee injury or an infection in your digestive tract, inflammation is essentially a big nudge to your body, letting it know something is not quite right and needs to be addressed swiftly. Inflammation is meant to be a short-lived process that resolves over hours, days, or, at worst, weeks. However, what we are witnessing in modern society is persistent, low-grade inflammation over longer periods of time, also referred to as "meta-inflammation."[77] Today we have a number of seemingly small and insignificant stressors that create subtle inflammation over long periods of time and can manifest in a multitude of symptoms. These range from the subtle and vague, such as fatigue, lack of mental clarity, and skin irritation, to the more pronounced, including pain, mood disorders, and heart disease.[78, 79] These symptoms will obviously overlap with other causes, but we are becoming more aware of the damaging effects of inflammation imbalance that is at least in part to be related to these and many other conditions.

Examples of stressors potentially causing low-grade inflammation include excess sugar consumption, psychological stress, sedentary behavior, accumulation of fat tissue, and nutrient deficiencies (including vitamin D, Omega-3, and different micronutrients). Depending on our ability to tolerate these factors, the result can be low-grade meta-inflammation. This culmination of seemingly insignificant stressors can potentially tip

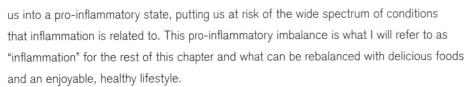

PRO-INFLAMMATORY	ANTI-INFLAMMATORY
Low fiber	Fiber
Nutrient deficiency	Quality fats
Excess sugar	Colorful plant foods
Stress	Mindfulness practice
Social isolation	Community
Antibiotic overuse	Sense of purpose
Sleep loss	Sleep hygiene
Sedentary behavior	Regular movement
Urban environments	Natural environment exposure

us into a pro-inflammatory state, putting us at risk of the wide spectrum of conditions that inflammation is related to. This pro-inflammatory imbalance is what I will refer to as "inflammation" for the rest of this chapter and what can be rebalanced with delicious foods and an enjoyable, healthy lifestyle.

While I want you to appreciate the importance of inflammation as a necessary mechanism in our body, when we examine the triggers of inflammation in modern life using this diagram, it becomes obvious why the balance of inflammation has become skewed towards the pro-inflammatory side of things. This meta-inflammation, as I've alluded to, has a role in many conditions including mental health disorders such as depression,[78] high blood pressure,[80] and insulin resistance, which is linked to the development of poor sugar control and ultimately Type 2 diabetes.[81, 82] With this in mind, it's important to try and find effective ways to prevent this imbalance from occurring, and the diagram gives us an idea of what we can do to restore the equilibrium.

STOP THE TRIGGERS

The reassuring fact is that we can manage inflammation effectively and simply with changes to what we eat and how we live. It's not expensive, it doesn't require excessive interventions or huge modifications, and I'm here to guide you through this process. We have many solutions within our control that we can broadly categorize into two steps. The first is to stop the pro-inflammation triggers in the first place. The second is to introduce diet and lifestyle changes to actively reduce inflammation; we possess the ability and mechanisms to purposely reduce the inflammatory response as well.[83]

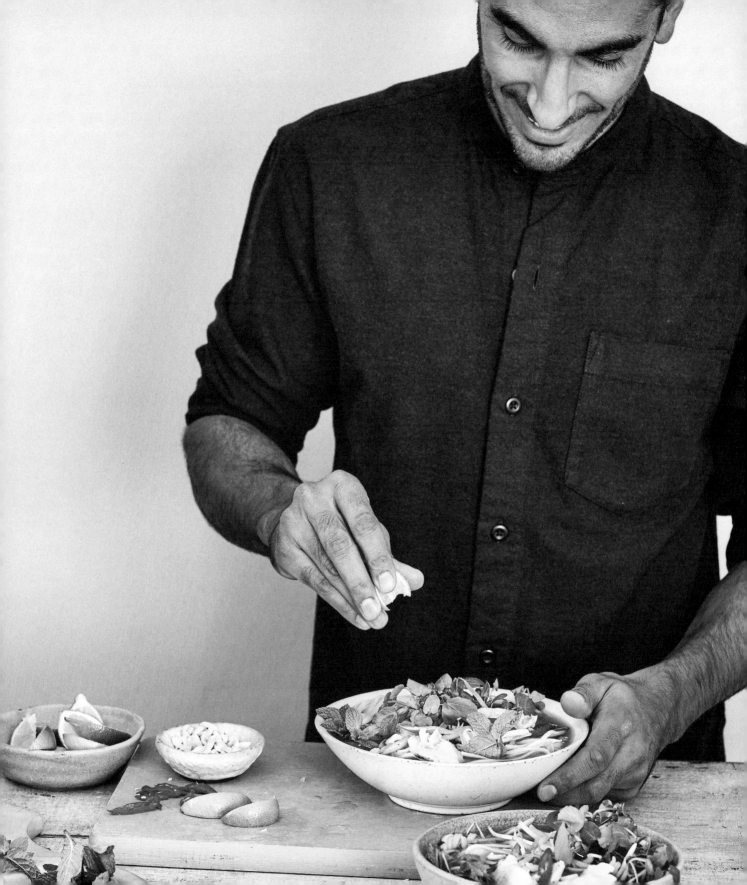

The most effective way to *stop* inflammation in its tracks is by assessing our diet, which in many cases is the most obvious and clear trigger. Looking at a number of large population studies, the benefits of eating a largely vegetarian diet, from the perspective of reducing inflammation, is undeniable. A number of researchers have demonstrated that eating a western diet made up of refined sugars and carbohydrates, large amounts of animal protein, processed foods, and poor-quality fats is related to higher amounts of inflammation signals when measured in the blood.[84]

Conversely, putting more plant foods and fiber in your diet, including good-quality fats that we obtain from nuts and seeds, and eating less animal protein, is linked to significantly lower measures of inflammation.[85, 86] Essentially, it is a fairly Mediterranean-style of eating, and we can reasonably infer from these studies that reduced inflammation is related to less disease and general health protection.[85]

EXCESS BODY FAT

Fat, also known as adipose tissue, is a very useful part of our bodies that we have required during our evolution. Without fat, we wouldn't have survived long periods where food was scarce. This explains why those who have a genetic predisposition to putting on fat, particularly around their organs and waists, may have actually been at an evolutionary advantage when it came to harsh winters, famine, and lack of nutrition for energy.[87] Essentially, it would have acted as a storage form of energy that was readily accessible when food was not available.

Today, however, the ability to put on and retain fat is a clear disadvantage considering our current food environment full of "convenient," energy-dense, and nutritionally poor options. With no famine around the corner, there isn't any need to carry fat on our body, and we do not end up burning it for energy. To add insult to the situation, if we do accumulate fat predominately around our organs and waistline, it is "metabolically active." That is to say, it promotes inflammatory signals that can contribute to the burden of diseases we've mentioned.[88] This is why the scientific community promotes "weight loss" and reducing one's body mass index (BMI) as a strategy to counter the effects of excess fatty tissue.

While I agree that fat tissue is pro-inflammatory and people who lose fat can reduce their inflammatory burden,[89] a narrow focus on weight alone is sometimes a negative goal for a lot of people who struggle to understand the wider context. I believe health can be independent of weight. It is your lifestyle, mind-set, and diet that are the biggest determinants of a happy, healthy life. I'd rather you focus on building healthy habits with well-being as your main goal, rather than a number on a set of scales. When you adopt a diet that reduces refined sugars and carbohydrates and replaces them with fiber, largely plants and colorful vegetables, coupled with the lifestyle changes I discuss throughout this book, you are lowering

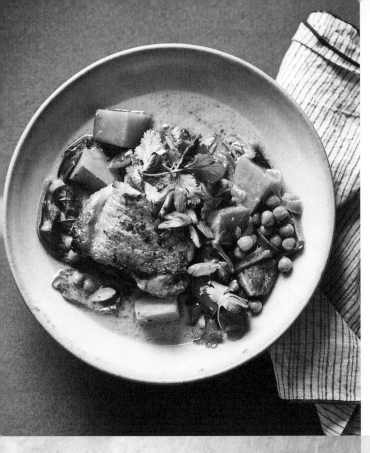

"Putting more plant foods and fiber in your diet, including good-quality fats from nuts and seeds, and eating less animal protein, is linked to significantly lower measures of inflammation."

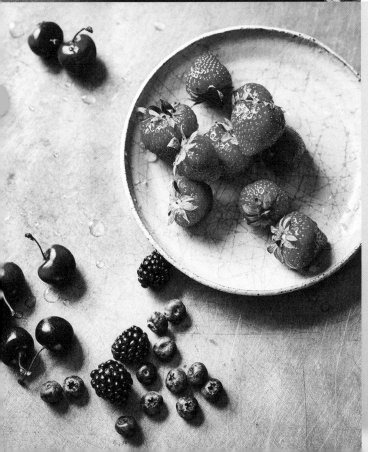

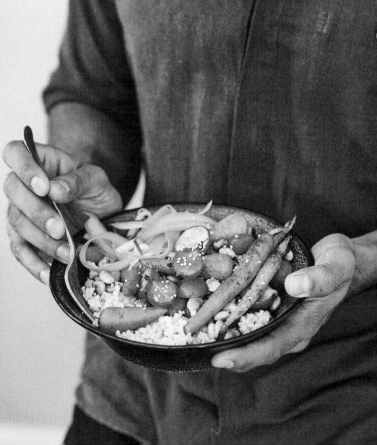

inflammation.[90] These are also the habits that can protect against the dangerous type of fat accumulating around our body's organs (known as visceral fat) that promotes inflammation and leads to health problems. Before we naively use our scale as a measure of success, I implore you to embrace healthy habits and the subjective measurement of how you feel as a better marker of health.

SUPPORT YOUR GUT

We are in constant communication with our environment via our digestive tract, and so it should come as no surprise that inflammation is heavily influenced by the microbes living in our gut.[91] Our microbiota, the different types of microbes such as bacteria and fungi living mostly in our gut, is an important modulator of inflammation. A diverse and healthy population of microbes is associated with lower levels of inflammation, and there are a number of mechanisms behind how they achieve this.

Your gut microbes support inflammation balance by increasing antioxidant production and reducing oxidative stress. They maintain the health of the tissues in your digestive tract to lower gut inflammation, which reduces the likelihood of foreign material inappropriately passing into your bloodstream, causing your body to react. Your microbes protect you from infections and improve your ability to control sugar in the blood, plus they actively secrete chemical signals that calm your immune system, preventing an inappropriate inflammatory response. These, and a number of other mechanisms, are why a flourishing, diverse population of microbes is so important from the perspective of balancing inflammation,[92, 93, 94, 95, 96, 63] and as you'll discover as you read on, the most effective way of nurturing a healthy microbiota is with your food.

There is huge scope for introducing specific bacterial strains to counter the ill effects of inflammation, and some studies have had promising results using probiotics (live bacterial strains in supplemental form).[63, 97] But before you reach for specifically designed strains of bacteria that are formulated with "anti-inflammation" claims, let me remind you that your microbiota is best served by a diverse, plant-focused diet with plenty of fiber and a variety of colors. This is the easiest and most effective way to support your microbes' anti-inflammatory ability.

What follows is a description of lifestyle changes and foods that support your bugs, prevent fat accumulation, and balance inflammation through a variety of pathways.

+ **Good-quality fats** It's long been thought of as a hindrance to health and wellness to have any fats in your diet because of fears of weight gain and risks to your heart, but once again it comes down to the quality of the fats in your diet rather than purely the amount.

"A diverse, plant-focused diet with plenty of fiber and a variety of colors is the easiest and most effective way to support your microbes' anti-inflammatory ability."

Dietary fatty acids from oily fish and nuts can positively impact inflammation by changing the expression of your genes, influencing the inflammation pathways within cells. They're also the building blocks of molecules that are used to signal your body's anti-inflammatory response.[98, 99, 100] Whole sources of fats from plants such as walnuts, macadamia nuts, pumpkin seeds, sunflower seeds, and of course extra-virgin olive oil[101] have been shown to be anti-inflammatory. These contain more of the Omega-3 fats that can balance inflammation, as we learned about in the chapter on heart health (pages 22–33). I tend to use olive oil liberally in cooking, and I use the highest quality, cold-pressed varieties where possible for flavor as well as function.

+ Polyphenols These are a category of health-promoting chemicals that we find in food, and there are literally thousands of them. In general, the colored vegetables lining our supermarket grocery aisles are great sources of these potent compounds, which can target processes related to inflammation. These targets have long and confusing names like the protein complex "nuclear factor-kappa B (NF-kB)"[102, 103] and the enzyme "cyclooxygenase (COX),"[104,] which also happen to be molecular targets for medications that we prescribe for things like arthritis and pain. This isn't to suggest that we can or should replace drugs with food, but the polyphenols you find in a crisp apple, humble pea, or vibrant butternut squash all possess the ability to modulate inflammation by impacting these and many other processes involved in inflammation.[105, 106] A rainbow diet is the easiest way to guarantee a collection of polyphenols that can lower the inflammatory burden.[103]

+ Green foods Of particular mention are undoubtedly the greens. The impact of brassica vegetables including broccoli, arugula, kale, bok choy, and sprouts are absolutely incredible, which is why I try to eat these daily, if not at most mealtimes . . . and yes, that includes breakfast (try my One-Pan Greek Breakfast on page 119 or Watercress, Walnut, and Crayfish on page 121). These ingredients contain many chemicals, including some well-studied compounds called sulforaphane and indole-3-carbinole that prevent oxidative stress.[107, 108] These are some of the most technologically advanced "drugs," and they're only available in grocery stores. Get them on your plate.

+ Red foods Deep red-colored foods contain a particular type of flavonoid called anthocyanin that is well known to be a potent anti-inflammatory chemical.[109] We get these from cheap accessible ingredients such as red cabbage, blue- and red-colored berries, and chard as well as more exotic ingredients such as black rice, red carrots, and purple potatoes. The benefits of red foods are complemented by other colors in your diet. I am by no means suggesting only eating red and green foods for inflammation, but discovering how and why these foods reduce oxidative stress and balance inflammation is exciting enough for me to include these in my diet regularly.

+ **High-fiber foods** Higher glycemic index (high GI) foods that release sugar into the bloodstream rapidly are associated with greater inflammation measures in the blood.[110, 111] Regular consumption of these high GI foods, such as refined cereals and grains, breads, pasta, cakes, and cookies (no matter whether they are labeled "healthy," "whole-grain," "gluten free," or anything else that has an apparent health connotation), is associated with a higher inflammatory burden. This is not a call to remove these foods entirely from your diet. I would never want to rob someone the pleasure of enjoying delicious freshly prepared pasta or a warm, fluffy doughnut with sticky jam. But greater awareness of why these are not the best foods to eat regularly will mold your daily choices and heighten your understanding of what health-promoting food means for you. A simple way to reduce inflammation is just switching from carbohydrates that quickly release sugar into the blood to foods that are higher in fiber and thus release sugar more slowly.[112] Examples include split peas, artichokes, onions, whole apples, black beans, and yellow lentils. In addition, these foods positively enhance the population of gut microbes by giving them a food source to flourish on.

+ **Spices** Exotic spices, such as turmeric and cloves, have become a popular topic among those trying to lead a healthier lifestyle. While I welcome greater research into the exciting compounds found within these spices, especially as they may have a role in treatment of inflammatory disorders such as osteoarthritis, psoriasis, and rheumatoid arthritis,[113, 114, 115] they are by no means the only ones. As a general rule of thumb, a wide range of spices contain dense concentrations of phytochemicals and micronutrients, which provide a variety of antioxidants that have the potential to reduce inflammation.[116, 117] Rather than concentrating your diet around specific spices that you may not even enjoy or have access to, a simple strategy is to use those that you appreciate the flavor of. You'll notice all of my dishes use plenty of spices and herbs, and there is a clinical as well as culinary reason behind this. I've purposely included a section dedicated to making fresh pastes and spice blends from scratch (pages 244–247), and I hope they will encourage you to enjoy the process of using these amazing ingredients, ranging from mint, basil, and marjoram to sumac, cinnamon, and cayenne.

LIFESTYLE 360

These changes to the diet can serve to improve our balance from a state of pro-inflammation to one that is more harmonious with the intended function of our bodies. Your lifestyle, however, is important, and these practices are just as impactful.

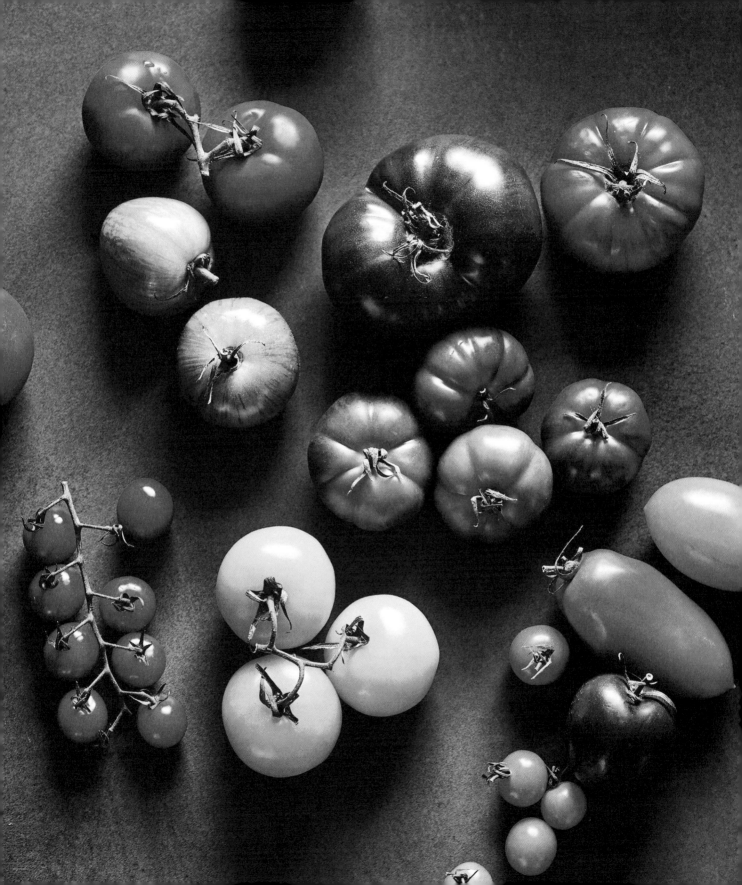

+ Slow down your eating   I used to find myself running from appointments across the city with a snack in my hand, eating at my desk while sifting through mounting paperwork during office hours or squeezing meals into a 10-minute break on an ER shift. Many of my colleagues and patients relate to this. Even when we're not rushed, we eat in front of screens, we scarf down our food, and hardly ever take time to appreciate the ingredients themselves. A measurement of stress in the body is a hormone called cortisol that is shown to be lowered if food is eaten slower and more mindfully.[118] The state in which food is consumed can be just as impactful on the body as the food itself. As a simple practice, I recommend patients take a few gentle breaths before starting to eat, and remove screens, in an effort to slow down the process so they can give their full attention to the food and perhaps the conversation around them.

+ Mind–body interventions   Mind–body interventions, like Tai Chi and meditation, have been shown to reduce the expression of genes that code for proteins that lead to inflammation.[119] In many studies, different types of stress-relieving and relaxation techniques have demonstrated significant anti-inflammatory effects.[120] There should be no doubt that stress and psychological ill health are associated with inflammation and that, conversely, stress-relieving techniques are anti-inflammatory.[121] When appropriate, I discuss these studies with patients, and I find that describing the clinical research underpinning my belief in the utility of mind–body interventions is really motivating for them. Think of mind–body interventions as any practice that encourages inner calm, whether that be the simple act of reading in a quiet space or meditation and yoga practices.

+ Walking   If the thought of joining a yoga class or even deep breathing is too overwhelming, you'll be pleased to hear about the mountains of research that consider the effectiveness of simple walks in nature. The Japanese practice of *shinrin yoku,* which literally translates as "forest bathing," has a large body of evidence examining the physiological as well as mental health benefits of this practice.[122, 123] Along with a reduction in heart rate and blood pressure and improvements in mood, forest bathing practices have reduced laboratory measures of inflammation such as cortisol and inflammatory proteins measured in the blood. Taking yourself to a park or forest at least once a week for a relaxing stroll could be one of the most hassle-free and effective ways to reduce your inflammatory burden without having to adjust your diet or do much at all.

+ Sleep   Given the number of homeostatic mechanisms that occur during sleep, it's unsurprising that even a single night's lack of shut-eye increases inflammatory signals

"If we can harness the incredible effects of not only our food, but the anti-inflammatory potential of our lifestyle, we could drastically reduce the problems that excess inflammation poses to our health."

in the body.[124] During sleep, our blood pressure lowers, our temperature drops, and rejuvenating hormones like melatonin, which have powerful antioxidant effects, rise to their highest levels. In his book *Why We Sleep*, the sleep medicine expert Professor Walker has warned that a lack of sleep puts us at greater risk of diabetes, cancer, and cardiovascular disease. It's often noted that people with high inflammation, as a result of conditions such as arthritis, diabetes, or obesity, often have disturbed sleep. It appears that inflammation and the proteins that signal inflammation have an interconnected relationship to sleep and may even regulate our need for slumber.[125] The advice for now is to at least allow yourself the opportunity to enjoy about 8–9 hours of rest per day. Put your electronic devices away a couple of hours before bed, eat early if possible, and give yourself potentially the best dose of anti-inflammatory medication available to us.

If we can harness the incredible effects of not only our food, but the anti-inflammatory potential of our lifestyle, we could drastically reduce the problems that excess inflammation poses to our health. What this chapter represents is a medicinal package for many patients without the need for strong drug interventions. We will always need pharmaceuticals, and as a doctor I do not hesitate to use them where appropriate. But the primary consideration should always be what we put on our plates and the way we live. These should be the first therapeutic interventions before we entertain more invasive measures that can carry a greater risk versus benefit.

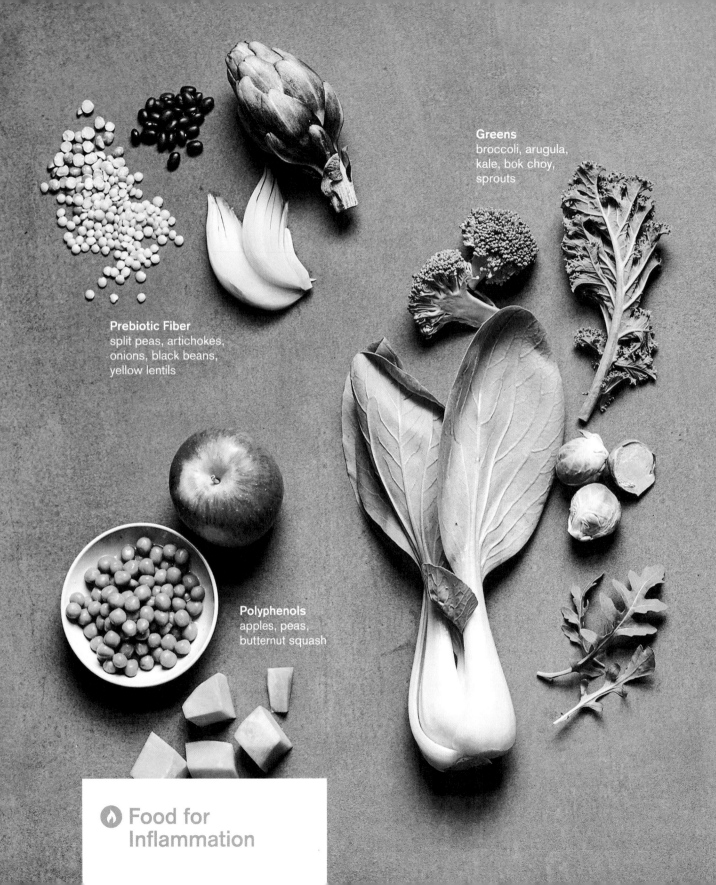

Greens
broccoli, arugula,
kale, bok choy,
sprouts

Prebiotic Fiber
split peas, artichokes,
onions, black beans,
yellow lentils

Polyphenols
apples, peas,
butternut squash

Food for
Inflammation

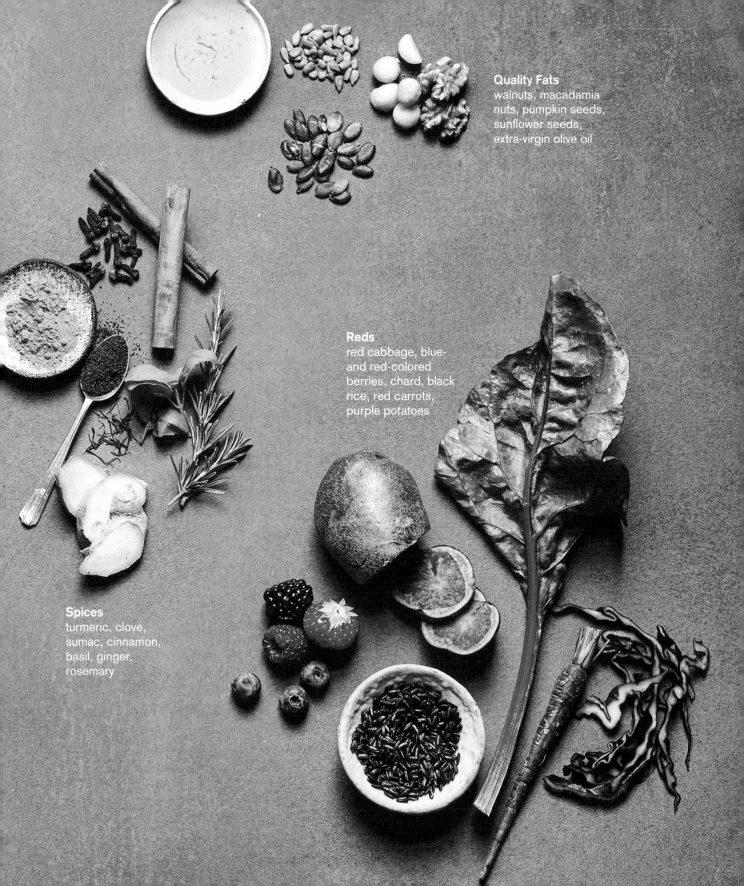

Quality Fats
walnuts, macadamia
nuts, pumpkin seeds,
sunflower seeds,
extra-virgin olive oil

Reds
red cabbage, blue-
and red-colored
berries, chard, black
rice, red carrots,
purple potatoes

Spices
turmeric, clove,
sumac, cinnamon,
basil, ginger,
rosemary

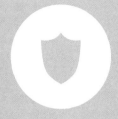

Eat for **Immunity**

The purpose of this chapter on immunity is to get you thinking about immune health in a different way. Rather than thinking of immunity as an isolated system that requires "boosting" with individual ingredients, think about it from the perspective of making healthy lifestyle choices to build your metabolic and energy reserve. This strengthens all of the specialized cells and organs needed to support your body's natural immunity and homeostatic mechanisms.

Your immune system is a collection of proteins, organs, and parts of the body that work in unison to protect us from harm. This includes everything from the acid found in your stomach to prevent harmful bacteria invading your gut, to the thick protective protein layer of your skin that physically keeps harmful microbes out. Immunity also includes the complex network of specialized cells that work in superb coordinated sequences to maintain the harmony of your internal ecosystem.

We need a resilient immune system to protect us from infective organisms like viruses and bacteria, but we also rely on this complex network to protect us from the malfunctioning of our own cells. Immunity is traditionally thought to be just our defense system, protecting us from harmful microbes that live in the external atmosphere, but it also ensures the correct functioning of our internal environment. Our immune system is responsible for identifying and appropriately clearing away mutated or malfunctioning cells that can lead to, for example, inflammation and uncontrolled growths that can become tumors.

Trillions of times a second, chemical reactions are occurring in your body, and as a product of normal metabolism and sheer probability, some cells are created that are malfunctioning or damaged.[126, 127] In addition, normal radiation from the sun or environmental pollution from smoke inhalation can also damage your skin and lung cells, respectively, and this needs to be dealt with. We rely on our body to clear these damaged cells effectively, so they don't lead to further negative effects. This is the job of our wonderful immune system. It is what we depend on to carry out these processes, and it does so with beautiful precision and efficiency without us having to think about it.

The wonderful thing about our immune system is that it is everywhere. You might think of our detoxification system as our liver and kidneys, or our mental activity center as our brain, but our immune system has to be prepared to step into action at any site in the body. Whether it's to protect us from a skin cut to the leg that could be an entry point for bacteria invading the bloodstream, or recognizing a malfunctioning cell in an organ and clearing it away so it doesn't develop into a growth, your immune system is ready.

I hope this gives you a broad idea of the magnitude of immunity and why simply eating or medicating to "boost" it is a misnomer. I appreciate it's a nice idea and an easy-to-understand concept; you eat something, it "boosts your immunity," and you become a common-cold-kicking superhuman. But in reality, our bodies do not work like that. Our vast interconnected systems of cells do not simply respond to one element like echinacea or zinc. It is called your immune system because it is an incredibly complex network of cells that require balance and harmony, and for this reason alone I hope you can already appreciate that there is no "silver bullet" nutritional supplement or pharmaceutical product that magically improves your immune health.

GUT HEALTH

There are particular sites in the body where immune cells interact with each other and are developed, including the bone marrow, the spleen in your abdomen, and lymph nodes dotted around your body such as the neck and groin. Of particular anatomical significance, however, is our gut. Our digestive system is the closest contact to the outside world. Everything we eat and drink from our environment is covered in microbes, and we have been in constant communication with them in our environment throughout our evolution via this 30-foot-long tube. But rather than being fearful of them, it's important to realize that most of the microbes that live in our digestive tract are integral to our health. Our microbiota, the population of microbes including viruses and fungi but predominantly bacteria, is mostly situated in the large intestine. As we have discussed, this huge population of foreign cells is responsible for digesting food, releasing vitamins from ingredients, and maintaining our health[128] (see page 40). The lining of the gut has to be super thin so the products of digestion and metabolites from gut microbe activity can pass through into the blood in order to be transported around the body.

The thin gut lining facilitating transfer of nutrients is necessary, but it's also a route for harmful microbes and products to pass into our blood, which could lead to damage; therefore, our immune cells need to be constantly assessing and recognizing friend from foe in these areas. It is relentless work to keep our human cells in harmony with foreign microbes, as well as detecting which of these organisms we need to get rid of. This is why so many immune cells are concentrated in our digestive tract, and it explains why the gut has the largest amount of "lymphoid tissue," which contains cells of the immune system.[129]

So, instead of simply using the analogy of an aggressive military force to describe our immune system, I like to see our immune cells as having just as much of a peacekeeper role in the complex world that is your human body. This is because the majority of cells contained within the body don't actually belong to us. Microbial cells outnumber our own human cells, and our health, particularly our immune health, depends on us keeping this population of microbes thriving. This objective is best served with a diet and lifestyle that nurture them.

Having a robust and well-functioning gut population protects and bolsters our ability to deal with infections on several levels. Specific gut microbes maintain the integrity of the gut wall, preventing harmful pathogens or materials inappropriately entering the bloodstream. They secrete their own antibiotic and anti-fungal chemicals that attack harmful microbes, preventing them from colonizing the gut. Beneficial microbes support an anti-inflammatory environment, which again is why good gut health improves cardiovascular disease and diabetes. The microbes themselves produce and release micronutrients that support our immune cells as well as protecting us from harmful environmental toxins.[130] Keeping our microbiota in shape improves our immune health and involves eating colorful vegetables, fiber, and a wide variety of whole foods. Dishes such as the Ethiopian Berbere Curry (see page 213) or the Pea Orecchiette (see page 169) are great ways to achieve this.

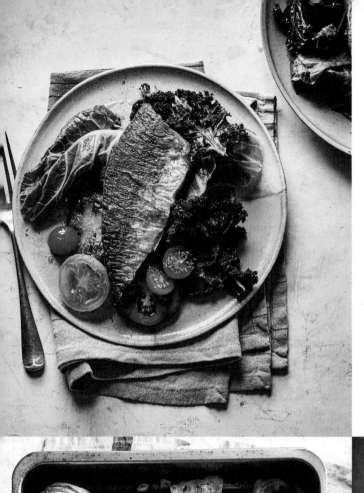

"Having a robust and well-functioning gut population protects and bolsters our ability to deal with infections on several levels."

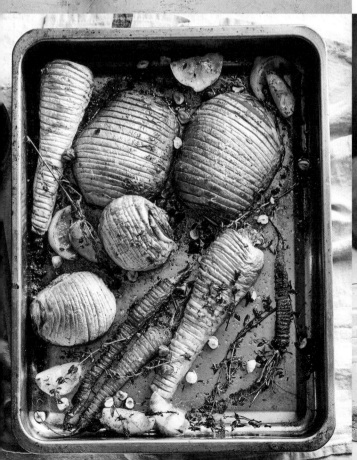

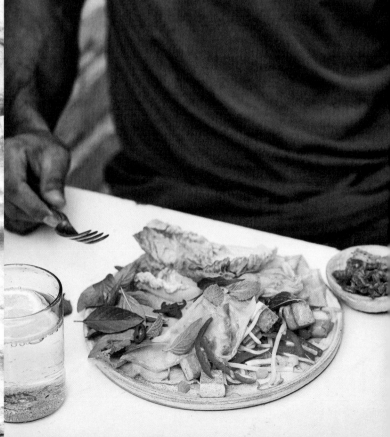

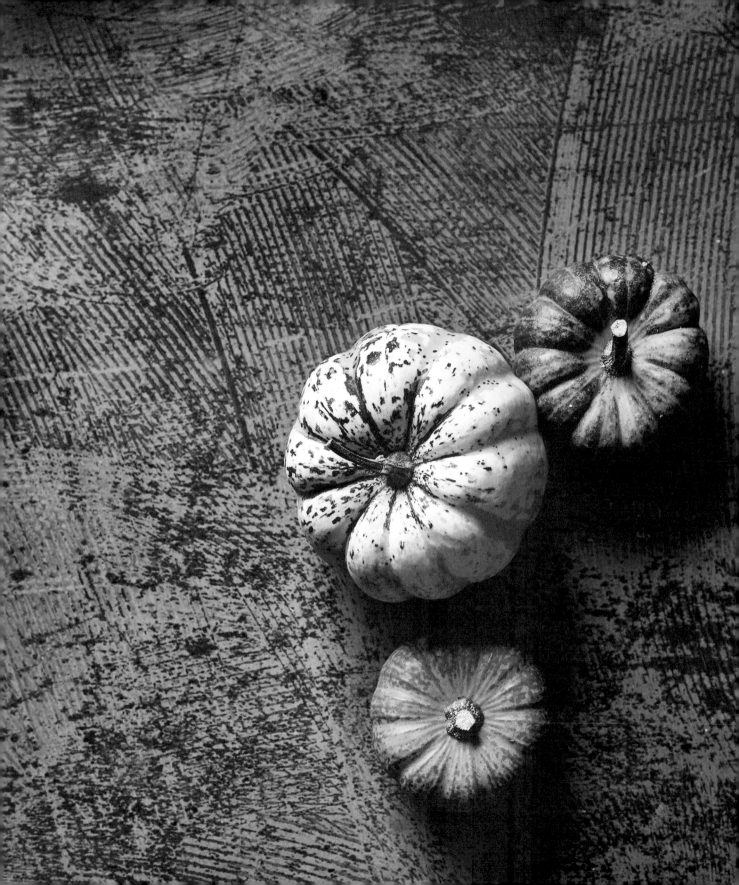

Because of a general recognition of the importance of the gut microbiota in immune-related diseases, researchers are increasingly looking at gut-focused treatments for problems related to imbalances in our immune system. Sometimes our immune cells can inappropriately send signals to fight infection or attack normal human cells that are perceived as foreign. This is a simplified explanation of autoimmunity, which differs from something like hay fever or dust-mite allergy, which is an exaggerated immune response.[131]

It's recognized that those who suffer from autoimmune conditions including psoriasis and rheumatoid arthritis tend to have imbalances in their gut populations.[132] The research is still in its early stages, but we also recognize that those who suffer from exaggerated immune responses, like in the case of asthma and eczema patients, may lack certain populations of gut bacteria that harmonize the body's immune response.[133, 134] This has led to the hypothesis that repopulating the gut microbiome with beneficial microbes may improve symptoms.

A theory gaining popularity to explain one of the causes of some autoimmune (AI) diseases is that the immune cells have been exposed to products that have entered directly into the bloodstream via "gaps" in the lining of our digestive tract.[135] These products have not been properly processed and identified by the immune system cells within the gut and thus trigger an aggressive response that leads to harm of the normal tissue. It's still under a lot of debate, but it's interesting to note that gut-focused treatments for AI disease, where potential triggers have been removed allowing the gut wall to repair itself, have led to some remarkable results.[136, 137] I don't have the space to dive into a full discussion of such a nuanced topic in this cookbook, but there is some interesting research on the horizon as well as a lot more we have to learn about process behind AI conditions and therapeutic dietary strategies. I suspect that it is more complicated than just nurturing the microbiome, but ensuring a healthy and thriving gut population using food could be a good starting point for helping with these illnesses, and a lot of well-respected scientists in the field are in agreement on this.

ELIMINATION DIETS It's my responsibility to be honest about the validity of these interventions and assess whether you could benefit from them. There has been a lot of speculation regarding AIP (autoimmune protocol) diets, and although these appear to be restrictive and eliminate perfectly healthy items from your food, there have been some interesting and significant outcomes gained from their use. Depending on the condition, these short-term therapeutic dietary interventions may be beneficial, but I hasten to add that they should be undertaken with the guidance of an experienced practitioner. I'm mindful of the scaremongering tactics surrounding components of food: gluten in flour, lectins in beans, and other common ingredients. My advice is to maintain a high suspicion of anyone blatantly brandishing a single food as harmful for everybody and making outlandish and unhelpful claims. It makes no scientific sense to suggest gluten is bad for everyone, for example, and I discussed the many reasons behind this in my first book. But I do believe there is a case for some patients to try out dietary strategies, and many rheumatologist and immunologist colleagues are starting to use them carefully with interesting anecdotal successes.

MITOCHONDRIAL SUPPORT

In recent years, we've also begun to recognize the profound importance of a component of our cells called mitochondria. These are found in all of our cells and have been traditionally referred to as the "powerhouses." These incredible batteries provide energy for all normal cell functions, but they're also critical for recognizing when an immune response is required.[138, 139] Cutting a long-winded biology lesson short, we require healthy, functioning mitochondria for a robust immune system that can boost its metabolic activity to adapt to the increased demands of when your immune system needs to be more active. Whether it's fighting an infection or balancing oxidative stress, your immune cells require more energy, and mitochondria are key to this. Supporting your mitochondria by preventing damage and providing them with fuel is therefore an essential immune-supporting strategy. Things that damage mitochondria include high-sugar diets and stress, and this gives us one explanation as to why poor diet and mental pressure appear to have detrimental impacts on our immunity.[140]

This is a very new area of research, so the evidence base behind what to eat for mitochondrial support is lacking, but that shouldn't stop us from being able to make reasonable, educated adjustments to our lifestyles that we can be sure are safe. Even if we cannot accurately determine that they are specifically supporting mitochondria, they are certainly beneficial to your body in many other ways.

However, diet related to immunity is a difficult topic to tackle. Unlike cardiovascular disease or diabetes, there aren't many studies examining the effects on immunity nor biomarkers that we regularly test to check someone's immune capacity.[141] However, the suggestions below encompass the entire ethos of this book: to give you reasonable evidence-based suggestions, with a good dose of common sense, about how your lifestyle can enhance the functioning of your incredible body. These delicious ingredients will get you thinking about how nutrition is exceptionally important to building your immunity.

+ Orange, yellow, and green foods Bright orange and yellow foods, including winter squash and sweet potato, as well as dark greens such as kale contain vitamin A precursors called carotenoids. These plant chemicals are essential to our immune system and have a role in maintaining our gut barrier, the functioning of specialized immune cells, as well as the cells involved in the immediate response to stressors.[142] We also find different sources of vitamin A in animal products such as fatty fish and organ meats we don't tend to consume much of, such as liver. Try the Fennel Sardines with Pine Nuts (see page 180) or the Butter Beans, Butternut Squash, and Spicy Couscous (see page 165).

Along with vitamin A, brightly colored foods also contain vitamin C, as do a number of green vegetables including broccoli, parsley, spring greens, and Brussels sprouts, and by lightly steaming them (a technique I use regularly in my recipes), we can maintain this vitamin content. It's long been recognized that vitamin C is important for immune cells.[143] It can aid your "first response" immune system activity, and vitamin C itself is a strong antioxidant that is important to protect your immune cells and limit the oxidative stress within your mitochondria.[144, 145]

For these reasons, many of my patients have bought into the advertising for vitamin C supplements. Although I believe these are fairly safe and well tolerated, there are added benefits of obtaining vitamin C, plus the abundance of other vital micronutrients, from whole foods rather than supplements in isolation. There are a huge range of other nutrients contained in dark leafy greens and citrus fruits beyond just vitamin C. For instance, a pile of steamed greens with olive oil, salt, and lemon (like my Horta recipe on page 182) would be a fantastic accompaniment to most meals as it doesn't just offer vitamin C; it delivers sulforaphane, magnesium, and added fiber to your diet. I encourage people to think of their food as a wonderful collection of thousands of micronutrients and plant chemicals rather than just one or two vitamins.

+ Nuts and seeds Nuts like cashews, almonds, and Brazil nuts, as well as sunflower seeds and flaxseed, contain good sources of zinc, selenium, and vitamin E. These three micronutrients have individually been studied in clinical trials using larger doses than found naturally with some positive results on immune health, which is why they're labeled "immune boosting" in many stores.[146, 147, 148] However, I believe using supplements of individual micronutrients in large quantities is unjustified for the majority of people. Certain populations that may be at risk of deficiency and have lowered immune health, such as the elderly, may benefit from supplemental forms, but we can obtain reasonable amounts of these essential

> "There are added benefits of obtaining vitamin C, plus the abundance of other vital micronutrients, from whole foods rather than supplements in isolation."

nutrients from wholesome, delicious food. Not only do I use nuts and seeds to add texture to food, but they're fantastic sources of protein and fiber that additionally contribute to immune health. Try the Herby Walnut and Cashew Roast (see page 195) for a great way of using more quality fats.

+ **Fiber** An effective strategy to improve our immune system would be anything that helps our gut environment; specialized prebiotic fibers including chicory, endive, Jerusalem artichoke, and garlic provide your microbes with a source of food. When digested, they're able to make a fatty acid chemical called butyrate, which helps maintain the lining of the gut wall.[149] A well-fed microbiota is better equipped to carry out its immune-modulating role of reducing inflammation and preventing pathogenic microbes from colonizing in the gut, causing ill health.

+ **Herbs and spices** A variety of vegetables, like the colorful ingredients described above, also provide a fantastic food source for the microbes, and there is also a rationale for using plentiful herbs and spices. Ginger, turmeric, fennel, and some botanicals like peppermint may have a role in immune support as they have been shown in some small studies to reduce gut inflammation.[150] I think regularly including herbs and spices in our food for a culinary as well as functional purpose is an important aspect of our diets that we should embrace. Try the Ras el Hanout (see page 245) or the Laksa Paste (see page 246) for ideas.

There are some specific botanicals and herbs that have shown "immune-modulating" capacity, in that they may stimulate the production of cells of the immune system.[151] There is also a tradition of using different herbs for immune support across many cultures, including elderberry, echinacea, mushroom varieties, and probiotics. However, I would rather we focus on accessible diet and lifestyle aspects that serve to build your immune reserve rather than relying on immune-modulating plants for general sustenance. Improving your lifestyle and diet are much more powerful strategies than relying on a special flower or fungi for support.

LIFESTYLE 360

Nutrition has a huge role in maintaining robust and balanced immunity, but if there is any system that exemplifies why total coordination of lifestyle factors, such as exercise and sleep, is necessary for universal functioning, your immune system is the poster boy. By harnessing the power of a variety of lifestyle factors, you can greatly enhance your metabolic energy and the ability of your immune system to perform at its peak. It will not only improve your resilience to common viruses and pathogens but also aid inflammation balance under the control of immune cells.

+ Exercise For everyone there is an exercise sweet spot. Regular moderate exercise has been shown to universally benefit immunity. Aerobic exercise actually encourages your body to be more resilient to stressors and therefore has an overall benefit, despite the short-term effects of exercise being inflammatory.[152] Aerobic exercise can actually improve your mitochondrial function, which may also be why regular exercise builds a resilient immune system.[153, 154]

Persistent over-training, however, is associated with reduced immune reserve. There are recognized health risks of putting high amounts of strain on your body by over-exercising that researchers have observed in endurance athletes like cyclists.[155] A balance of training is what we should be aiming to achieve, and there are specific types of exercises that may be particularly good for immune health.

+ Yoga Described as both a mindfulness technique as well as a form of exercise, recent studies on yoga have examined a fascinating effect on immune cells.[156] Researchers have demonstrated that yoga practices can impact the expression of genes to one that positively improves immune cell function. Similar effects have been shown with other practices such as qigong and tai chi.[120] Combined with the physical benefits of the exercise, yoga could be one of the best all-round immune health–promoting activities we know of. The best advice I have is to mix it up. I have developed my own yoga routine from watching online yoga sessions that are very accessible and easy to follow, as well as attending classes now and again to get some pointers. But I would also encourage HIIT (high-intensity interval training) sessions, too, to improve aerobic capacity, as well as endurance training such as cycling and swimming for their additional benefits.

+ Meditation The gradual deterioration of our immune capability as we age, known as immunosenescence, may be closely related to both psychological distress and stress hormones.[157] It would stand to reason that techniques to reduce stress effects may be beneficial from an immune perspective. Combined with the many positive effects of mind–body interventions, practices such as deep breathing, transcendental meditation, or simple walks in nature are a no-brainer for me to advise. I was pleased to read a paper about the positive effect of walking in nature, specifically on cells of the immune system.[158] So perhaps the most immune-system-enhancing of activities could be a yoga session in a park followed by deep breathing in natural sunlight. And this brings me nicely to the subject of vitamin D.

+ Vitamin D More than a vitamin, vitamin D acts as a master hormone that regulates a multitude of genes involved in a huge number of processes. Beyond its well-recognized

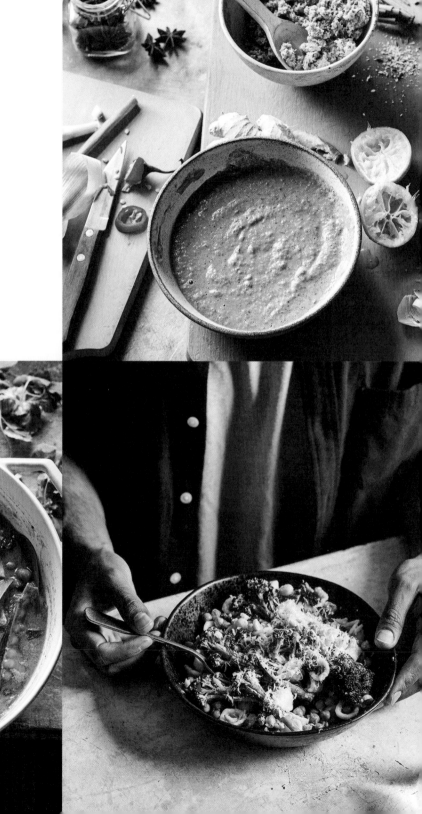

"By harnessing the power of lifestyle factors, you can greatly enhance your metabolic energy and the ability of your immune system to perform at its peak."

involvement in bone health and calcium regulation, vitamin D has a very important role in immune health.[159, 160] In both the initial "innate" response to infections and the more specific "adaptive" responses, scientists are researching the role of vitamin D and its importance to auto-immune conditions. There are very few sources of vitamin D in the diet, and thus medical practitioners have taken to recommending vitamin D for the whole population during winter months and for those with darker skin colors. The best advice is to get adequate sun exposure outdoors, have regular tests by your GP if you're at risk, and take a supplement during the darker months of September to March.

+ Sleep deprivation It will come as no surprise to many people that sleep deprivation drastically lowers a person's immunity. Your immune system is very likely to be regulated by routine and the 24-hour sleep-wake cycle that influences all other cells in your body.[161] This is why sleep is integral to a healthy immune system. As a GP, I've lost count of the number of people turning up on a Monday suffering acute tonsillitis directly attributable to late nights on the weekend or travel. But this is just the tip of the iceberg. Persistent sleep loss significantly disrupts your immune system, increasing inflammation, which drastically raises the risk of chronic illnesses like heart disease, Type 2 diabetes, and even cancer. As you can probably appreciate by now, these are all conditions related to an ill-performing immune system. Achieving 7–9 hours of sleep a night could be considered one of the most potent therapies for improving one's immune system, and it's definitely on my prescription pad.

To sum up diet and lifestyle strategies to improve immune health, we simply need to remember a few facts: gut health is exceptionally important; there are well-recognized detrimental effects of a western diet on immune health[162] (high in sugar and refined carbohydrates, low in fiber, and lacking in micronutrients); certain micronutrients are critical for the adequate functioning of our immune cells; and the importance of supporting our mitochondria cannot be underestimated. Although this may sound complicated, the reality is that these additions to your diet and routine are accessible and straightforward. I'm confident that it is achievable for you, as it is for many of my patients, and my recipes will set you on the right path.

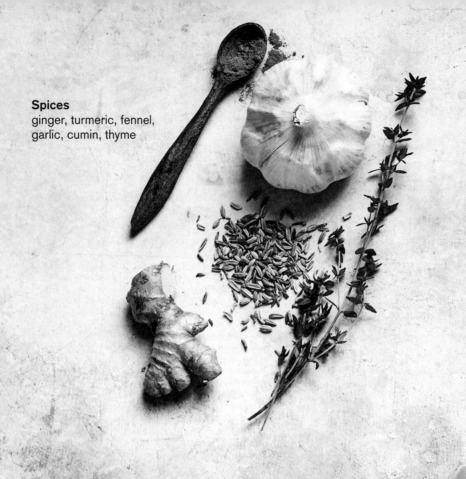

Spices
ginger, turmeric, fennel,
garlic, cumin, thyme

Prebiotic Fibers
chicory, endive,
Jerusalem artichokes,
garlic

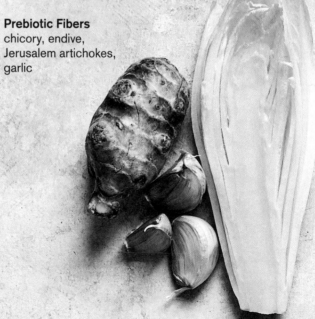

Food for Immunity

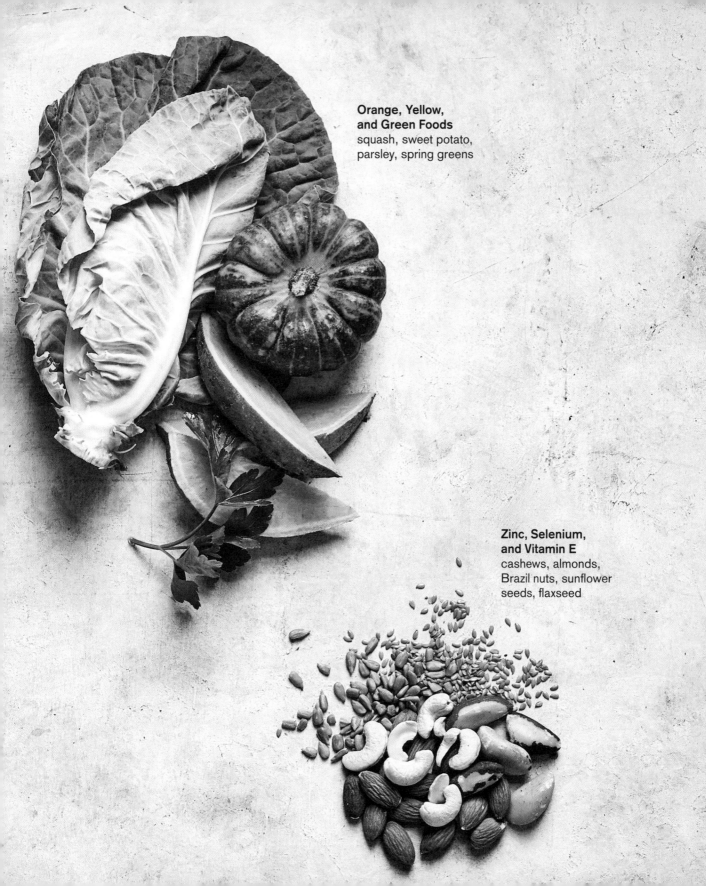

Orange, Yellow, and Green Foods
squash, sweet potato, parsley, spring greens

Zinc, Selenium, and Vitamin E
cashews, almonds, Brazil nuts, sunflower seeds, flaxseed

Eat to Beat Cancer

This was by far the most difficult chapter to write. Not least because it is a complicated topic to tackle, but also because it is an emotive subject matter and therefore the most controversial. However, I believe it is our responsibility as medical professionals to educate ourselves, appreciate the wealth of literature surrounding this complicated topic, and share it responsibly with the public.

Our understanding of cancer biology is continually evolving, and the deeper one goes into the literature, the more complex the systems that underpin this life-changing disease appear to be. Cancer can be loosely defined as a series of mutations that have spun out of control, leading to uncontrollable growth of cells. It's really an umbrella term to describe lots of different types of cancers that can be caused by different things (like bacteria, viruses, or UV radiation) and affect different parts of the body. Some cancers are the result of inherited genes, but most of them occur as we age and acquire more mutations. The processes that prevent these mutations from developing into cancer become less reliable with age, which is why we see most cancers in patients over 50.

Apart from the classic "eat a balanced diet" advice, we, the medical profession, have traditionally been reluctant to delve into meaningful discussions about the role of food and lifestyle as chemopreventative. A chemopreventative is a natural or synthetic substance that reduces the risk of cancer (examples included drugs like Tamoxifen to prevent certain types of breast cancer[163]), but food is generally not accepted as one. The argument against labeling food as potentially cancer protective is that there are simply not enough clinical trials yielding irrefutable, large-scale evidence. But considering how much we already know about the impact of diet and lifestyle, I sincerely hope this will change.

The lack of dialogue has created a vacuum of information that has, on occasion, been willingly filled by unqualified health commentators who have led people astray. It is this taint that continues to mark cancer and nutrition as a taboo subject. But it is time to redress the balance and normalize the conversation around food and cancer. In my opinion, it is simply inexcusable to say "nutrition has no role in cancer prevention or management." This chapter is by no means comprehensive, but it should give you an idea of why I'm so passionate about this subject matter and the need for more robust nutrition and lifestyle advice within the field of oncology.

For anyone to suggest that they have the "cure for cancer" shows a complete lack of understanding about how diverse this illness is, and it is the opposite of what I am trying to emphasize in this chapter. There are so many different types of cancer, different stages of the disease process, as well as the added complexity of cancer cells being able to mutate and change their function to avoid detection. Every cancer patient requires a tailored approach to treatment unique to them, which is why cancer treatments are discussed in multidisciplinary meetings with different specialists weighing in with their thoughts about management.

There are many diet and lifestyle strategies being explored as both adjuncts to traditional treatment and ways to reduce the chances of recurrence, but it would be naive of me to try and squeeze an explanation of all of these into a cookbook. Instead, this chapter is a succinct review about what we know in regard to preventing cancer from occurring in the first place, and I encourage everyone to always work with their practitioner.

I also want to make it clear from the outset that no one should be thought to be at fault for suffering cancer. Ever. We can live the healthiest lifestyle with minimal exposure to well-known carcinogens in our environment, eat and exercise well, live a happy fulfilled life, and despite this, a random mutation that gets out of hand can strike anyone at any time. Such is the frustrating and inexplicable randomness of cancer biology.

64   From the trillions of processes that are occurring in your body as you read these words, it is understandable that despite leading the healthiest life, despite eating the right foods, despite performing all the best lifestyle-enhancing activities, out of sheer probability some of us will experience cancer. However, diet and lifestyle change is not futile, and what this chapter will detail are changes within our control that reduce the chances of this happening and put the odds more in our favor. It is my job as a medical practitioner to discuss the mountains of information about what the best protective practices are, and to give my patients the best odds of avoiding cancer. The most encouraging thing about these protective practices is that they benefit you in more ways than avoiding cancer risk. They are key to living a healthy and happy life.

MOSTLY PLANTS

What I can say with utmost certainty from the start is that you can reduce your overall risk of cancer by concentrating your diet around a wide range of colorful fruits and vegetables.[164, 165] A number of studies demonstrate this, and I have no reservation putting it on paper. It's something that everyone needs to know and take action on. Research specifically examining the Mediterranean diet has found it is one of the best at lowering the risk of cancer.[166] The Mediterranean way of eating is one that focuses on higher intakes of fruits, colorful vegetables, nuts, seeds, and whole grains. When we examine the effects of these types of foods and their chemicals on our cellular biology, we can begin to understand how they can protect us.

ANTIOXIDANTS

Micronutrients such as vitamins C and E that we find in colorful foods such as peppers, radishes, beets, and squash directly block DNA damage caused by carcinogens in our environment as well as oxidants as a result of normal metabolism in our cells.[167, 168] Most notably, foods rich in vitamins C and E have been shown to be exceptionally good for reducing oxidative stress in cells and balancing inflammation. This has led to an explosion of people using high-dose vitamin C tablets and intravenous drips in treatment, but your food should always be where you obtain nutrition in the first instance. Concentrate on consuming colored vegetables and greens, and you'll be taking in adequate amounts of vitamin C.

ENZYME PROCESSES

Plants also contain micronutrients that act as co-factors, or "helper molecules," that are required for a number of processes in the body. These co-factors include B vitamins, magnesium, and co-enzyme Q10, which we find in broccoli, spinach, cauliflower, and

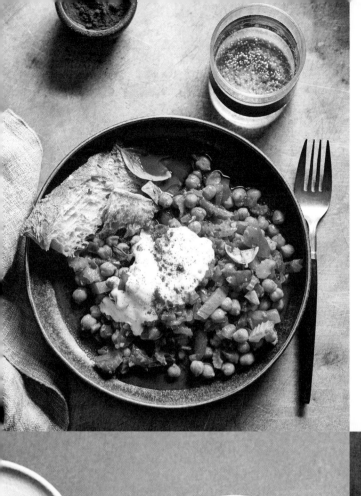

"What I can say with utmost certainty from the start is that you can reduce your overall risk of cancer by concentrating your diet around a wide range of colorful fruits and vegetables."

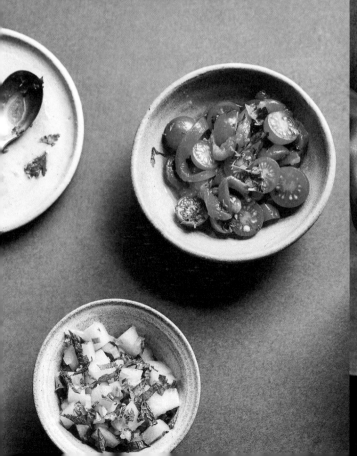

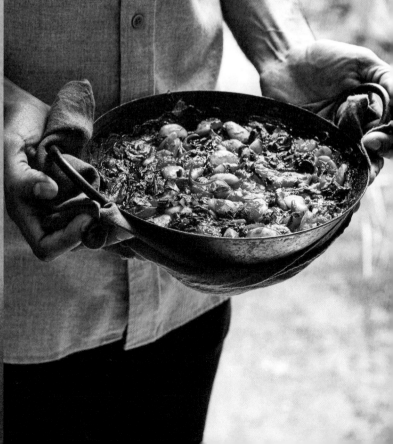

mushrooms. Some of these co-factors are necessary to facilitate your body's natural ability to remove environmental carcinogens.[169] For example, your liver requires a number of different micronutrients that we obtain from food to allow it to filter harmful substances, render them innocuous, and remove them from the body. Providing your body with these key nutrients allows it to perform this function optimally,[170, 171] and the principles of healthy eating that I describe provide plenty of these nutritionally dense ingredients without the need to eat "prescriptively."

GENETIC EXPRESSION

Nutrigenomics is the study of how nutrition affects the expression of our genes, and it has been shown in a number of studies to have utmost importance in the field of cancer.[172] There are crucial links between components in our diet and their role in preventing DNA damage via gene expression. Certain foods increase certain genes' activity while decreasing others, which can lead to an overall anticancer effect.[173] Examples of these types of "cancer protective" foods that I find in the literature include broccoli, green tea, and cauliflower, which contain plant chemicals including sulfurophane, epigallocatechin gallate, and indole-3-carbinol. This is not an exclusive list, however, and I imagine we have a lot to learn about many other foods when we begin to study their plant chemicals and their impact on genetic expression. What I want you to take away from this is that our food can communicate with both our cells' molecular mechanisms and genetic information to limit damage from internal and environmental stressors. Food is quite literally information.

FIBER

Plant-focused diets, like the Mediterranean diet, tend to contain more fiber from ingredients such as nuts, seeds, pulses, and whole grains, and dietary fiber has been shown to have a strong protective effect on certain types of cancer.[174] There are a number of reasons why increasing fiber in your diet is cancer protective. High-fiber foods release sugar slowly into the bloodstream, therefore reducing sugar spikes and insulin release, which reduces the risk of fat accumulation around our organs and thus lowers cancer risk.[175] Fiber improves digestive transit time, which reduces the exposure to both environmental pollutants and excess hormones that need to be cleared from the body via the intestines.[176] As we've covered extensively in previous chapters, varied sources of fiber feed your gut microbes and improve their activity. Your microbes are critical to the protective capability of your body's immune system, and part of its role is to identify and rid the body of malfunctioning and damaged cells. Researchers are also looking at the effect of certain microbe populations and the response to cancer treatments,[177] and there is mounting evidence supporting the role of the microbiota in response to cancer therapy. I'm sure that in the future, "microbiota-focused therapies" alongside chemotherapy will become normal practice. But while we don't have definitive evidence of what the ideal microbe population looks like for anticancer properties, it is clear that nurturing this population with diet and lifestyle is going to be key for promoting health and reducing cancer risk.[178]

Although there is no such thing as a "silver bullet" for cancer prevention, there are many foods that are demonstrating a protective role against many forms of cancer.[179] Vegetables are key. In fact, the National Cancer Institute has identified 35 plant-based foods that possess cancer-preventive properties, including garlic, ginger, onion, turmeric, tomatoes and cruciferous vegetables, which we'll be discussing.[180] These are just some of my favorites from both a culinary and scientific perspective:

+ **Red Foods** Lycopene, a chemical found in tomatoes and exotic fruit like guava and watermelon, has been shown to inhibit several types of cancer by interfering with cell signals that effectively stop the cells from growing.[181] While it's hard to prove direct effects on cancer outcomes, these ingredients are accessible and could be part of a diet that protects against cancer. There's been lots of interest specifically with prostate cancer, but the overall benefits of antioxidants found in red-colored foods are phenomenal.[182] For inspiration, try my Spanish Chickpea Stew (see page 170).

+ **Berries** The bitter polyphenols found in blackberries, blueberries, cherries, and strawberries are shown to inhibit cancer cells in lab studies by interfering with their ability to grow vessels.[183, 184] In addition, plant chemicals called anthocyanins encourage cancer cells to "commit suicide," a normal cellular process known as apoptosis.[185, 186, 187] Berries are concentrated sources of antioxidants that can reduce oxidative stress in human cells, making them universally beneficial for health.[188] I tend to use berries in smoothies, I top desserts with them, and I always keep frozen packages at hand. Try them in my Banana Berry Scoops (see page 238).

+ **Greens** Brassica vegetables are perhaps my favorite of all the cheap and widely accessible ingredients that line our supermarket shelves. They contain an abundance of plant chemicals, including glucosinolates and sulfurophane, that have incredible anticancer properties.[180] These compounds have been shown to aid your body's ability to remove environmental pollutants and balance inflammation.[189, 190, 179, 191] Large studies examining eating habits have also shown that populations that consume more brassica vegetables than others significantly reduce their cancer risk. You'll notice cauliflower, broccoli, arugula, Brussels sprouts, and cabbage are frequent ingredients in my recipes. We all need to be eating more of these delicious and health-promoting foods.

+ Herbs and spices Garlic, ginger, turmeric, and a number of other ingredients are commonly cited as "anticancer" foods. While I'm not a fan of prescriptively labeling ingredients, there is some exciting research examining why these, and many other herbs and spices, could be preventative for cancer. The phytochemical curcumin, found in turmeric, is one of the most extensively studied in the literature. But along with gingerols, found in ginger, and quercetin, found in onions and apples, these chemicals have been shown in experimental models to have activity that reduces the growth potential of cancer cells.[179] Essentially, plant chemicals that are found in a variety of herbs and spices interfere with the process of normal cells turning into cancer cells. Some interact with genetic material, others modify cell signaling, and some prevent the formation of blood vessels being formed that help tumors grow. In many cases, like in the case of turmeric, herbs and spices do many of these things simultaneously.[192] In fact, the same processes that these foods impact are those that are targeted by cancer drugs. This isn't to suggest that we should be thinking of replacing drugs with food, but it highlights the significance of what we put on our plates as a cancer preventative. Increasing our use of herbs and spices could be a key cancer-preventing strategy. Whether you add mint to a dressing or thyme to heighten the flavor of root vegetables, you'll notice how spiced my dishes are for flavor and functional processes.

+ Fiber Varying your sources of fiber is key to encouraging a healthy microbe population, which is why I encourage eating garlic, chicory, leeks, and whole fruits such as apples and peaches (which also contain their own protective phytochemicals). I like to focus my meals around plant proteins, which is why the majority of the recipes in this cookbook contain delicious whole sources of beans, legumes, nuts, and seeds, which are fantastic for improving the microbiome population.[193]

+ Flaxseed, extra-virgin olive oil, and green tea You'll find a number of ingredients being given a lot of attention in the media as potential cancer-preventative foods, but I think these in particular deserve a mention. Omega-3, which we find in flaxseed, cold-pressed olive oil, walnuts, chia, and wild fatty fish, may be beneficial from a cancer perspective. Not only do these ingredients contain an abundance of other micronutrients like vitamin E and selenium that can reduce oxidative stress, Omega-3 itself may elicit a protective effect in part due to its anti-inflammatory properties.[194, 195, 196] Green tea contains different types of polyphenols, called catechins, which have been studied for their chemopreventative effects.

"It's without reservation that I believe we should be encouraging people to consider our diet as cancer protective."

While green tea can be an expensive ingredient to acquire (and a flavor you need to develop a taste for), the biological mechanisms behind why this ingredient may be protective are fascinating.[171]

The issue with nutrition and oncology is that the efficacy of diet-derived chemo-preventative agents has not been established conclusively. Most of what we know about food and cancer properties comes from animal experiments or those done in a petri dish. However, we can appreciate that diets made up largely of colorful vegetables have protective functions, and robust, large-scale studies of nutrition in humans will always be difficult to conduct.[165] These foods I've mentioned above are generally considered to be safe additions to our diet and have enormous potential in the fight against the cancer process. For these reasons, it's without reservation that I believe we should be encouraging people to consider our diet as cancer protective.

LIFESTYLE 360

As part of a holistic cancer preventative package, there is evidence for certain lifestyle factors that can further reduce our risk of cancer in addition to food. These practices have been shown to be beneficial during treatment as well as reducing the risk of recurrence. If you are undergoing cancer therapy, work with your practitioners to see which of these are appropriate for you.

+ Exercise Movement is pure medicine. The benefits of outdoor exercise in green spaces,[197, 198] the inflammation-reducing effect of movement, and its ability to enhance your immune system[199] are all reasons why exercise is so healthy—especially during cancer treatment. Gone are the days where we would advise all cancer patients to rest, in the same way we, within reason, no longer advise post-surgical patients or heart attack sufferers to lie in bed for weeks after the event. The benefit of movement during cancer therapy has been shown to reduce treatment side effects, fatigue, and mental stress and to lower recurrence rates.[200] We are really at a stage where the evidence is telling us that exercise is beneficial as a preventative measure, during management, and to lower the risk of recurrence.

As well as the impact on immunity, inflammation, and mental health, movement improves circulating hormone levels and reduces fat tissue accumulation around our organs, which is metabolically active and has been shown to promote cancer. Instead of turning to scaremongering tactics and simply stating the link between obesity and cancer, I'd rather bring attention to the positive aspects of lifestyle. Despite having a raised body mass index and despite not being an ideal weight, it is the summation of your health habits that determine your risk. If you can move every day, do something that raises your heart rate, and importantly something you enjoy, you can drastically lower your risk of cancer. Focus on well-being habits, and worry less about the number on the scale.

+ Vitamin D Vitamin D crops up as a subject time and time again because it is such an important regulator of multiple processes in your body, extending beyond just calcium balance. Vitamin D has been shown in both animal and lab studies to be an agent that inhibits the growth of cancer cells through a variety of molecular targets. Whether this is true in humans remains to be seen, but there is a lot of evidence looking at population studies to demonstrate a relationship between adequate vitamin D levels and lower rates of cancer.[201] Considering it is relatively safe, a pragmatic approach to cancer prevention is to discuss vitamin D tablets with your practitioner—it is something I talk to many patients about.

+ Stress A lot of attention has been given to stress and its role in many conditions beyond mental health. Nobel laureate Dr. Elizabeth Blackburn and her colleague Dr. Elissa Epel studied the relationship between stress and telomeres and cited many of this fascinating research in their book *The Telomere Effect*. Telomeres are found at the end of your chromosomes and protect the genetic material housed in every cell in your body. Telomeres are also used as a biological marker of aging in research.[202] Emotional stress can cause "shortening" of your telomeres, which can negatively impact their protective effect and increases the risk of mutations that can lead to cancer.

We know, by looking at population studies, that psychological stress has only a weak association with the incidence of cancer. But considering what we currently know about stress-relieving techniques, mindfulness meditation, and the general health benefits to be gained from this practice, I would argue that stress management is a pragmatic approach to reducing cancer risk and certainly has benefits during treatment.[203, 204, 205] I was lucky enough to visit an incredible cancer center in England, Penny Brohn UK, where mindfulness meditation and art therapy play a central role in helping clients manage their treatment.

There is no hard proof that stress-relieving techniques such as meditation and mindfulness reduce the risk of cancer. However, there is enough in the way of holistic benefits of mindfulness techniques for me to advise everyone that it's at least worth a try. It doesn't have to be a cliché or hard. Simple breathing techniques, walks in green spaces, or even listening to music is enough to give you some benefit.

I wanted to close this chapter by highlighting the work of Dr. Dean Ornish and colleagues from America, who in part inspired me on my own personal health journey.

They demonstrated, using elegant gene-mapping models, just how effective a combination of dietary and lifestyle change can be in low-risk prostate cancer patients. By introducing largely plant-based diets, exercise regimens, and meditation techniques, they were able to show how tumor suppressor genes were switched on, while tumor promoter genes were switched off.[206] Beyond gene mapping, the patients involved in the study improved multiple parameters of health, including inflammation and quality of life. The evidence behind each of these interventions may not be the strongest, but I believe it is this pragmatic and commonsense approach to health that we need to be more open-minded about.

Understanding the mechanisms of how comprehensive lifestyle changes can affect our biology is key to strengthening efforts to develop effective prevention and treatment of many diseases, including cancer. If we are genuinely trying to make an impact on the statistic that 1 in 3 of us will experience this devastating disease, we need to get real about the power of lifestyle. The knowledge gained from investigations into the role of diet in cancer and cancer prevention should be integrated into lifestyle modifications in order to reduce the occurrence of this emotionally and physically draining condition. I sincerely hope this chapter has given you some confidence and motivation about how much control we really have.

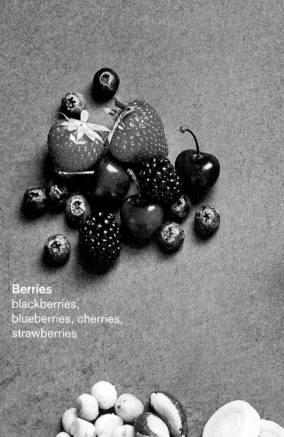
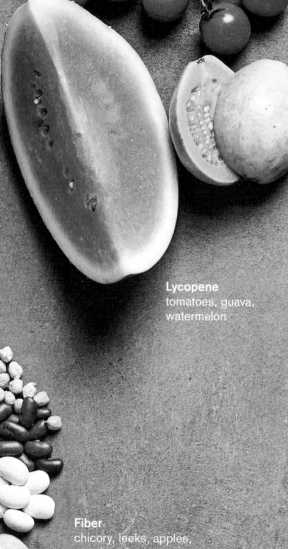

Berries
blackberries,
blueberries, cherries,
strawberries

Lycopene
tomatoes, guava,
watermelon

Fiber
chicory, leeks, apples,
peaches, beans,
legumes, nuts, seeds

🎗 Food for Cancer

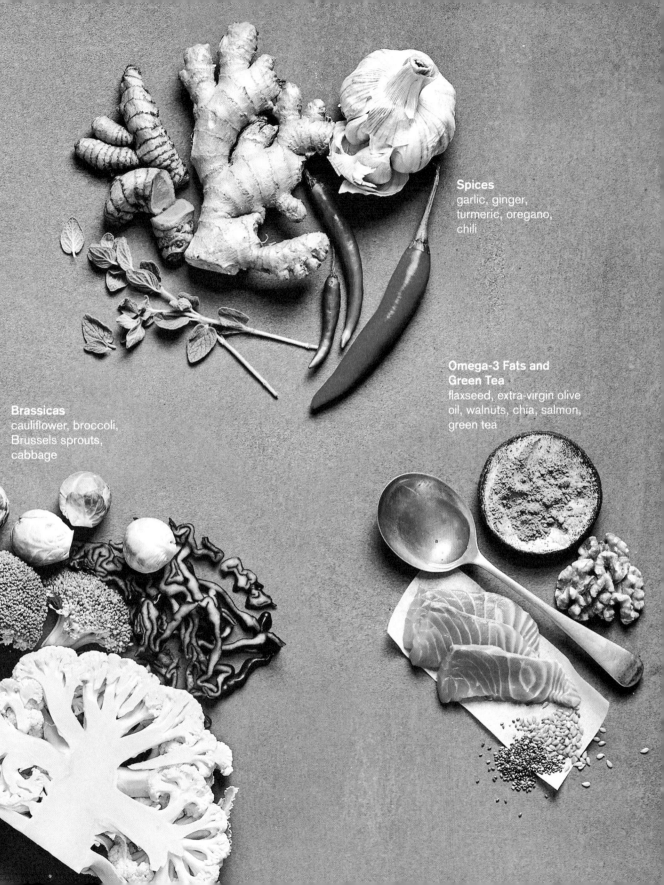

Spices
garlic, ginger, turmeric, oregano, chili

Omega-3 Fats and Green Tea
flaxseed, extra-virgin olive oil, walnuts, chia, salmon, green tea

Brassicas
cauliflower, broccoli, Brussels sprouts, cabbage

Eat for Your Mood

Mood disorders, including depression and anxiety, are now one of the most common causes of disability in the industrialized world. More people will be diagnosed with major depressive disorders in the next generation than before. It is quite literally a public health crisis.[207] Both as a GP in my practice and at public speaking events, I'm often asked, "What can I eat to help my mood?" It's a reasonable question. Many people have been led to believe that pills, in the form of antidepressants and other psychiatric medications, can effectively treat mood disorders, and perhaps there is a more "natural" route with food?

However, I beg you to think differently about how to treat something as complicated as
mental health. Rather than using food or drugs alone to treat symptoms, instead start with
the question, "Why do I have these symptoms in the first place?" When we attempt to look
for the root cause of mental health problems, or any condition for that matter, we can tailor
more effective treatments and stand the best chance of achieving resolution.

As a doctor who works in both general practice and emergency medicine, I witness just
how common and complex mental health problems can be. It would be naive to think that we
can reverse our symptoms of depression or anxiety, for example, with one intervention alone,
be that diet-led or pharmaceutical. In many cases patients require more than a collection of
foods with particular compounds and a holistic attitude to treating mental health disorders.
It is not simply a case of neurochemical imbalance that needs "boosting" with drugs or
ingredients, and it's really important to keep sight of this. Making sure you get the right help
and interventions from your doctor is key. Psychotherapy and support groups as well as
pharmaceutical interventions can all have a role.

I'm a firm believer in having open, honest conversations with patients about how
potentially effective and safe lifestyle interventions can be at preventing and managing
common mental health problems. I was pleased to discover a recognition from the
professional psychiatry community about the link between food and mental illness in a 2015
Lancet paper.[208] Since then, interest in using nutrition alongside conventional treatments
has snowballed as psychiatrists scramble to find complementary ways of treating the rising
number of patients who need help. I address diet and lifestyle with all of my patients, and I'm
confident that these interventions will have positive effects for most people. This chapter will
introduce you to the important role of food and lifestyle that should always be thought of as
an adjunct to mental health treatment.

MANAGING INFLAMMATION

It's not a coincidence that conditions related to inflammation, such as heart disease,
diabetes, and autoimmune conditions (including rheumatoid arthritis) are all correlated with
high rates of depression,[78] and there is great interest from the psychiatric medical community
in determining why this is the case.[209] It is a relatively new discovery that the brain has
a lymphatic system, which is a network of vessels that carry water, waste products, and
immune cells around the body. Previously, it was thought that the brain was shielded from
microbes and inflammation by something called the blood-brain barrier and therefore did
not require an immune network. But the discovery of this system suggests that it is not as
protected as we once thought and that the brain relies on these "glymphatics" to facilitate

the transport of inflammatory proteins out of the nervous system[210] to maintain balance. As the brain is exposed to inflammation, it's speculated that reducing overall inflammation in the body could therefore prove useful in the treatment of mental health conditions.[78, 211, 212]

While many practitioners might immediately think of using a pharmaceutical to reduce inflammation, like an anti-inflammatory drug, it's actually your diet and lifestyle that can have an incredible impact. I talk about inflammation and what this actually means in more detail on pages 34–47, but eating a nutrient-dense and varied diet with vegetables of many colors can significantly reduce inflammation in our bodies.[110, 75] This could be the reason why diets that contain less processed and high-sugar foods and more colorful, largely plant-based ingredients are correlated with lower rates of mental health issues.[213, 214, 215, 216]

HELPING THE GUT

There are not many topics that concern nutrition and health where gut health does not deserve a mention, and especially so when it comes to mental health. The microbiota is the collection of bacteria, fungi, and viruses that live in and around your body, largely concentrated in your gut. In my first book, I discussed how a diet that incorporates fiber-rich foods and a variety of largely plant-based, colorful ingredients can nurture this population, which is closely intertwined with our health. We are learning so much more about how this population of organisms has a role in regulating blood sugar, reducing inflammation, and manufacturing micronutrients from our food.[217]

Along with a multitude of other functions, our gut microbes are involved in creating hormones and neurotransmitters that can impact our mental health.[218] There are a number of theories as to how this population is able to do this, but none have been proven conclusively. What we do know is that the gut–brain axis is real, and it will be revolutionary for many specialties, especially mental health. Treatments may include transplanting bacteria directly into the gut, consuming specific antibacterials to alter the microbe population, and even a new class of therapeutics called "psychobiotics"—particular types of bacteria and fibers that are known to improve mental health.[219] There is accumulating evidence that these psychobiotics have the potential to treat a number of psychiatric conditions, including low mood and even anxiety.[220, 221]

The current issue is a lack of rigorous human clinical trials to definitely prove which microbes are doing what, and there is a lot of work in this area still to be done. In the interim, the best advice is to eat and live according to a lifestyle that nurtures your microbes.[222] I think it's definitely worth being mindful of how our diet can affect our microbiota, and my recipes will make this an easy task for even the least confident of cooks.

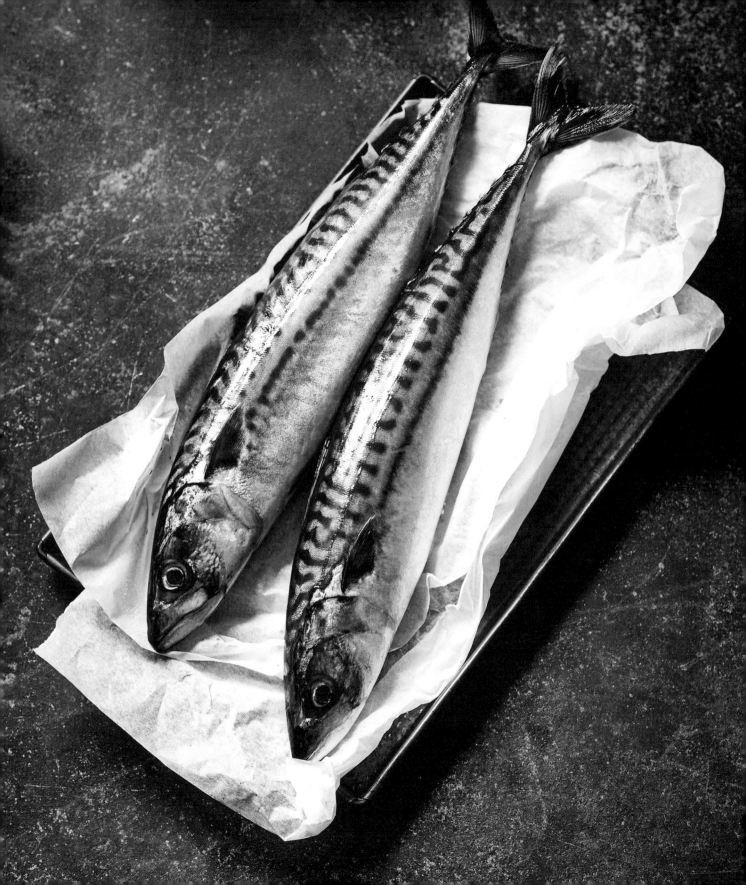

We now know that it is certain types of fat (commonly found in processed foods and deep-fried products) that cause ill health, especially the combination of poor-quality fats and high-sugar products.[223, 224] But contrary to what you may have heard, sugar is not the devil. It is the *excess* of sugar in our diets that is one of the many causes of health problems plaguing industrialized nations. Excess sugars are found in soft drinks, alcohol, and refined carbohydrates such as white bread and pasta, cakes and cookies. These can raise inflammation levels, put us at greater risk of obesity and diabetes (which themselves have links to mental health problems), and are best consumed only on occasion.

Instead of suggesting we radically remove foods from our diets, I would rather focus on ingredients that we should be introducing into our diets. What I think is lacking in many of my patients' diets are good-quality fats from a variety of sources. Delicious, wholesome foods such as walnuts, sunflower seeds, and avocado are heart healthy and contain special types of fatty acids that have been shown to improve behavior and mood.[225, 226]

Omega-3 fatty acids are one of the only types of fats that have been shown to clearly improve mental health outcomes when taken as a supplement. While I'm not a fan of supplementing in isolation, Omega-3 does appear to have a number of potential psychiatric benefits with minimal side effects.[227] Omega-3 fatty acids also reduce inflammation, which is another reason why good-quality fats are essential in a healthy diet. You'll notice my recipes regularly include different nuts, seeds, and extra-virgin olive oil and a focus on Omega-3 fats for this reason. Try looking at the Spicy Peanut and Lime Stir-Fry (see page 172) for inspiration.

Eating to improve and harness the power of your brain and mood means eating an abundance of foods with high nutrient density. There is huge potential for nutritional psychiatry, and I'm excited about the future applications of food and even dietary adjuncts in this specialty.[228] For now, these are my suggestions for food that could benefit mental health using the evidence available.

+ **Color** Eating a rainbow of foods has the potential for positive effects on mental health, and eating naturally colorful foods is the easiest way to secure those ingredients with a varied collection of phytochemicals that have an anti-inflammatory effect. My favorite ingredients include beets, parsley, rosemary, spinach, and purple sprouting broccoli. The colors are sure to put a smile on your face, and the variety of polyphenols will benefit your overall health.

+ **Herbs and spices** Spices, including cloves, turmeric, and star anise, may have additional benefits for inflammation, and I tend to use these particular ones often. Although "adaptogens" like ashwagandha and maca root are becoming popular, simple spices and herbs such as rosemary and thyme are just as impressive from the perspective of balancing inflammation, plus they are much cheaper, and your supermarket is more likely to stock them. Try the Spinach and Sorrel Borscht (see page 161) for a delicious recipe using more accessible herbs.

+ Fiber Feeding your microbiota involves having a large variety of foods on your plate, but also a good selection of fibers. Garlic, chicory, and Jerusalem artichoke are fantastic vegetables that contain specialized fibers called prebiotics that are specifically good for the gut microbes. In addition to the positive impact on the microbiome, lentils, beans, and other pulses are less likely to spike your sugar levels. Get used to using lots of garlic, have fiber with every meal, and experiment with pulses. My go-to fiber-rich ingredients are oats, chickpeas, puy lentils, and peas, and you'll see they're included in quite a few recipes throughout the book, including my Celeriac and Broad Bean Rendang Curry (see page 229) and Black Bean Goulash (see page 167).

+ Probiotics These are ingredients that contain live bacteria and other microbes and are thought to potentially benefit the gut by introducing different microbe strains into the mix. There is a lot of research to be done on the exact strains of microbes and how these may or may not have an effect on mood, but regardless, these are delicious ingredients that add a wealth of flavor to cooking, and there are some interesting studies on the horizon. For now, I recommend experimenting with traditionally prepared sauerkrauts, kimchis, and probiotic yogurts, which can positively impact the gut bacteria in your digestive system.

+ Good-quality fats Increasing the amount of fats containing Omega-3, as well as a multitude of other nutrients, is easily done by adding walnuts, chia, good-quality olive oil, and oily fish like mackerel to your diet. These are really easy to incorporate into recipes, even if it's as simple as lightly toasting some nuts and tossing them into a pasta dish (see page 169) or combining them with some whole fruit. Another consideration is that those who are depressed are more likely to be deficient in key micronutrients such as folate, zinc, and selenium.[229] That doesn't necessarily point to the exact mechanism for how depression is caused, but it's reassuring to note that a diet consisting of a variety of ingredients, including nuts and seeds, contains good levels of these micronutrients.

+ Protein This is a vital constituent of our diet. During the process of digestion, large protein structures are broken down into their building blocks made up of amino acids. These are used to make cell structures, enzymes, and also hormones that include neurotransmitters that impact our brain health and mood. We generally have enough protein in our diets, and deficiency is

"Delicious, wholesome foods such as walnuts, sunflower seeds and avocado contain special types of fatty acids that have been shown to improve behavior and mood."

unlikely to be an issue, but improving the quality of your protein and varying your sources are good ways of ensuring a variety of amino acids. Instead of relying on just meat and fish products, try pumpkin seeds, sunflower seeds, whole grains like rice and quinoa, eggs, and tofu.

LIFESTYLE 360

Coupled with diet, our lifestyle can have exceptionally positive effects on our well-being. I wouldn't be doing this mental health chapter justice without bringing to your attention the wonderful impacts of lifestyle on your brain and mental health.

+ Movement Exercise is one of the most powerful and well-recognized interventions for preventing and managing depression and anxiety. Increasing the production of certain hormones known to induce a calm state as well as stimulating muscle fibers to create anti-inflammatory signals are just a few of the mechanisms that suggest why exercise is so effective at improving mental health.[230, 231, 232]

In particular, high-intensity interval training (HIIT) has been shown to significantly increase mitochondrial function, the battery powerhouses of your cells, which may explain the improved mood, cognition, and euphoric effects experienced after

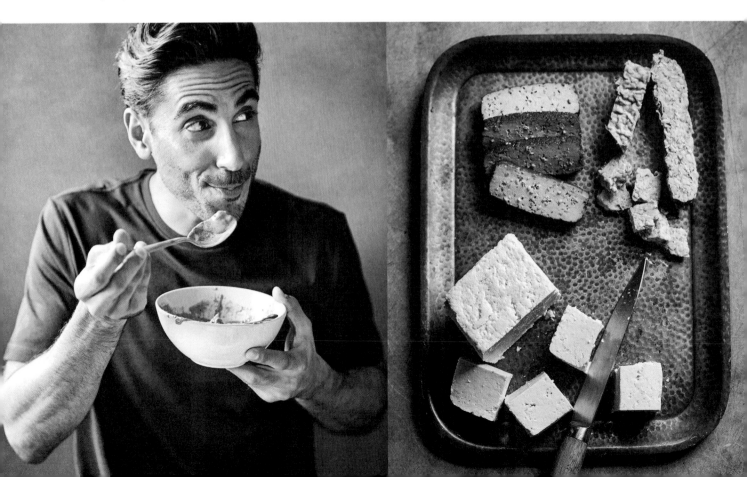

exercise.[154, 233] But you don't need to do strenuous, lengthy endurance or intense HIIT sessions. Just taking time to do some simple stretching, mobility, and flow exercises at home or during your working day is a great start to becoming more active. Making this a daily habit can improve the resilience of your mind.

+ Sleep Eating late at night, using electronic devices just before bed, and generally not recognizing our bodies' need for quality sleep has effects on so many aspects of our health. In the modern era of fast-paced living, hyper-connectivity, and instant gratification, sleep appears to have slipped down the list of priorities. There are multiple studies that demonstrate a clear link between poor sleep, disruption to our normal routine from shift work or travel, and a greater likelihood of mental health problems.[234, 235, 236] Achieving quality sleep of 7–9 hours a night could be the best thing we could do when it comes to a holistic approach to mental health.

+ Meditation Patients are often surprised when I discuss meditation, mindfulness therapies, and breathing exercises in the context of depression, but there's actually a wealth of science explaining how these interventions can be effective. When we practice consciously breathing, even if it is only for a couple of minutes, we generally become more aware of the breath throughout the day. We're actually stimulating our parasympathetic nervous system, which can modulate inflammation in our bodies.[237, 238] Another mechanism that has been proposed is meditation's influence on the expression of our genes to promote changes that reduce inflammation.[120]

In light of this evidence and the fact that mindfulness is very safe and accessible, I tend to use a few simple techniques with those suffering anxiety and low mood. Box breathing (also known as square breathing) and grounding practices are tools to bring your body into a calmer, more relaxed state and may result in a physical change of inflammation in the body[239] (I have some examples of how to do these on my website, www.thedoctorskitchen .com). I find the benefits of meditation are far more effective in a preventative context, so we can create a more resilient mind that can endure the inevitable stresses of life.

+ Cutting alcohol consumption Forgive me for being the bearer of bad news, but if you have symptoms of low mood, alcohol is not your friend. While many patients use alcohol as a relaxant and some even to aid sleep, it is well known to be a depressant, which is why many people who drink excessively suffer with low mood and anxiety. It is incredibly difficult to treat. Patients often find themselves in a vicious cycle when trying to cut down on their alcohol use while simultaneously balancing their anxiety and low mood symptoms. Always get help and speak to your doctor.

+ Psychogenic environment Our obesogenic environment has been given greater attention over the last few years as our population is gaining weight at an incredible rate. We need to be aware of not only how our environment can dictate poor food choices, but also how it affects our mental health. It's something I refer to as the "psychogenic environment," an environment that would predispose a person to having mental health problems.

We've evolved to live in tribes of people, where members of the community support and look after each other and where every person has a role. In the context of modern living, and a targeted drive towards consumerism, our sense of purpose has been lost. The entrapment of these external pressures as well as a lack of "belonging" creates an incredible storm of emotions that can tie many of today's generations to anxiety and mood disorders.[207] The constant bombardment of products you need to have, clothes you must wear, places you have to be seen at, and people you should aspire to look like, driven by mass-market advertising, social media, and mainstream platforms, are ironically creating an epidemic of loneliness and lack of fulfillment. I certainly don't think the sole solution lies in a bowl of food, an exercise program, or a better sleep schedule, but rather a systemic change in our physical and emotional environments that can be shaped with better understanding of our evolutionary needs and mental design. Once we accept what creates a psychogenic environment, we'd be in a stronger position to make positive, impactful changes.

Food is just one part of the prevention and management of a very complex problem. Don't fall for any marketing traps or sensationalist headlines that promote a magic "superfood" that is going to reverse all your anxiety issues. That is simply not how our bodies work. Your body is a magnificent and complicated machine. When we put it in the best environment and implement simple lifestyle strategies, it can work wonderfully.

The reason we're seeing a host of mental health issues growing in prevalence, of which anxiety and low mood are just a couple, is likely to be multifaceted. I'm not tempted to blame just one element of our lifestyle, but my guess is that it's an interplay of hyper-connectivity, excess stimulation, record levels of stress, and social isolation, combined with poor diets, sedentary lifestyles, and an over-reliance on pharmaceuticals. This could be creating a perfect storm for lots of health issues, but I want you to understand that you have more control over this than you may realize. We all have the ability to change this effectively and simply, and there are many services via your doctor that are available to help you.

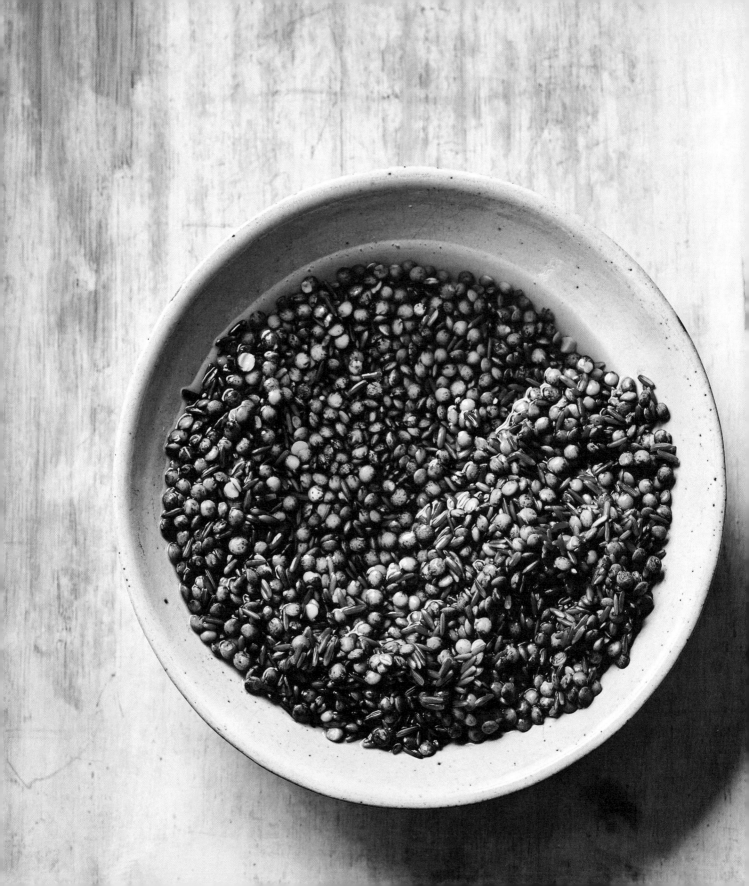

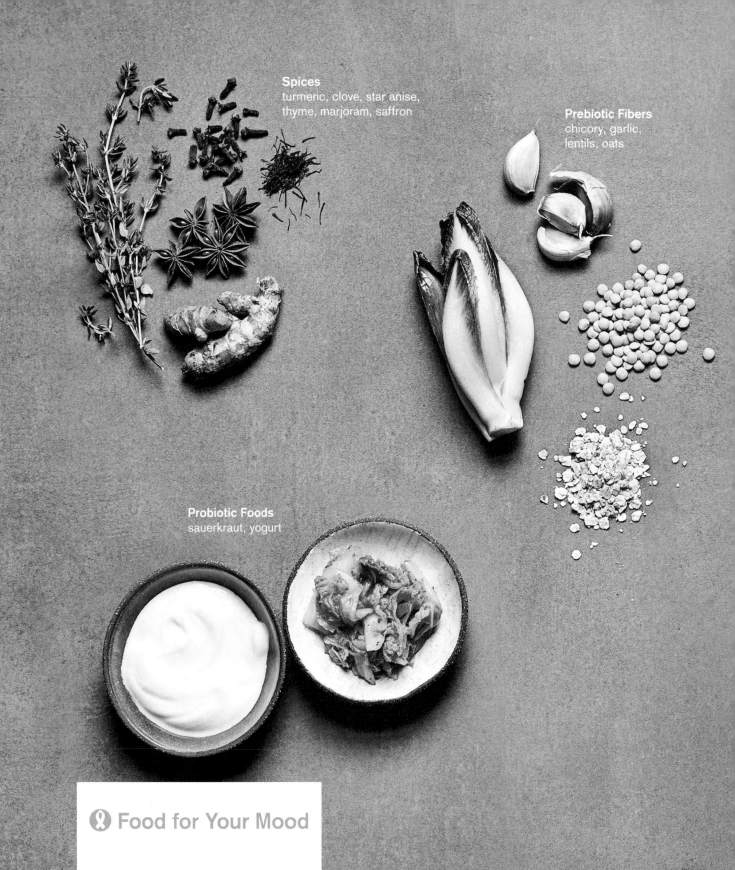

Spices
turmeric, clove, star anise, thyme, marjoram, saffron

Prebiotic Fibers
chicory, garlic, lentils, oats

Probiotic Foods
sauerkraut, yogurt

Food for Your Mood

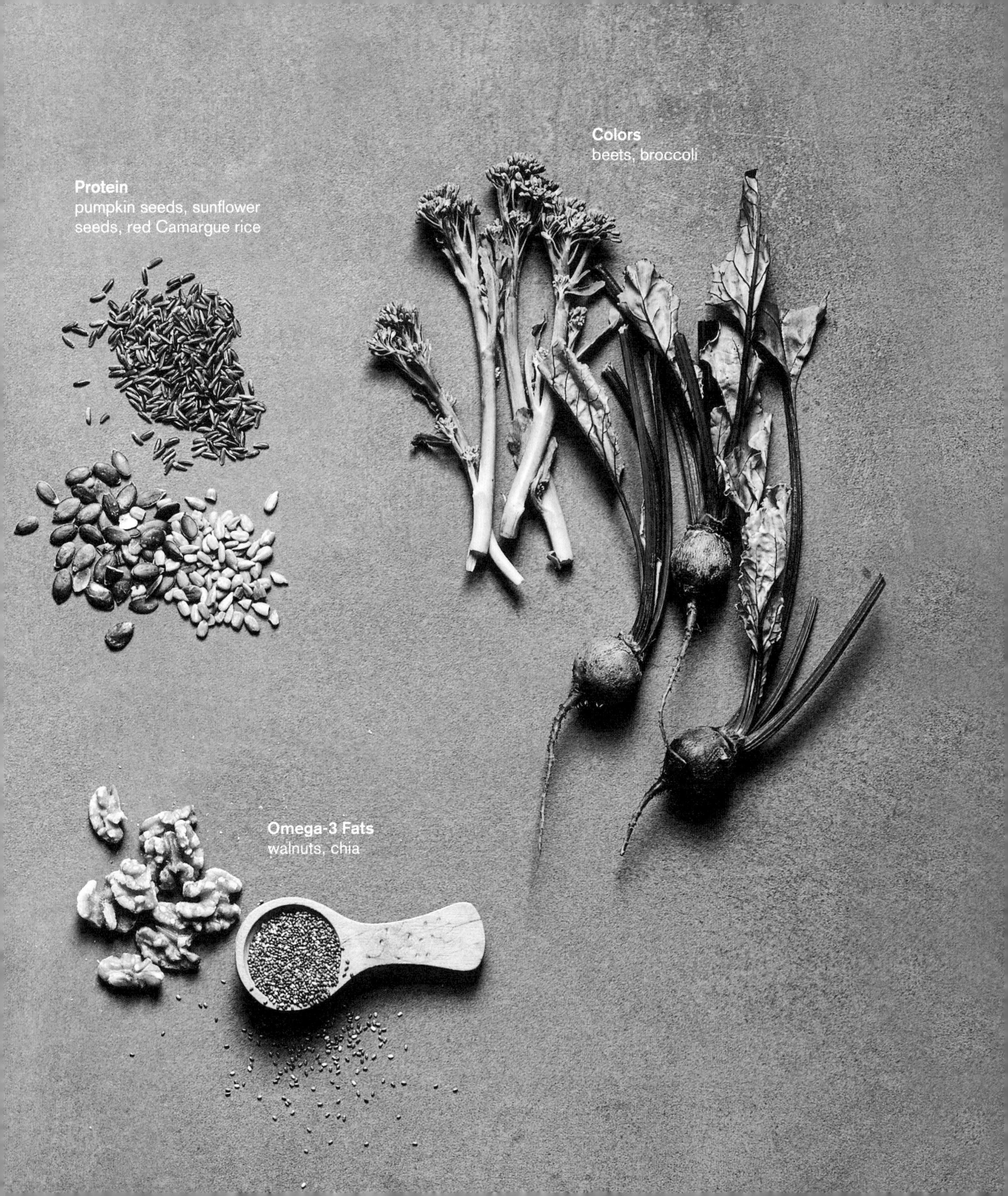

Protein
pumpkin seeds, sunflower
seeds, red Camargue rice

Colors
beets, broccoli

Omega-3 Fats
walnuts, chia

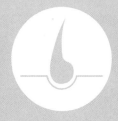

Eat for Your Skin

The skin covering your entire body is a collection of different specialized cells, working in a coordinated fashion to protect you from excessive light and harmful microbes in your environment and to regulate your temperature. It is a vital part of your immune system and the location of vitamin D production, yet the appreciation of your skin's health rarely goes beyond the aesthetic.

Most people aspire to have glowing, wrinkle-free skin without any flaws, and they try to achieve it by any means necessary. This desire has fueled a multibillion-dollar global industry that capitalizes on people's beauty ambitions or a belief that there is some sort of hidden beauty secret that only those "in the know" have access to. Before you save up to buy yet another anti-aging cream, let me make it clear to you: harnessing the power of diet and lifestyle is the most effective way to improve the look and feel of the largest organ in your body: your skin. I believe skin health should be thought of as beyond beauty.

As you will discover, the health of this complex, protective layer is heavily influenced by food, micronutrients, and how you live your life,[240] and hopefully I can convince you that we should aspire for more than blemish-free, perfect skin and encourage you to think deeper about the vital role that this organ is performing for you.

When you focus on eating for the health of your skin, rather than trying to prevent or rid yourself of a particular condition, you're actually working to create the perfect environment for your skin cells to thrive. In doing so, you allow your cells to do their job. Feed your body the right collection of nutrients, and you will be surprised at its ability to look after itself.

Nutrients in our diet can protect us from harmful sun rays and reduce inflammation that can lead to premature aging and potential mutations in cells that cause cancer. They promote the building blocks of skin, the extracellular matrix between cells, which may have an impact on wrinkle appearance. More so, they enhance the functioning of this vital organ, which has an essential role beyond simply appearance.

A lot of people assume that when I approach the subject of diet and skin, I'm going to be telling them what to cut out of their diet—sugar, dairy, fat, meat … the list appears endless. Conversely, I believe the initial focus should be what can you put into your diet to help your skin cells flourish. I want you to be interested in how amazing skin is and what it requires to perform its essential function of protecting us. Like everything else, it starts on your plate, but your lifestyle is also a critical determinant.

SKIN AGING

One of the most well recognized environmental insults that can negatively affect the health of our skin and lead to premature skin aging and cancers is harmful over-exposure to UV rays from the sun.[241] Many public health campaigns have focused on promoting the use of sun creams and raising awareness of this issue. While I agree that sun safety is of utmost importance, what these promotions noticeably lack is advice about diet. Studies have been examining the potential role of food as "photoprotective" (protective against harmful UV rays).[242, 243] One of the ways in which sunlight can be damaging is that it can penetrate deep into the layers of the skin, creating reactive oxidative species (ROS) that disrupt proteins, fats, and DNA, causing inflammation and potentially cancers.[244] The antioxidant capacity of colorful vegetables and fruits could provide additional whole-body protection from sunlight due to the vitamins and phytonutrients contained within them that can scavenge these damaging oxidative species, thus reducing their negative effects.[240] While most of the skin-protective effects of nutrient-dense vegetables can be explained by their antioxidant capacity, there may be some other fascinating biological mechanisms at play. Some micronutrients, such as beta-carotene, which we consume in the form of red- and orange-pigmented plant foods like papaya and squash, may have the physical ability to absorb harmful light.[245] Not only do these foods perform a valuable service by reducing damage from oxidation, they could also be physically protecting components of the skin and improving its repair. I want to make it clear that sun protection using physical barriers like screens and blocks is essential, but what we put on our plates could provide additional defenses to harmful sunlight exposure.[246] The damage from sunlight can be seen in the skin as early as your twenties (depending on your skin tone) and is a common reason for rough skin texture and poor moisture retention.[241] Try the 5-Spice Sticky Eggplant Bake (see page 175) as a way of loading up on delicious colored vegetables that may preserve skin quality.

INFLAMED SKIN

Some of the most common conditions that I see in my medical practice include dermatitis, psoriasis, and dry skin. In my experience, the root cause of these issues can be multifactorial, including stress, food sensitivity, essential vitamin deficiency, and diet. Inflammation, a topic we cover on pages 34–47, can be a factor in the development of many skin conditions. Whether it's caused by poor food choice, excess exposure to sunlight, or psychological stressors, inflammation plays a significant role in many skin complaints, and it's important we target it.

Good-quality fats from nuts, seeds, and fish contain beneficial Omega-3 fatty acids and have been shown in some studies to improve inflammatory skin conditions such as psoriasis.[247] This could be due in part to their immune-modulating properties, as eating a variety of fats from plants or fish oil is known to balance inflammation.[247] A number of small studies have demonstrated the benefit of including more good-quality fats in the diet with specific regard to dry skin and psoriasis. At a biological level, these fats suppress the release of inflammatory proteins and increase anti-inflammatory signals, which may in some part explain their benefits.[248] Extrapolating some of the findings from studies to clinical practice is difficult, but the benefits of eating more good-quality fat sources extend beyond skin and may prove worthwhile for a lot of people.

ACNE

While academics, dermatologists, and dieticians continue to debate and research the potential relationship between diet and acne (an inflammatory skin condition characterized by excess sebum production and hormone imbalance resulting in pustules and scarring), in my clinical experience, I've found the best approach is to address each person as an individual. Many patients are disinterested in the idea of dietary change for their skin condition, but the

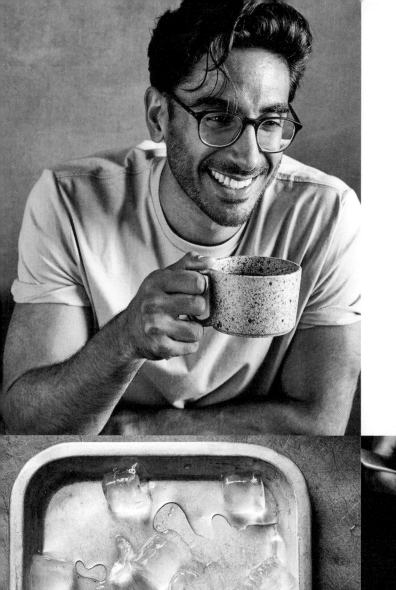

"Sun protection using physical barriers like screens and blocks is essential, but what we put on our plates could provide additional defenses to harmful sunlight exposure."

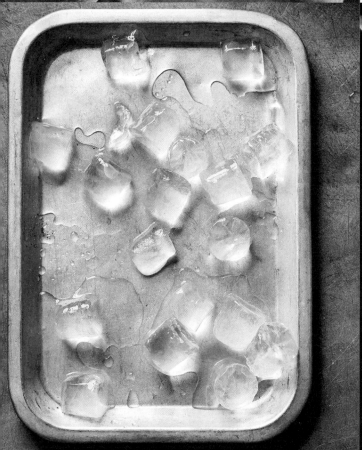

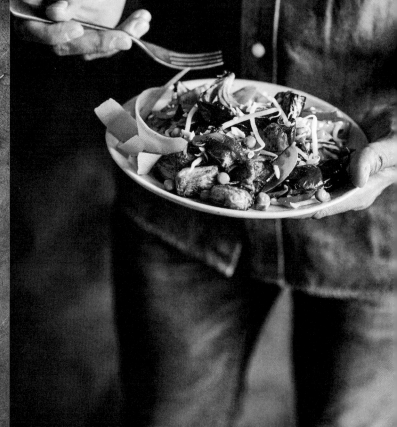

role of the clinician in modern healthcare is to explain their choices and come to a decision together. While there is contention in this category, I still think dietary change could be advised as at least one component of treatment. Within this field you will find mountains of conflicting evidence promoting supplements and restrictive diets, but I encourage a simple approach in the first instance. As I said at the start, it's more important to focus on what your body needs rather than arbitrarily cutting things out without a clear strategy.

The best evidence we have for a diet that reduces the incidence of acne is one that reduces refined carbohydrates, which are found in typical western foods including white bread, pasta, and quick-releasing sugars in cookies and sweets.[249] This could in part be explained by their effect on spiking insulin levels in the blood, causing hormonal changes leading to spots. In some further studies, skimmed milk and other dairy products appear to share a similar mechanism causing acne.[250] This isn't to suggest that we should radically remove all dairy from our diets, because these products contain a lot of valuable nutrition for many people. But as a short-term trial, some practitioners have carefully removed and replaced dairy with good effect for skin complaints like acne. I say this with a lot of caution, however, and I would always suggest consulting your practitioner before trying it, especially as the evidence is limited.

What you'll find in many studies, not just those related to skin or acne, is that dietary interventions are performed in isolation to test the theory that a particular supplement, ingredient, or ratio of macronutrients (carbohydrates to protein to fat) in meals has had an effect. It doesn't take a scientist to realize how impractical and unrealistic this is. We do not eat regimented diets in this way, and when you change components of your eating and living habits (such as exercising more, eating a variety of nutrient-dense foods, and perhaps improving your sleep habits), you are changing a multitude of factors that could be having a positive or negative effect. It is near impossible to tease these nuances out using the research tools available, and this is where I believe a commonsense approach should be employed. It might not be dairy that is the problem, but instead what else is lacking in your diet that could be more culpable. When we exclude or limit certain ingredients, we may end up replacing them with nutrient-dense ingredients that are lower in sugar and thus may improve the original skin complaint. As frustrating as this is, biology is not an exact science.

There is potential for specific micronutrients such as vitamin E, zinc, selenium, and Omega-3 to benefit acne. But rather than consuming supplements of these, if we encourage principles of healthy eating that include consuming nuts, seeds, good-quality fats from oil and fish, plus a large selection of colorful vegetables, we naturally obtain these nutrients from our food.[251, 252] Particularly noteworthy foods with these characteristics include Brazil nuts, pumpkin seeds, and legumes such as chickpeas. Not only do they contain zinc and selenium, but their higher fiber content reduces blood sugar spikes that are thought to potentially exacerbate acne. Essentially, it is a Mediterranean style of eating, with perhaps a greater focus on nuts and seeds, that provides good amounts of these micronutrients. These principles are employed throughout all my recipes, and with this in mind I want to showcase some ingredients as part of a varied diet. These are particularly fascinating from the perspective of skin health and may benefit a number of the skin conditions mentioned above.

+ Red and yellow vegetables As well as preventing inflammation and cancer caused by sun damage,[253] the carotenoids found in red, orange, and yellow vegetables like beets, carrots, and squash may improve the appearance of skin due to their ability to prevent extracellular matrix breakdown.[254] This is responsible for keeping the structure of the skin firm. Tomatoes, red fruits, and papaya also contain lycopene, considered to be one of the most effective antioxidants that prevent damage to cells. Mangoes, papayas, and root vegetables all contain a special type of carotenoid called beta-carotene, which inhibits free radicals and could give rise to their sun-protective effects.[255] We cannot make our own carotenoids, so it's important that we obtain them through food,[256] and my recipes will show you how to easily incorporate them into your diet. Try out the Glazed Asian Vegetable

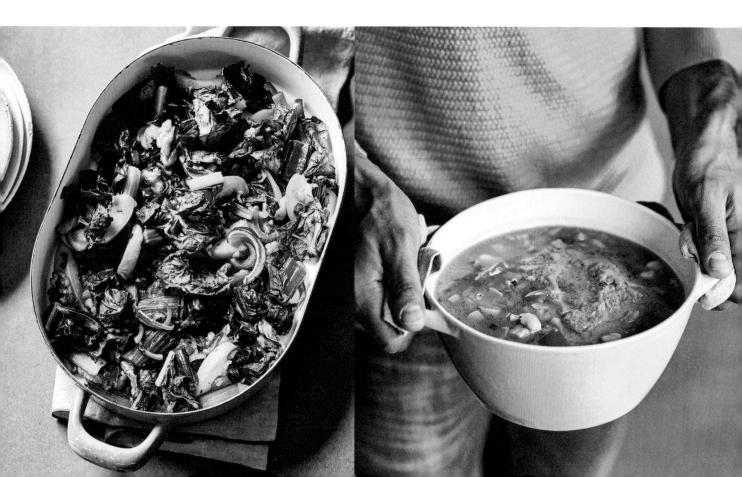

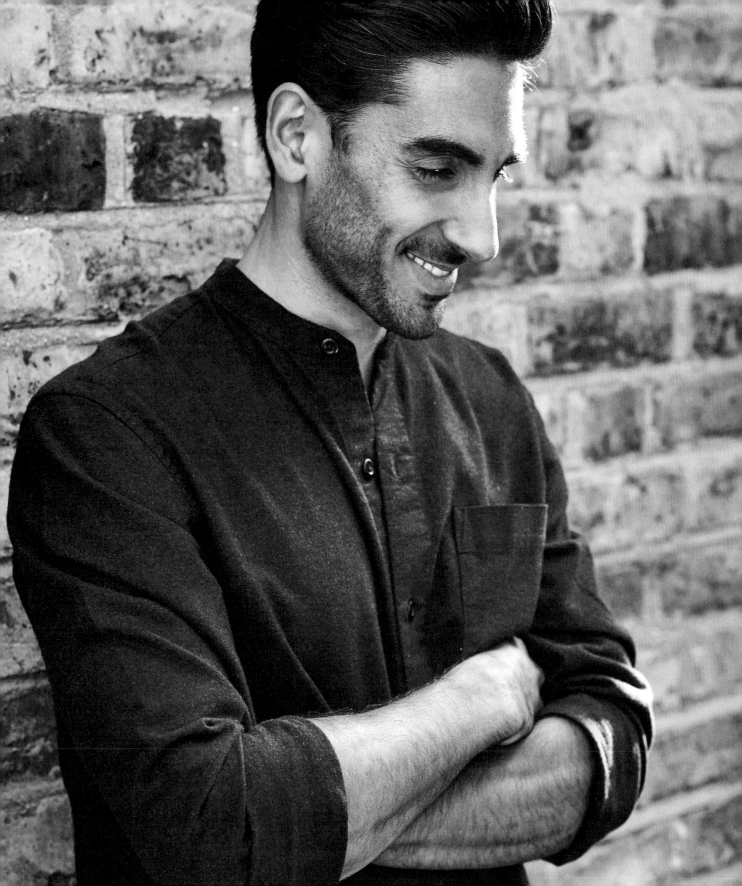

Rice Bowls (see page 193) or even the Radicchio, Peach, and Fennel Salad with Balsamic Croutons (see page 148).

+ **Greens** Dark, leafy greens such as kale, cavolo nero, cabbage, and spring greens are the richest source of the plant chemical lutein, but it can also be found in foods such as broccoli and peas. This phytochemical from the carotenoid family has been shown to prevent the breakdown of the skin's matrix, which is essentially the scaffolding that maintains the skin. Dark greens are also a great source of vitamin C, which inhibits a particular enzyme that breaks down the skin's structure and therefore could decrease the appearance of wrinkles.[257] Not only is this encouraging from an aesthetic point of view but it enhances your skin's resilience to harsh environments. The Split Green Pea and Pearl Barley Pan (see page 223) is one of my favorites for getting in greens like spinach, but you could also use Swiss chard and kale.

+ **Whole grains, beans, and nuts** Whole grains, beans, and nuts are a source of copper, which encourages skin rejuvenation and wound repair through its collagen crosslinking properties.[258] Almonds, Brazil nuts, and sunflower seeds all contain a wide variety of micronutrients, including good amounts of vitamin E that scavenge pro-oxidants in your skin layers.[55] These can mitigate the effect of inflammatory particles produced from both normal cell metabolism and damage from sunlight. Nuts and seeds are also a source of selenium, which works by increasing the production of enzymes that remove damaging oxides formed during oxidative stress (a topic we cover on pages 34–47), and these can stabilize cells and prevent DNA damage that could prevent mutations leading to cancer.[254] The zinc and selenium content of nuts and seeds may also reduce the redness and inflammation associated with acne.[259] Polyunsaturated fats from nuts, good-quality oils, and fatty fish serve as an important structural component within the epidermis as well as having an anti-inflammatory role. These fatty acids add structural integrity to the skin and reduce redness and inflammation, which is why they may be useful in helping to treat inflammatory skin conditions.[260] Try the Seasonal Soup with Red Pesto (see page 186) for an interesting way of using both nuts and beans.

+ **Plant fiber** As with most medical specialties, there is definitely a connection between your skin and the health of the microbiota (the population of microbes, largely bacteria, found concentrated in your large intestine). A specific gut–skin connection may exist with dermatitis and other inflammatory skin conditions that have an immune component.[261] A lifestyle that nurtures the gut microbiota is essentially one focused on a variety of plant fibers like leeks and chicory and artichokes, plus lots of color in the diet. This explains why some people find that improving their diet in this way improves these particular skin complaints.[262] I examine the role of this fascinating population of gut bugs, which are inseparable from health and specifically inflammation, on pages 34–47.

+ Water Considering this organ is largely made up of water and regulates temperature using perspiration mechanisms, hydration is a key component of skin health. As well as the benefits of adequate hydration to brain health, digestion, and transport of nutrients through the bloodstream, water maintains the structure of your skin cell walls. The elasticity of skin is something we use in clinical practice to determine hydration status, and it demonstrates how essential water is to this organ. Focus on drinking around 5–8½ cups of plain water per day rather than black teas or coffee, as these can have dehydrating effects.

LIFESTYLE 360

When we consume whole food ingredients that are good sources of particular micronutrients, we benefit from the additional nutrients these contain such as folate, iron, phytosterols, and a host of other health-promoting compounds. But in many cases, it's not a simple micronutrient deficiency in isolation that manifests as a skin complaint. Your lifestyle is an important determinant of overall health as well as skin quality, and these are some important factors to be mindful of.

+ Mindfulness We now understand that psychological stress can produce higher amounts of free radicals and inflammation, which fragment and degrade collagen and elastic fibers.[263] On an anecdotal level, stress appears to be a trigger in many of my patients' skin conditions. It's not uncommon to see stressful episodes trigger flares of eczema, psoriasis, and autoimmune conditions such as inflammatory bowel disease.[264,265] Finding a mindfulness strategy has benefits beyond mental well-being, and I think it's very worthwhile investing a few minutes of your day for a mindful walk, simple breathing exercises, or a meditation practice. It may or may not benefit your skin health, but it will certainly benefit your overall well-being.

+ Sleep It's obvious when you are burnt out and not getting enough sleep. Your face cannot hide the detrimental impact of poor rest. Sleep is an essential mechanism by which we repair and restore our bodies. It mellows inflammation and helps ameliorate the buildup of free radicals that could disrupt skin cell function.[266] With the additional benefits of achieving good-quality sleep, and at the very least 7 hours of shut-eye a night, getting enough sleep is an important all-round habit to get into, especially for good skin health.

"I would rather empower you to enjoy delicious, colorful food that can not only prevent skin problems, but also correct any potentially underlying conditions."

I like to examine healthcare through the lens of patient experience and the principle of "first do no harm." Being offered a harsh topical ointment, cream, or—even worse—an oral pharmaceutical drug before any assessment of how a patient's lifestyle could be driving their condition is inexcusable. High-sugar diets, poor sleep, lack of phytonutrients that protect the skin, and stress all have considerable effects on the health of this vital organ. Using a reductionist approach and simply adding a drug to the cataclysm of issues as a result of poor lifestyle may serve to worsen patient outcomes. Before even thinking about reaching for a prescription, we need to have a conversation about the basics. Pharmaceuticals are necessary in many cases, but we need to get to the root of what could ultimately be the cause of your problems. Lifestyle can be a contributing factor in many of them.

The lack of rigorous nutritional science studies prevents healthcare practitioners from being able to make specific recommendations, but this is where I believe common sense should prevail. Many of my patients are interested in alternatives to existing approaches for maintaining long-lasting healthy skin that potentially improve acne and other skin conditions. Using sound clinical judgment, I often assess and recommend dietary changes as a preliminary, evidence-based tool for tackling skin disorders alongside other treatments. The diet and lifestyle recommendations I've discussed represent the most healthy and safe methods to maintain youthful-appearing skin but also prevent and manage common skin complaints.

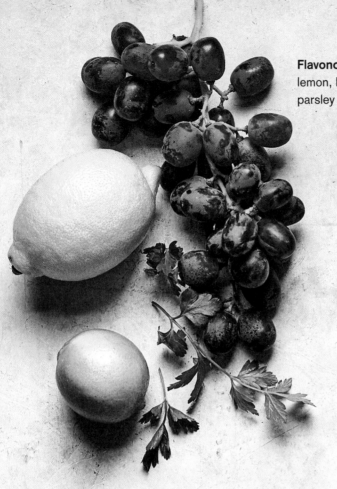

Flavonoids
lemon, lime, grapes, parsley

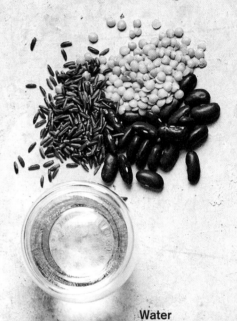

Whole Grains and Legumes
red kidney beans, Camargue rice, yellow lentils

Water

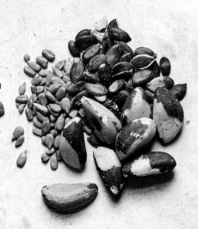

Selenium, Zinc, and Vitamin E
sunflower seeds, Brazil nuts, pumpkin seeds

Food for Your Skin

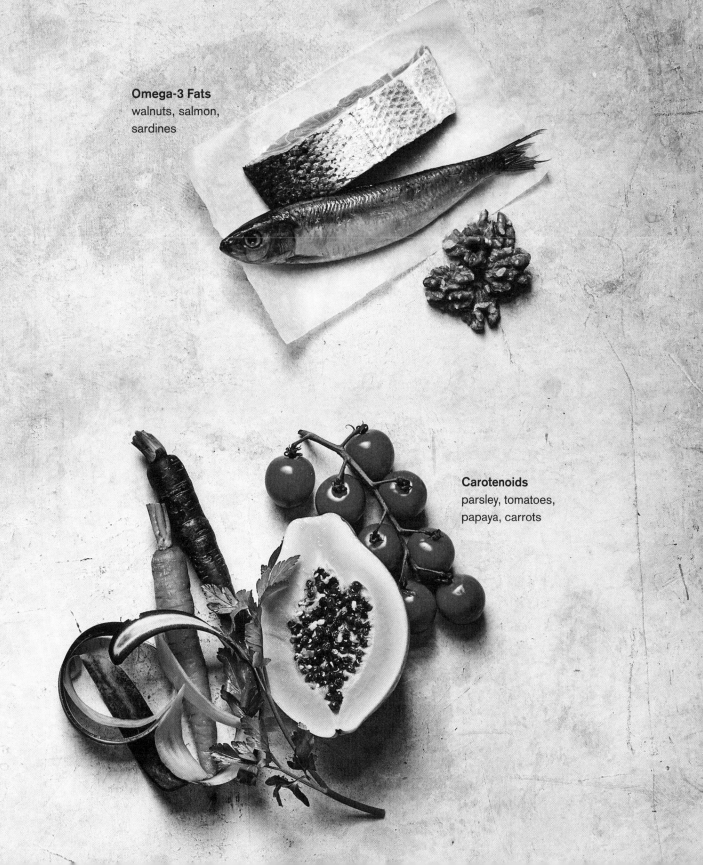

Omega-3 Fats
walnuts, salmon, sardines

Carotenoids
parsley, tomatoes, papaya, carrots

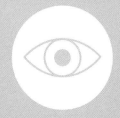

Eat for Your Eyes

Your eyes are the most wonderful and precious part of your body. Considering their compact size, they contain the most dense and intricate networks of vessels and receptors that produce our spectacular vision.

The degree of biological technology that enables us to have a constant live stream of our environment is staggering, yet most of us don't pay any attention to preserving our eye health until something goes wrong. In reality, these delicate organs are the window to our overall health as well as our soul.

Our eyes give us an early indication of when our general health is poor, which is why diabetes and cardiovascular disease are correlated with visual problems. Often the first signs of uncontrolled blood sugar or blood pressure are changes in the fine layers at the backs of our eyes.

As exemplified by the increasing prevalence of eye problems such as cataracts and retinopathies (damage to the retina at the back of the eye commonly related to vascular disease and diabetes), it's clear to see that our eyes have become as unhealthy as our bodies. However, lifestyle changes have been shown to protect our eyes and other delicate organs from damage, and as ever, good nutrition is at the core of it. This chapter discusses the role of eye health through the lens of nutrition.

CATARACTS

The most common eye surgery performed in the US is for cataracts, a condition where the lens of the eye, which is normally clear, becomes cloudy with clumped proteins. The surgery is a relatively quick procedure for a problem that has many causes but is largely related to normal aging, affecting people most commonly over the age of 50. There isn't much in the way of evidence for lifestyle and dietary change to prevent or treat cataracts, but we do know that diabetes, smoking, and high alcohol consumption will likely increase the risk of this condition.[267] One strategy to prevent the likelihood of cataracts is therefore to quit smoking and maintain sugar control. But what is also interesting is a suggestion in the research that antioxidants from a variety of sources (both food and supplements) may have the potential to prevent cataracts from forming, too.

The equilibrium between oxidants (damaging products of metabolism or from the environment) and antioxidants (substances that prevent damage) is very important in the eye and something that is lost due to normal aging, which can lead to changes in the lens causing a cataract.[268] It's speculated that during the process of cataract formation, the balance of eye antioxidants versus pro-oxidants diminishes, and it is that imbalance that can cause an issue in the lens.[269] The question we still have is whether a nutrient-dense diet, abundant in varied antioxidants, can maintain the balance of pro-oxidants versus antioxidants in the eye and prevent cataracts. Some large studies looking specifically at vitamin C and E supplements have so far not provided evidence of benefit.[270]

However, a lot of these studies simply involved adding an isolated supplement to the diet of people who could have been nutritionally deficient in other ways.[271] In my opinion, adding a supplement in isolation, without really focusing on the overall nutrient and antioxidant density of a person's diet, let alone lifestyle, is unlikely to be beneficial. There are a few studies that have shown that an increase in dietary antioxidants from greater fruit and vegetable intakes, rather than supplements, could potentially be protective against cataract formation, but more research is required.[272] What we can say for sure is that a diet that contains an abundance of different antioxidants is certainly going to benefit your health in many ways. Ensuring you eat foods low in sugar and high in fiber, and avoid refined carbohydrates, will also improve your metabolic health and may potentially have a preventative effect on cataract formation.[273]

RETINAL HEALTH

The Royal National Institute of Blind People predicts that the number of people living with sight loss will increase by 30 percent, yet despite this worrying projection, not many of us have regular eye exams.[274, 275] My first suggestion is to have regular checkups with your eye doctor. But in addition I'd like you to consider some powerful lifestyle and diet interventions for vision that may protect your sight from ever being robbed.

The retina, a thin layer of cells at the back of the eye, has the highest rate of metabolic activity of any tissue. Because of the retina's unique photo receptors, it is constantly renewing cells and requires the highest amount of oxygen to convert light energy into electrical impulses transmitted to the brain, creating vision. With such high cellular activity and oxygen demand, it is particularly vulnerable to the damaging products of normal metabolism, which create free radicals. Free radicals are unstable molecules that are produced as a normal by-product of metabolism and cause "oxidation" and "oxidative stress," which is harmful. Your cells have the ability to stabilize these free radicals (also known as "oxidants") using their own internal "antioxidants," but foods rich in antioxidants from plants can also help protect against free-radical effects.

The most common cause of blindness in industrialized countries is macular degeneration. It's a condition that we see mostly in people over 50 years old and one that is characterized by blind spots appearing in the center of vision. This particular condition has received a lot of attention in nutrition research since studies have demonstrated the ability of certain micronutrients, found in common fruits and vegetables like parsley and bell peppers, to significantly slow the progression of this disease.[276, 277] As well as recommending that patients with macular degeneration stop smoking, control their blood pressure, and limit alcohol intake, doctors are now able to consider recommending supplements for managing the progression of the condition.

In some landmark studies, they used supplements (known as the "AREDS formulation") that included specific plant chemicals, lutein and zeaxanthin, which are components of the macula pigment in the eye.[278] This pigment has an uncertain role, but it's thought to protect your eyes by limiting the damaging effect of UV light and reducing "oxidative stress." This type of stress (discussed further on pages 34–47) is a result of normal aging and cell metabolism that produces free radicals, and our food has a central role in scavenging free radicals, making them harmless.

The possible protective role of antioxidants found in the AREDS formulation could be attributed to the fact that they mitigate against this oxidation effect, scavenge free radicals,[279, 280] and limit oxidative stress, therefore slowing the progression of the disease. There is some disagreement among scientists about the benefits of supplementation and whether it's beneficial for everyone with macular degeneration, and I'm personally wary of supplementation for large numbers of people.

My opinion on these studies is that it's going to take a while before we can state with absolute certainty that specific supplementation is beneficial. But the benefits of a colorful diet, with a focus on ingredients that improve the pigments found in the eye, are undeniable.[281] There is consensus that a balanced diet rich in fruits and vegetables, with particular attention to dietary sources of lutein, zeaxanthin, and vitamins E and C, could be beneficial and slow the progression of this disease.[278] Without a doubt, it is worth considering dietary change as an adjunct to treatment for eye conditions like macular degeneration and certainly for prevention. There is simply no reason why we shouldn't be recommending food as medicine in this scenario; it's safe, potentially effective and promotes overall health. Recipes like my Heirloom Tomatoes, Horta, and Mackerel (see page 182) will help you include these specific phytochemicals, like lutein and zeaxanthin, into your meals easily.

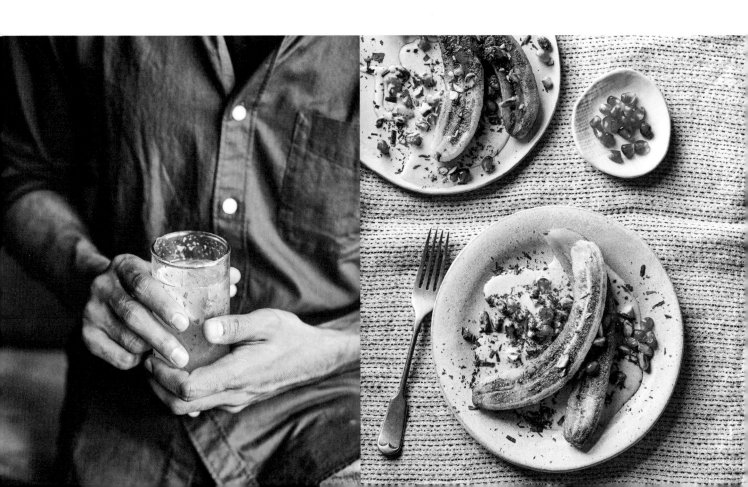

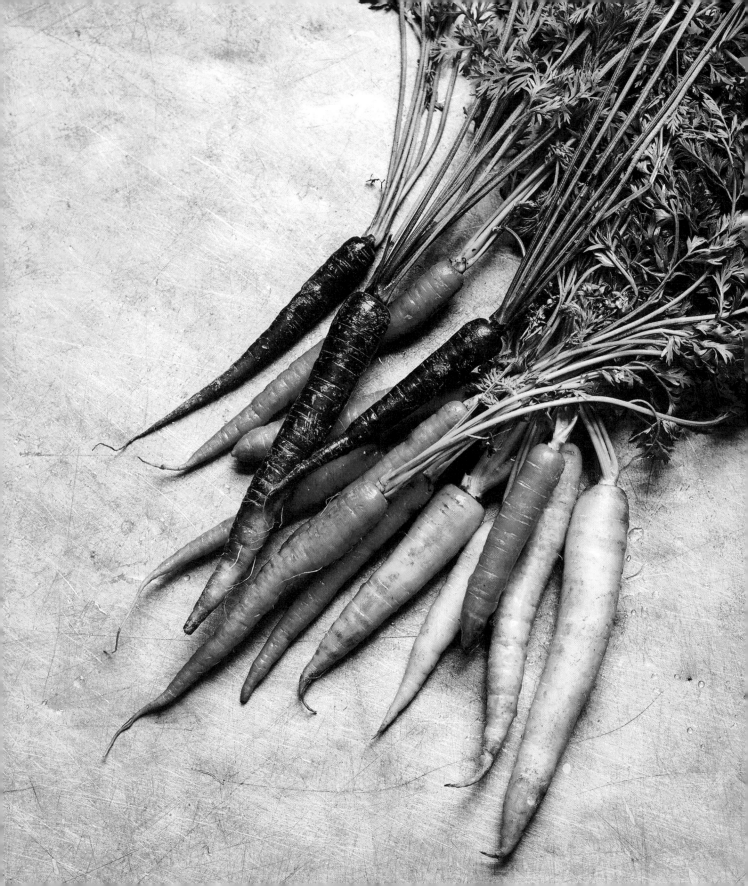

Shortsightedness, known as myopia, is the most common eye disorder in the world, and it is growing rapidly.[282, 283] The inability to see objects clearly from a distance is something that I have personally suffered with since the age of 6, yet nobody in my family from previous generations has ever needed glasses from childhood. It's a common anomaly that I see in patients' families, and there are many hypotheses as to why this may be the case.

It's generally agreed that the intensity of schooling from a young age is associated with this condition.[284] It's partly the reason why we see many new and younger cases of myopia in countries with better access to schools as well as countries with a strong culture of high academic achievement, but education alone cannot fully explain the phenomena.

If you think about shortsightedness from an evolutionary perspective, it would have been exceptionally hard to live in the wilderness foraging for food and running away from predators with poor vision.[285] When analyzing traditional civilizations that have lived outside of industrialized societies, we can demonstrate that the prevalence of myopia is 1 in 1,000. It's not common. But when people from the same population are integrated into industrialized society, the rates of myopia rapidly increase to rates similar in the western world.

For this reason, there is an argument that myopia may not only be linked with higher rates of education but also higher amounts of sugar in the diet, as those from a traditional culture adopt more westernized foods. It's known that there is a greater likelihood of shortsightedness with higher levels of sugar in the blood, hence why we see this correlation between diabetes and poor visual acuity. The potential mechanism is due to changes in the lens brought about by high sugar intake leading to higher insulin levels, but these have yet to be fully investigated and proven.[286]

Although diet is just one of many potential contributors to shortsightedness, knowing it may play a part should encourage us to eat less processed food and refined carbohydrates in an effort to maintain more stable blood sugar levels. Eating more fiber (pulses, lentils, and beans) may have protective effects on your vision, but we know it certainly helps our general metabolic health and improves the functioning of our gut.

The foods that I encourage from the perspective of improving eye health are colorful and diverse. These are some of the ingredients that could specifically benefit your vision:

+ Red and yellow vegetables Looking for these colors is the easiest way to spot sources of beta-carotene on supermarket and grocery shelves. Beta-carotene is a type of plant chemical that is concentrated in the eye and serves as a strong antioxidant, which is essential for the health of the retina.[287] Pumpkin, red pepper, carrots, and sweet potato are all examples of foods that contain beta-carotene and also help with immunity. Try the Carrot and Zucchini Laksa for a delicious recipe using these ingredients (see page 158).

+ Citrus fruits and berries These have been suggested as important for eye health, in part due to their strong antioxidant capacity, which could balance oxidative stress in the retina.[288] Lab studies have also shown that plant chemicals in berries, such as anthocyanin, can directly interact with visual pigments in the eye to improve vision.[269] We're a long way from being able to prove this definitively, but the health-promoting effects of flavonoids in berries and citrus fruit make it certainly worth including them in your diet. Blackberries, blueberries, pomegranate, grapefruit, oranges, and lemons are delicious ingredients to get into desserts or even cut into segments to finish salads. Try my Citrus and Pineapple Asian Salad (see page 142) or the Cod Bites with Lemon and Seaweed (see page 176).

+ Green foods Kale, spinach, cabbage, and parsley (and other green foods) are sources of the plant chemicals lutein and zeaxanthin, which are the predominant carotenoids found in the retina and form a protective pigment. Even though there are over 600 types of carotenoids, lutein and zeaxanthin are the only ones to be found in the eye, and they've received much attention since studies demonstrated their ability to slow the progression of blindness (caused by macular degeneration). There is a misconception that you would need huge quantities of these ingredients to get the necessary levels of these chemicals in your bloodstream. But due to the variety of foods that contain these chemicals, it's quite easy to get adequate amounts through dietary means. The added bonus of consuming these ingredients in their dietary form, found in spring greens and spinach, are the additional micronutrients such as vitamin C that can also scavenge free radicals and improve eye health.[289]

+ Garlic, onions, and brassicas Vegetables like broccoli and sprouts, as well as garlic and onion, all contain sulphur compounds that are necessary for the production of a compound called glutathione in your cells. This is the most abundant intracellular antioxidant: an antioxidant that is produced by your own cells. Considering how vulnerable your retinal cells are to oxidation, having good amounts of glutathione could also help prevent damage.[290]

+ Good-quality fats A lot of the plant chemicals beneficial for the eye are fat soluble, so they need a source of fat to transport them around the body.[291] Luckily, a lot of good-quality fats contain further beneficial components for eye health. Egg yolks, pistachios, and flaxseed contain a mix of lutein and zeaxanthin, as well as Omega-3 fatty acids and vitamin E, which combine to further enhance the functioning of your eyes as well as boosting the delivery of carotenoids for eye health.[287] Omega-3 is a major structural component of the retina and may also play a role as a precursor to signaling molecules with the ability to influence retinal function.

"Spending time outside and exercising outdoors rather than purely indoors (particularly among children) have been associated with better visual acuity and could prevent early-onset short-sightedness."

Apart from smoking cessation, limiting alcohol, and optimizing our food choices, I'd like to bring attention to having regular eye checkups (especially if you're shortsighted) and lifestyle practices to positively impact eye health. These are a few simple strategies that can enhance and help preserve your vision.

+ Screen breaks One of the many mechanisms behind myopia could be the continual physical strain on the ocular muscles that stretch and compress the eyeball during reading or when using smartphones and laptop screens.[292] Since learning more about the theory behind resting our eyes, I've decided to take regular breaks and give myself time away from the screen. It's not unusual for people to be stuck behind a screen (or a book during schooling) where your eyes are in an unnatural position for hours at a time. This is a practical suggestion that could help minimize the strain on our precious organ.

An ophthalmology colleague of mine suggests practicing the 20-20-20 rule. Every 20 minutes, look away from your screen for 20 seconds and to a distance of 20 feet. This may also help with symptoms of dry eye and headaches that are related to excessive screen time.

+ Natural light There are so many benefits of exercise to the vascular system, which will also positively impact your eyes. Researchers have found that those living more active lifestyles outdoors are much less likely to suffer macular degeneration.[279] Spending time outside and exercising outdoors rather than purely indoors (particularly among children) have been associated with better visual acuity and could prevent early-onset shortsightedness.[284, 293] The theory is that natural light intensity improves the depth of vision and stimulates the retina to release dopamine, which can prevent changes to the eye's structure causing nearsightedness.[294] It's a simple strategy with limited side effects that could reduce the risk of myopia and progression in children and young adolescents.[295] Put this book down and get outdoors.

I sincerely believe that having a holistic view of eye health can reduce the growing burden of eye disease. Movement, nutrient density, smoking cessation, and regular eye checkups are critical. My recipes will demonstrate how to get the right ingredients on your plate. The rest is down to your motivation, and hopefully this will spur you in the right direction.

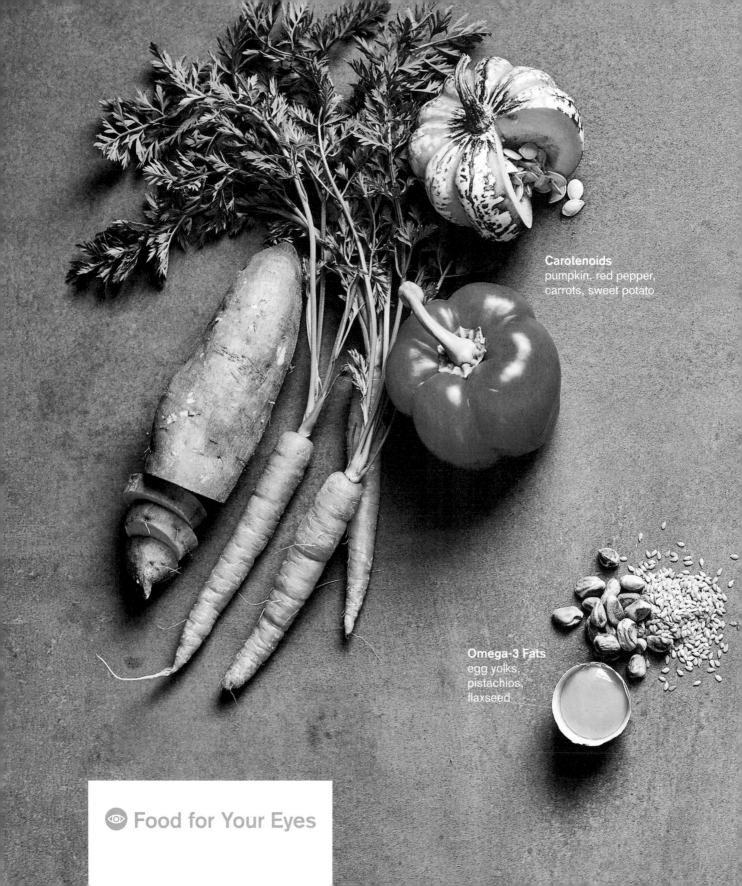

Carotenoids
pumpkin, red pepper,
carrots, sweet potato

Omega-3 Fats
egg yolks,
pistachios,
flaxseed

Food for Your Eyes

Glutathione
garlic, onions, brassica
vegetables like broccoli and
Brussels sprouts

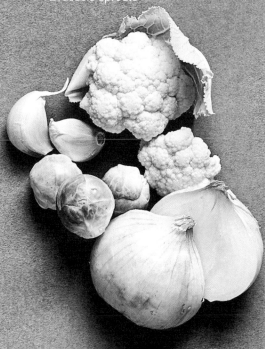

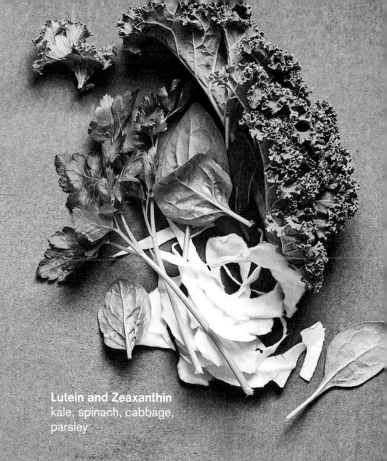

Lutein and Zeaxanthin
kale, spinach, cabbage,
parsley

Citrus Fruits and Berries
blackberries, blueberries,
pomegranate, grapefruit,
oranges, lemons

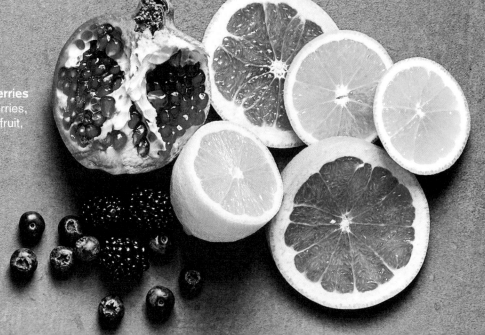

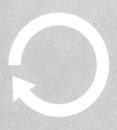

Eating and Living for
Ultimate Health

My idea, to help you understand the complex unit that is your body, was to zoom in on different topics and give you an understanding of why nutrition and lifestyle have a significant impact. Now I invite you to zoom out and appreciate the wider context. Your body is a wonderful ecosystem that operates as a perfectly functioning unit rather than as individual components.

In these final pages I want to bring everything together. At this point, I hope you've noticed a common theme throughout each chapter: the secret behind a high-functioning brain, strong bones, flourishing skin, a resilient heart is . . . not a secret. We do not eat for just one part of the body or even one condition. We eat to fuel the incredible internal ecosystem that is our body, and it already knows how to maintain itself.

Time and time again I plead with patients to understand and appreciate that we do not eat for specific problems. It simply does not make any sense to eat prescriptively when our food has a multitude of effects on our biology. Instead, what I try to encourage is eating with the perspective of trying to improve our internal environment. And for this purpose, whole foods are quite literally the most technologically advanced "drugs" we could ever introduce into our bodies. By focusing on wellness, feeding our bodies with incredible nutrition, and putting them in the right environment using lifestyle factors, we can naturally optimize every aspect of our health.

When we eat and live with this motivation in mind, we improve our brain health, skin quality, and mood and balance inflammation simultaneously. The effects of one dish are far beyond the reach of just one bodily system. The interconnectedness of our mind and physical health is difficult to fathom initially, but when we break it down system by system, as I have done over the course of these chapters, we begin to see the patterns and similarities emerge.

To quote Voltaire: "The art of medicine consists in amusing the patient while nature cures the diseases." While this isn't necessarily true of the many cases that I come across in the emergency department, I do believe there is a lot we can learn from this observation. I consider that one of my responsibilities as a physician is to help my patients put their bodies in the right environment to allow our innate mechanisms of self-healing to achieve a state of equilibrium. Although this may sound unscientific, the body has an incredible ability to look after itself, and we can enhance this with food and lifestyle. Repeatedly, I see patients improve their internal environment and report enhanced mental clarity, better pain management, and improved mental health, as well as looking and feeling better.

Through personal experience of reversing my own heart condition, and inspired by the thousands of other patients across the globe who have achieved similar successes, I was driven to try to retrospectively understand how this was possible. I dug deep into the literature in an attempt to comprehend the mechanisms behind the effectiveness of lifestyle medicine. What I present in this book is an extraction of all the research examining the theory and science behind plant-based diets, chrononutrition (defining when we eat), nutrigenomics, sleep medicine, exercise physiology, inflammation, and the microbiome, to name just a few. I have condensed this huge body of knowledge into actionable principles of eating and living well that you can use right now.

I don't present these principles as a panacea, but as a recognition of just how precise, interconnected, and engineered our bodies are and what we can do to encourage thriving health. These reflect the best of what we currently understand about how to harness our internal mechanisms to protect and support our health as best we can. We all have the ability

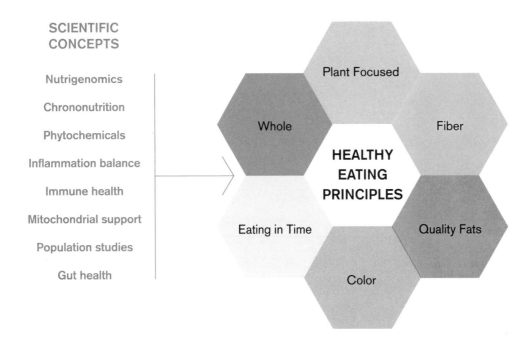

SCIENTIFIC
CONCEPTS

Nutrigenomics

Chrononutrition

Phytochemicals

Inflammation balance

Immune health

Mitochondrial support

Population studies

Gut health

Plant Focused

Whole

Fiber

**HEALTHY
EATING
PRINCIPLES**

Eating in Time

Quality Fats

Color

to live happier, healthier lives, and by offering these simple principles I hope to support and facilitate your journey.

+ Whole Food exists on a spectrum, from raw uncooked vegetables to packaged, refined foods with added sugar, salt, preservatives, color, refined oils, and flavoring. Instead of scaring you away from having a chocolate bar or fries ever again, we simply want as much of your diet to be as minimally processed as possible. Also, cooking, steaming, and sautéing foods can heighten the availability of nutrients when we consume them, so this isn't a suggestion that we should only have a raw diet. As a general guide, choosing most of your ingredients from the fresh grocery aisle, and reducing refined carbohydrates made from flours like breads, cakes, pasta, and products with added sugar, is the best way to eat "whole."

+ Plant focused I introduced the concept of a plant-focused diet in my first book, and I'm reiterating it here. For most people, a diet made up of vegetables, with judicious inclusion of animal products as luxury items (ones that you'd have once or twice a week at most), is the healthiest starting point. Opt for the vegetables, and fill your plates with a variety of them at every meal.

+ Look for the colors Make sure you include at least two different vegetables at every meal, varying them throughout the week and experimenting with seasonal vegetables. Learn to complement foods with spices, which are concentrated sources of micronutrients and

phytochemicals. My recipes will show you how. I have a downloadable guide to seasonal fruit
and veggies at www.thedoctorskitchen.com to give you ideas.

+ Good-quality fats These are essential to our health. As we've learned, they're vital for
our immune health, skin cells, and inflammation pathways. Whole sources of fats from nuts,
seeds, and quality cold-pressed oils such as olive oil are delicious and should be encouraged.
Vary the types of them throughout your week, and invest in airtight containers to store
different nuts and seeds.

+ Fiber This key part of our diets is often lacking. When we focus our meals around a
variety of plant foods, we automatically obtain plenty of fiber, but pulses, legumes, nuts, and
seeds are key sources of this vital ingredient. Fiber feeds our microbiota, and by now you
understand just how critical it is to health and well-being.

+ Timing As a general principle, restricting your eating hours to a window of 10–12 hours,
and eating at regular times, is a useful guide that will prevent late-night snacking out of
boredom and regulate your daily rhythm. In reality, this means having an early dinner around
7 p.m. if you choose to have breakfast at 8 a.m. These practices have been shown in
numerous studies examining "chrononutrition" to have benefits on sleep, inflammation, and
metabolic control. This general rule of thumb is common sense, and many patients of mine
find it simple to implement and effective.

LIFESTYLE 360

The practices of a wholesome nutrient-dense diet, combined with lifestyle factors, are
exceptionally powerful. When we complement these eating principles with a lifestyle
conducive to well-being, it creates an optimal internal environment. Looking through
countless research studies examining the chapter subjects (and many other topics
that I haven't covered in this book, including autoimmunity, fatigue, gastrointestinal
issues, and women's health) I saw that these lifestyle recommendations essentially
form a medicinal package that allows your body and mind to perform at their best.
When we examine the science behind these individual lifestyle practices, we can
start to appreciate the interdependence of biological mechanisms and understand
why they're so impactful.

+ Sleep Respect your body's need to sleep as you would respect your body's need
to eat. Sleep is key to regulating hormonal rhythms, balancing inflammation, and
improving metabolic health. You may also find improved mental clarity, and a greater
capacity to work efficiently, and there is evidence that good sleep hygiene can protect

us against mental health problems. Seven to eight hours is the minimum for an adult, and I believe the effects extend far beyond physical health.

+ Exercise and outdoor activity You don't need to follow an intense exercise regimen. Variety, very much like food, is what your body thrives on. Try different modes of movement like running, resistance, yoga, Pilates, and flow. Each individual form of exercise has its benefits, and there isn't one "best" form. Try something you genuinely enjoy, and remember to mix it up. Move throughout the day: your body is beautifully designed to be in motion, so try to stretch regularly and take walking breaks from your desk.

+ Environment and community As well as being designed to move, we're also designed to be exposed to natural light and connected to nature. The Japanese research examining the health effects of forest bathing, the behavioral studies examining cognitive ability and mood after being exposed to natural environments, and the benefits of simple light exposure all point to this conclusion. Getting outdoors and spending time in green spaces have a positive impact on both your psychological and physical health. I also believe that we as human beings have an innate "tribal mentality." We have grown and adapted to live in communities with our sense of purpose largely entwined with survival and food. Considering how loneliness and isolation are a huge issue, which many doctors believe is related to rising rates of physical ill health, making time to meet with friends or simply spending time in the company of colleagues is something that we should prioritize.

+ Mindfulness My interest in meditation and breathing techniques started in my teenage years during exam periods and continued throughout medical school. The anecdotal experiences of meditation are interesting, but the mechanistic evidence examining how and why a mindfulness practice can lead to benefits is much more exciting to me. Forget the commercial interpretations of mindfulness, and concentrate on the core strategies that have underpinned ancient medicine for millennia. There are clear scientific reasons as to why different civilizations from across our world all have mindfulness as a core feature of medicine. Flicking through the chapters of this book, you'll begin to see that it's not just a mood enhancer and that there are many ways to achieve mindfulness. In our modern hyper-connected, over-stimulated lives, the need for incorporating a mindfulness practice into our daily routine has never been more relevant, and I encourage you to try a few different practices. Check out my website, www.thedoctorskitchen.com, for more examples of mindfulness and how to practice it in your daily routine.

"By employing these lifestyle factors with food as medicine, we create an ultimate package for well-being that is accessible, evidence-based, and effective."

This condensed list, in combination with our healthy eating principles, represents all the ways in which we can improve our well-being. These core practices, as determined by a mix of evidence, anecdotal clinical experience, and common sense, will give you the best chance at thriving. Lifestyle factors are beyond subjective feelings of wellness; these interact with your biology on multiple levels.

This book will help you gain a broader picture of how everything is linked and offers a process of how to achieve a healthier, happier life from here onwards. By employing these lifestyle factors with food as medicine, we create an ultimate package for well-being that is accessible, evidence-based, and effective. For more information on a course I'm developing to help you employ all these lifestyle factors, as well as plenty of YouTube videos, check out my website, www.thedoctorskitchen.com.

And now to the table. The focus of my recipes is speed, simplicity of ingredients, incredible flavor, and high nutritional value. grab your pans, pots, and aprons. It's time to get in the kitchen and experience a health journey, one delicious meal at a time.

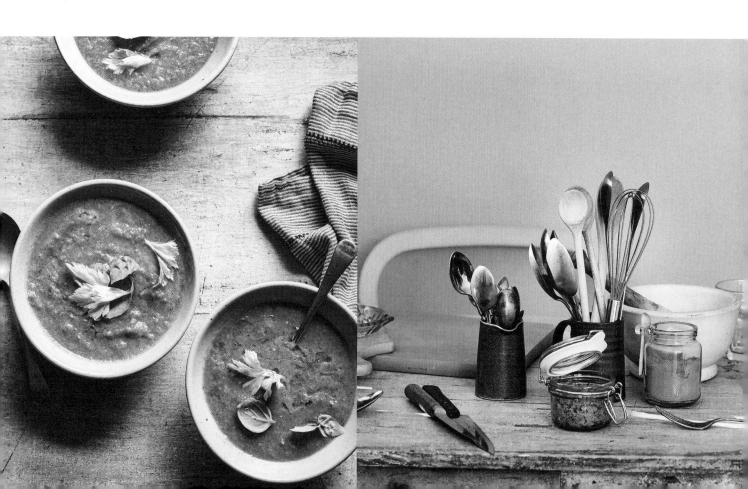

Simple, quick breakfast ideas are what most people need to get their day started in the right direction. Having a colorful mix of greens, lots of fiber, and quality fats in my breakfast is what keeps me going without having to snack midmorning. My favorites for when I'm limited on time are the one-pan meals. The more you practice making these, the easier and quicker they become.

Breakfast

Serves 2

2 tbsp extra-virgin olive oil, plus extra for drizzling

10½ oz sweet potato (unpeeled), cut into ½-inch cubes

2 oz spring onions, trimmed and finely chopped

4 eggs

1 tsp dried thyme

1 tsp dried oregano

1 tsp sweet paprika

½ tsp cayenne pepper, plus extra to serve

½ tsp ground black pepper

3½ oz curly kale, stems removed and leaves roughly chopped

3½ oz sweet corn kernels (fresh, frozen, or canned)

1 oz sunflower seeds, toasted and lightly crushed

sea salt and freshly ground black pepper

Cajun Sweet Potato Hash

When I have an extra 10 minutes for breakfast, this hash is what I often turn to. It couldn't be easier (chopping sweet potatoes and throwing them in a pan with a drizzle of oil is the hardest thing about the recipe). Using eggs adds extra protein to the meal as well as lutein and zeaxanthin, compounds that are important for eye health. Using the whole sweet potato with the skin on introduces extra fiber to the dish. The kale contains a good amount of folate and vitamin K, essential for the proper functioning of our genes, and its bitterness is mellowed by flavorful, nutrient-dense oregano and thyme.

Heat the oil in a large frying pan over medium heat, and add the sweet potato and spring onions. Cover and cook for 8 minutes.

Meanwhile, place the eggs in a saucepan of cold water and bring to a boil, then reduce the heat and simmer for 3 minutes (if you want a soft-boiled egg). Remove and transfer to a bowl of cold water to stop the cooking process (or cool under cold running water). Once cool, peel off the shells.

Combine the herbs and spices, and toss into the sweet potatoes with some salt and pepper; add the kale and corn kernels. Cook for a further 3–4 minutes, uncovered, until the potatoes are cooked through and the kale has wilted. Remove from the heat and transfer to plates.

Slice the eggs in half and place them on the sweet potato hash. Sprinkle with the sunflower seeds and some cayenne pepper, and drizzle with a little olive oil.

VARIATIONS

+ Try Swiss chard, spinach, or even arugula instead of kale.
+ Experiment by swapping the sweet corn for sprouted sunflower seeds or cooked puy lentils.

TIP

+ Use a simple Cajun spice blend instead of making the spice mix from scratch if you're short on time.

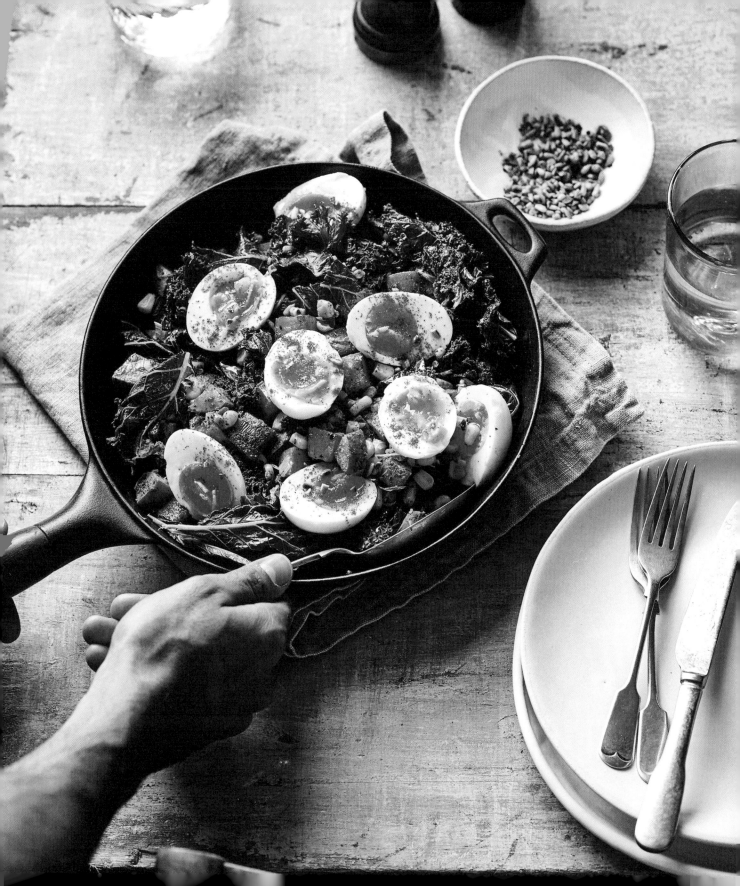

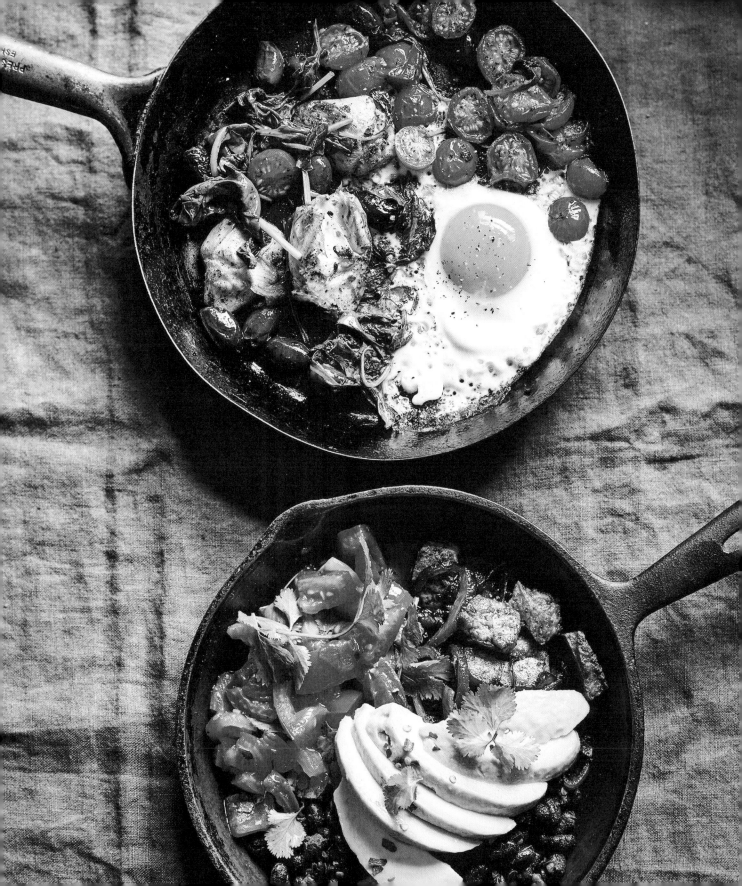

One-Pan Greek Breakfast

One-pan breakfasts for me are absolutely great when you're short of time, and they are a fantastic way to consume phytonutrient-dense ingredients first thing in the morning. This style of breakfast will fuel you throughout the morning so you won't need to rely on snacks to keep you satiated. It's a beautiful mix of proteins and unusual ingredients that work really well together. Simply use a bigger pan and double up the quantities if you want to cook for more people.

Serves 1

1 tbsp extra-virgin olive oil, plus extra for drizzling (if needed)
¾ oz drained preserved artichokes
¾ oz pitted kalamata olives
1 oz cherry tomatoes, halved
1 tsp dried oregano
1 oz spinach, roughly chopped
generous pinch of black pepper
1 or 2 eggs
½ lemon

Heat the oil in a frying pan with a lid over medium heat. Add the artichokes and olives to the pan, fry for a minute, stirring, then move them to a quarter section of the pan. Add the tomatoes, cut side down, to an empty section of the pan, scatter with the oregano, then move them to another quarter section, next to the olives and artichokes. Scatter the chopped spinach on top of the olives, and add the black pepper.

Drizzle a little oil in the remaining empty half of the pan (if needed), and carefully crack the egg (or eggs) into this section. Once the translucent part of the egg has turned white, cover and cook for 3–4 minutes until the egg yolk is cooked through.

Squeeze a little lemon juice over the artichokes, spinach, and olives, and serve. You don't need to add salt to this dish as the olives are salty enough.

One-Pan Cajun Scramble

Instead of having eggs in the morning, I sometimes scramble tofu. Tofu is a great source of protein for largely plant-based eaters like myself, but alone it can be quite bland. Cooking it with a Cajun spice blend and turmeric is a great way to flavor the tofu and make it visually appealing. This is a hearty, quick dish, packed with nutrient-dense spices and fiber that will set you up for a productive day.

Serves 2

3½ oz firm tofu, drained
3 tbsp extra-virgin olive oil, plus extra for drizzling
2 tsp Cajun spice blend
½ tsp ground turmeric
½ red onion, thinly sliced
14 oz canned black beans, drained and rinsed
½ tsp dried chili pepper
2 oz tomatoes, roughly chopped
½ oz fresh coriander, finely chopped
ripe avocado, stoned, peeled, and sliced
sea salt and freshly ground black pepper

Crumble the tofu into a bowl, and add half the olive oil along with all the Cajun spice blend and turmeric, and some salt and pepper. Mix thoroughly.

Heat the remaining olive oil in a frying pan with a lid over medium heat, add the onion, and sauté for 3–4 minutes until softened, then add the crumbled tofu to the pan, mix it with the onions, and cook for a further 4–5 minutes. Move it to a quarter section of the pan, add the black beans and chili, along with a little salt and pepper, to the empty part of the pan, and mix together. Move this to another quarter section of the pan. Add the chopped tomatoes and coriander to the empty section of the pan with a drizzle of olive oil, cover, and cook for 3–4 minutes to warm through all the ingredients.

Serve right away, with sliced avocado on top.

One-Pan Spicy Bean and Mushroom Breakfast

Serves 2

1 tbsp extra-virgin olive oil

3 oz chestnut mushrooms, thinly sliced

3½ oz zucchini, cut into ¾-inch dice

1 garlic clove, finely chopped

¼ oz fresh tarragon, finely chopped (or 1 tsp dried tarragon)

14 oz canned borlotti beans, drained and rinsed

¾ cup water

1 tsp tomato puree

½ tsp chili powder

2½ oz spinach, roughly chopped

1 oz sun-dried tomatoes in oil, drained and chopped

sea salt and freshly ground black pepper

Once you get used to making one-pan meals, it becomes so much easier to add vegetables to your diet. There are clear benefits associated with consuming more than 5 portions of fruit and vegetables a day, and this breakfast helps you tick off 2–3 portions in less than 15 minutes. Prepare the ingredients in advance so you're ready to cook in the morning, and you'll become a pro.

Heat the oil in a large frying pan with a lid over medium heat. Add the mushrooms, zucchini, and garlic, season with salt and pepper, and sauté for 3–4 minutes until softened.

Add the tarragon and push the mixture to one quarter section of the pan. Add the borlotti beans to an empty section of the pan to warm up while you bring the water to a boil. Add the tomato puree and chili powder to the boiling water in a small heatproof bowl to make a sauce. Pour the sauce over the beans, mix together, and gently push to an empty half section of the pan. Add the chopped spinach and sun-dried tomatoes to the remaining empty quarter of the pan, season lightly with salt and pepper, cover, and cook for 2–3 minutes until the spinach has lightly wilted and the beans are warmed through.

Serve right away.

TIP

+ If you prefer it less spicy, substitute sweet paprika for the chili powder.

Watercress, Walnut, and Crayfish

Serves 2

3½ oz watercress, roughly chopped

2 oz walnuts, roughly chopped

2 tbsp extra-virgin olive oil

5½ oz chestnut mushrooms, thinly sliced

5½ oz peas (fresh or thawed)

½ oz fresh tarragon leaves, finely chopped

1 tsp grass-fed butter

3½ oz cooked crayfish tails (or smoked salmon slices)

sea salt and freshly ground black pepper

I like to describe this as a brain-boosting breakfast. I was inspired to create this meal after doing a recording for my podcast with a good friend of mine, Dr. Panja, who's a colleague with a specialist interest in brain health. While we were talking about what foods are essential for cognition and reducing the likelihood of dementia, I visualized this beautiful platter of ingredients with its complementary flavors and textures. I try to use grass-fed animal products, including butter and milk, as they have been shown to have higher Omega-3 value.

Put the watercress on a large serving plate. Toast the walnuts in a dry pan over medium heat for 1 minute, then scatter them over the bed of watercress and drizzle with half the oil.

Heat the rest of the oil in the same pan over medium heat, add the mushrooms and peas, season with salt and pepper, and sauté for about 3 minutes until softened and cooked, then add the tarragon, butter, and cooked crayfish tails, and cook for a further 1–2 minutes. Spoon the mixture over the watercress and walnuts, using the residual butter and oil in the pan as a dressing.

VARIATIONS

+ Substitute dried herbs like oregano or rosemary for the tarragon.
+ To make this vegetarian, replace the crayfish with cooked broad beans or edamame beans.

Pimenton Oats with Poached Salmon

Serves 2

7 oz skinless salmon fillet

2 eggs

1 tbsp extra-virgin olive oil, plus extra for drizzling

4 garlic cloves, thinly sliced

1 tsp pimenton (or sweet paprika)

5½ oz oats

5½ oz peas (fresh or thawed)

¾ cup hot water

1 tsp dried oregano

1½ oz sun-dried tomatoes in oil, drained and chopped

2 oz spinach, roughly chopped

½ oz fresh flat-leaf parsley, finely chopped

sea salt and freshly ground black pepper

I love using oats in savory dishes. This, my take on a traditional kedgeree, uses this versatile fiber-rich ingredient with a dash of Spanish flair. Using whole-grain rolled oats instead of rice reduces the cooking time, and they also soak up the wonderfully hot pimenton flavor along with the vibrant red color of the spice. There are so many delicious greens in this breakfast dish, but you'd never guess it was jam-packed with health-boosting ingredients.

Bring a saucepan of water to a simmer. Place the salmon and eggs into the pan, and cook for 8 minutes. Remove the salmon with a fish slice and set aside; remove the eggs and cool them under cold running water to stop them cooking further. Flake the salmon, and peel and quarter the eggs and set aside.

Heat the olive oil in a medium saucepan over medium heat, add the garlic and sauté for 2–3 minutes, then add the pimenton and mix it with the oil before adding the oats and peas and seasoning with salt and pepper. Cook the oats and peas for a minute, then pour in the hot water and add the oregano and sun-dried tomatoes. Cover and cook for 4 minutes, adding more water if you prefer it creamier. When the oats are soft and cooked, stir in the spinach and flaked salmon.

Serve topped with the parsley, quartered eggs and a drizzle of oil.

VARIATION

+ You can leave out the salmon to make this dish vegetarian.

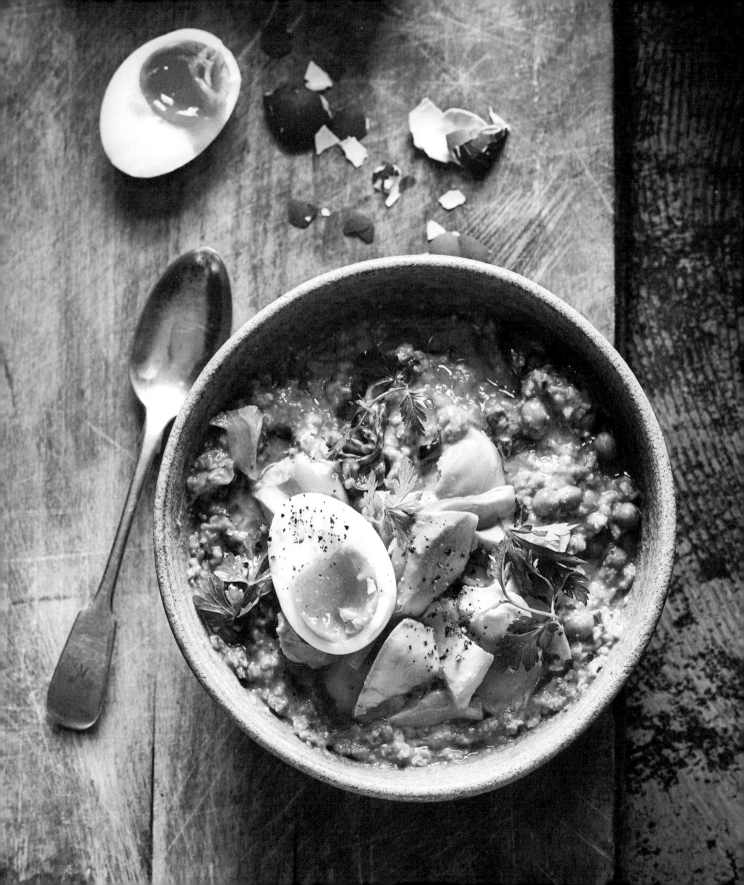

Wild Mushroom and Herb Frittata

Serves 6

12 large eggs

2 tbsp extra-virgin olive oil

1 oz dried wild mushrooms, rehydrated for 10 minutes in warm water and drained (or 50g fresh mushrooms)

3½ oz cooked chestnuts, halved

2 tsp dried oregano

2 tsp dried sage

1 tsp cracked black pepper

3½ oz peas (fresh or thawed)

2 oz sun-dried tomatoes (dry or in oil), roughly chopped

sea salt and freshly ground black pepper

I tend to make this delicious frittata at the start of the week and either eat it for breakfast or put it in my Tupperware box for lunch—it keeps well in the fridge for up to 3–4 days. It's packed with different types of vegetables, plenty of herbs for a nutritional kick, as well as one of my favorite high-fiber ingredients—chestnuts. Varying your ingredients is an easy way to ensure your gut microbiome has a variety of food sources. This leads to better inflammation control and sugar balance. A delicious slice of this sets me up for the day, and it's easy to experiment with different herbs to suit your taste. Dry herbs are just as beneficial as fresh, so don't be afraid to use these when you can't find fresh herbs in the shops.

Preheat the oven to 400°F.

Break the eggs into a bowl, and beat with a pinch of salt and pepper.

Heat the oil in a wide ovenproof pan over medium heat. Add the drained mushrooms and chestnuts, and sauté for 2–3 minutes, then add the herbs, pepper, peas, and sun-dried tomatoes, and stir for another 2 minutes. Add the eggs, and stir briefly so the egg coats the bottom of the pan and covers the vegetables. Stop stirring and let the sides set for 2 minutes before transferring the pan to the oven for 15 minutes until the frittata is set and cooked through.

TIP

+ Serve this frittata with wilted greens or fresh arugula salad and pine nuts to turn it into a full meal.

Oats and Butter Bean Breakfast

Oats are a wonderful addition to the diet. They contain a special type of fiber called beta-glucan that slows the release of sugars into the bloodstream, as well as a host of antioxidants that are also found in whole grains including barley and spelt. This meal is a fantastic way to start the day: it will keep you feeling satiated for hours and help stave off that 11 o'clock snack temptation.

Serves 2

2 tbsp extra-virgin olive oil, plus extra for drizzling

1 tsp butter

2 oz whole-grain oats

7 oz chestnut mushrooms, thinly sliced

2 tsp dried tarragon

2½ oz spinach, roughly chopped

7 oz canned butter beans, drained and rinsed

sea salt and freshly ground black pepper

Warm the oil and butter in a large saucepan over medium heat.

Add the oats and mushrooms, season with salt and pepper, and stir to coat in the oil.

Cook for 5 minutes, or until the mushrooms soften, then add the tarragon, spinach, and butter beans. Stir well to combine, cover, and cook for a further 3–4 minutes. The steam will lightly cook the oats and heat through the beans.

Serve hearty servings in bowls, drizzled with oil.

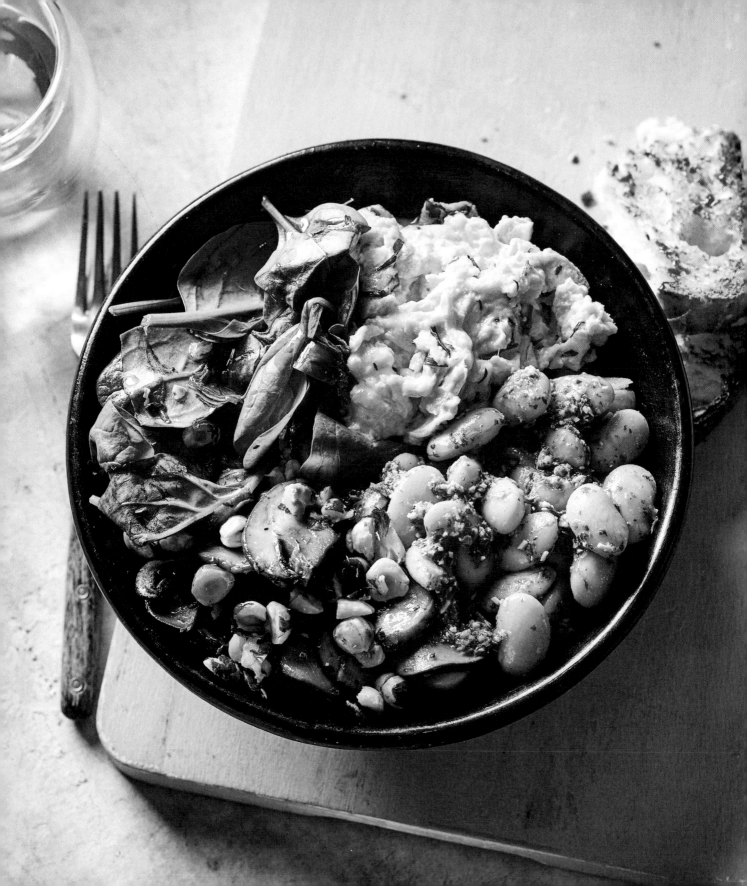

My Best Breakfast Bowl

Serves 2

2 tbsp olive oil

7 oz chestnut mushrooms, thinly sliced

½ tsp dried oregano

14 oz canned butter beans, drained and rinsed

2 tsp green pesto (fresh or store-bought)

3½ oz spinach, chopped or whole leaves

2 tsp grass-fed butter (see note on page 121)

2 tsp chopped fresh tarragon leaves (chives or dill can also work)

4 eggs, beaten

sea salt and freshly ground black pepper

To serve

2 slices of sourdough, toasted

Marmite, for spreading (optional)

¾ oz raw hazelnuts, lightly toasted and roughly chopped

I hardly ever eat sweet breakfasts these days. I love the feeling of having a hearty, nutrient-dense breakfast in the morning that will keep me satisfied throughout the day. This recipe combines two of my favorite things: bowl food and breakfast. The herb, mushroom, and nut combination is such a winner for me, and the eggs and tarragon are delicious. This is a collection of ingredients that will build up your gut bugs and reduce inflammation, and the sight of it alone will improve your mood.

Heat the olive oil in a saucepan over high heat, add the mushrooms and oregano, and sauté for 6 minutes. Divide the mushrooms between two serving bowls.

Put the butter beans and pesto into the empty pan, and put the pan back over medium heat. Cook, gently stirring, for 4–5 minutes to warm through the beans, then transfer the mixture to the serving bowls, keeping it separate from the mushrooms.

Put the spinach into the empty pan, off the heat, and cover for 1–2 minutes to allow the leaves to gently wilt in the residual heat of the pan.

Melt the butter in a small frying pan over medium heat. Add the chopped tarragon before the butter has a chance to brown, and stir for 20–30 seconds, then add the beaten eggs and scramble them with a whisk or fork, stirring them continuously. Take the pan off the heat when the eggs are almost cooked. They will finish cooking in the residual heat (this technique prevents them overcooking and maintains a creamy texture).

Put the eggs and spinach in the serving bowl, and season lightly with salt and pepper.

Serve the breakfast bowls with a slice of sourdough (spread with Marmite, if you like), and scatter the toasted hazelnuts over the mushrooms.

TIP

+ Any mushrooms will work here. Try chestnut, porcini, portobello, or even girolles if you're feeling fancy.

Preparing lots of little plates of food for sharing is my favorite way to entertain. It's also how I like to build healthy meals at home. A lot of what I tend to eat are small dishes combined to create healthy platters that are both delightful to look at and incredible for health.

Small plates

Greek Skewers with Tzatziki

Most vegetables will work in this recipe, and it's a great way to use up any you have languishing at the bottom of your fridge. I tend to cook a bunch of them in advance, for work lunches. You can cook them on a barbecue, but oven-baking them will remind you of summer times even in the depths of winter. The garlic and lemon marinade is another way to easily introduce delicious nutrient-dense ingredients into your diet. If you can't get hold of herb-marinated tofu, simply use more mushrooms instead.

Combine the garlic and lemon marinade ingredients in a large bowl. Add the tofu and vegetables, coat them in the mixture, and leave to marinate for at least 20 minutes (ideally overnight).

Preheat the oven to 400°F, and push the marinated vegetables onto skewers (soak wood or bamboo skewers in water for 20 minutes first, to avoid them burning). Arrange them on a baking tray, and bake for 15–20 minutes until golden.

To make the tzatziki, combine the yogurt, cucumber, and mint in a bowl, season with salt and pepper, and drizzle with the olive oil.

TIP

+ Serve the skewers on a bed of green salad leaves.

Makes about 6 skewers

10½ oz herb-marinated firm tofu, cut into ½-inch chunks

10½ oz brown mushrooms, cut into 1½-inch chunks

2 peppers (colors of choice), deseeded and cut into 1½-inch chunks

1 red onion, cut into 1½-inch chunks

1 white onion, cut into 1½-inch chunks

7 oz zucchini, cut into chunks

5½ oz lamb's lettuce or arugula, to serve

For the garlic and lemon marinade

2 tbsp olive oil

1 tbsp balsamic vinegar

grated zest and juice of 1 lemon

3 garlic cloves, grated

2 tsp sweet paprika

3 tsp mixed dried Mediterranean herbs (oregano, fennel, rosemary)

sea salt and freshly ground black pepper

For the tzatziki

3½ oz Greek yogurt (or dairy-free unflavored coconut yogurt)

3½ oz cucumber, grated

½ oz mint leaves, finely chopped

1 tbsp extra-virgin olive oil

sea salt and freshly ground black pepper

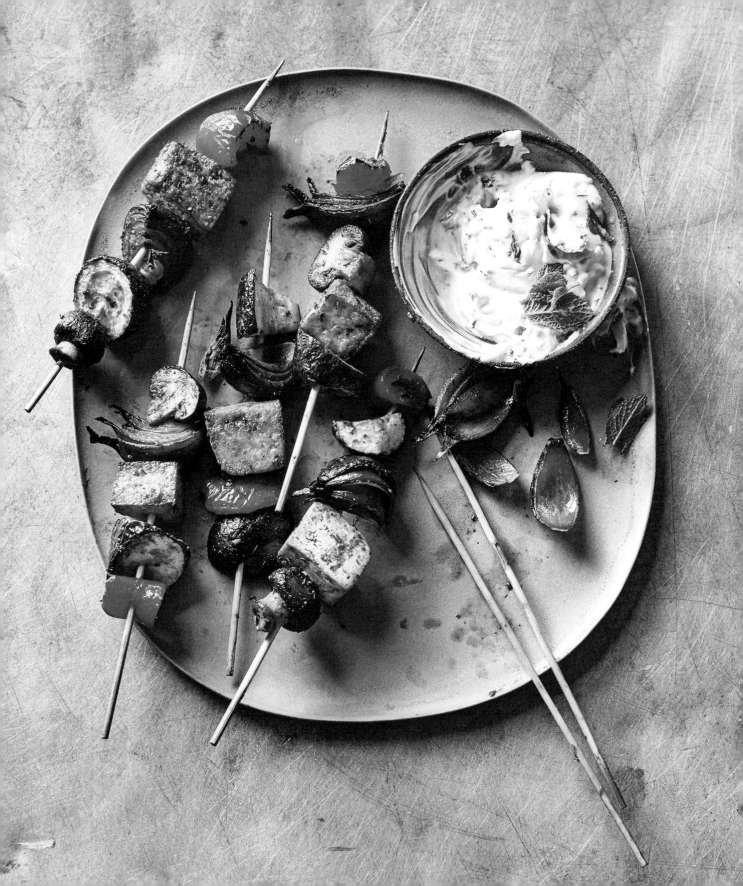

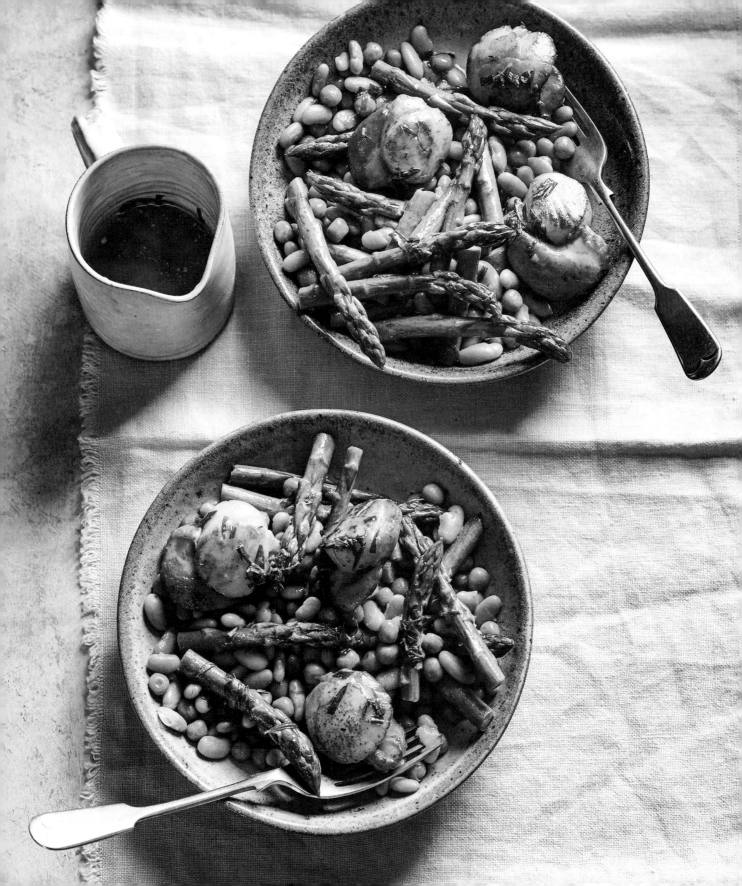

Spring Asparagus, Peas, and Scallops with Tarragon Butter

Serves 2

3 tbsp extra-virgin olive oil, divided

5½ oz asparagus spears, trimmed and cut into 1¼-inch pieces

3½ oz peas (fresh or thawed)

3½ oz canned flageolet beans, drained and rinsed

6 shelled and cleaned scallops (with the roe)

¼ oz fresh tarragon leaves, finely chopped

2 tsp grass-fed butter (see note on page 121)

sea salt and freshly ground black pepper

This is perhaps the most "cheffy" recipe in the book, but it's still easy to prepare. I want to show you that you can deliver an incredibly indulgent dish that is simple to make and has myriad health benefits. Fats are vital to help absorb those key fat-soluble vitamins in greens such as vitamins E and K. The roe from scallops often get discarded, but they're a source of long-chain fatty acids, EPA and DHA and vitamin B_{12}, which are essential for brain and heart health. I love this dish as it is, but it's also great served on a slice of toasted sourdough to soak up some of the flavors.

Heat 1 tablespoon of the olive oil in a large frying pan over medium heat. Add the asparagus to the pan, season with salt and pepper, cover, and cook for 5 minutes, then add the peas and beans. Cover again, and cook for a further 2 minutes, then set aside.

Heat a separate frying pan over high heat. Drizzle the scallops with half a tablespoon of the olive oil, and season them with salt and pepper, then add them to the pan. Sauté on each side for 60–90 seconds, or until just cooked through. Remove the scallops from the pan, and set aside.

Plate the asparagus, beans, and peas, then place the scallops on top.

Using the same pan used for the scallops, warm the remaining oil, and add the tarragon. Cook, stirring gently, for about a minute, then add the butter to the pan, and spoon the tarragon butter straight onto the scallops.

VARIATION

+ Swap the scallops for jumbo prawns.

TIP

+ If you can't source fresh scallops, look for frozen scallops and defrost them before use. Opt for hand-caught scallops where possible: they're much more sustainable and taste incredible.

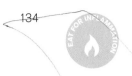

Sage Eggplant and Broccoli

Serves 2 as a side

2 small eggplants (about 12½ oz in total), cut into 1¼-inch cubes

7 oz Tenderstem broccoli, roughly chopped

2 tbsp extra-virgin olive oil

½ oz fresh sage leaves, finely chopped (or 2 tsp dried sage)

sea salt and freshly ground black pepper

This simple dish works really well as a side for dinner parties and gets you using eggplant, which a lot of people don't know how to cook. Sautéing it in a dry pan removes excess water from the eggplant that can otherwise ruin its texture. I've used a strong culinary herb, sage, to give these simple vegetables a satisfying flavor. Sage is a wonderful underused herb that has many medicinal properties that have been recognized since ancient times for their ability to aid digestion and fight inflammation. You don't need to eat it in large quantities, but getting more herb and spice onto your plate is the goal.

Heat a saucepan over medium heat, add the eggplant, and let it toast gently for 3–4 minutes (without any oil), tossing it and taking care not to burn the flesh.

Season the eggplant with salt and pepper, and add the broccoli, olive oil, and sage. Sauté for another 2–3 minutes in the oil, then cover the saucepan and allow the ingredients to gently steam in the heat for a further 2–3 minutes before serving.

VARIATION

+ Try adding different herbs (or spices) and preparing the dish in the same way: oregano, fennel, or even garam masala will work well.

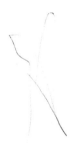

Sri Lankan–Style Oats

Serves 2

1 tbsp coconut oil

½ red onion, thinly sliced

1 tsp black mustard seeds

2 tsp Sri Lankan masala spice blend (or garam masala)

1 green chili, deseeded and thinly sliced

1 tsp ground turmeric

7 oz oats

2 cups boiling water

3½ oz spinach, finely chopped

½ oz fresh coriander, finely chopped

sea salt and freshly ground black pepper

One of the most amazing discoveries for me on my brief travels to Sri Lanka were the spice blends and how different they were to Indian blends. Pandan leaf, lemongrass, and kaffir lime, as well as clove, cinnamon, and asafoetida, are combined in a typical Sri Lankan crab curry masala. The spice blends are incredibly potent and like nothing else I have ever tasted. Oats are used in lots of savory Sri Lankan dishes, and this is a wonderful way of using this fiber-rich ingredient that we tend to only associate with sweet breakfasts.

Melt the coconut oil in a large, wide-based pan with a lid, add the red onion and mustard seeds, and sauté for 5–7 minutes until the onions have softened, then add the spice blend, chili, turmeric, and oats. Season with salt and pepper, and cook, stirring, for another 2 minutes.

Add the boiling water to the pan of oats, cover and simmer gently for another 6 minutes, then remove from the heat, fold in the spinach, cover, and leave for 2 minutes to allow the greens to wilt. Stir in most of the coriander, reserving some for garnish.

Divide between two bowls, and garnish with the remaining coriander.

TIP

+ You can find Sri Lankan spice blends in an Indian store or online.

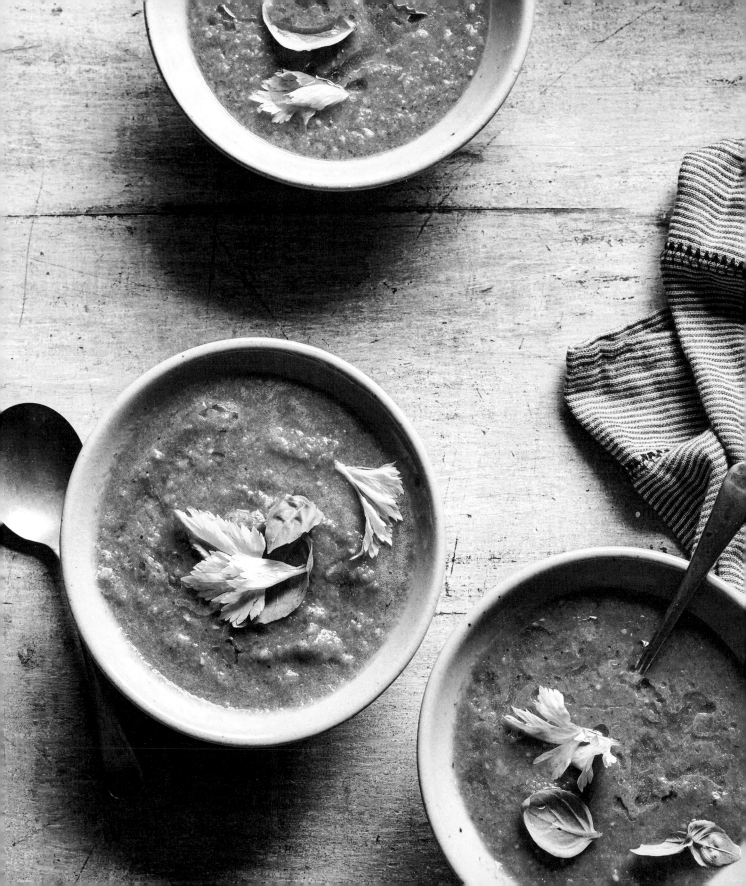

Speedy Gazpacho

Serves 4

1 cucumber, roughly chopped

6 medium tomatoes (heirloom variety if possible)

½ oz basil leaves, stems removed

1 celery stalk, roughly chopped

½ red pepper, deseeded and roughly chopped

2 garlic cloves, grated

juice of 1 lemon

1 tbsp extra-virgin olive oil, plus extra for drizzling

1 tbsp red wine vinegar

sea salt and freshly ground black pepper

This is the quickest dish in the book, best enjoyed on a hot day. I ate it first when I was staying in Bristol, teaching the UK's first culinary medicine course to medical students. Professor Trevor Thompson and Dr. Elizabeth Thompson are incredible clinicians who both work at Bristol Medical School and embrace all different types of medicine. Elizabeth made us this exquisite soup from simple locally grown ingredients while we sat outside in the balmy July heat and discussed the interplay between art and medicine. It was probably one of the most pleasant evenings I've had, highlighted by a poetry recital of Mary Oliver's "Wild Geese."

Put all the ingredients in a food processor and blitz until smooth, then season to taste with salt and pepper.

Add some water to loosen the soup if needed, then divide it between bowls and drizzle some more oil on top to serve.

Lemon, Thyme, and Hazelnut Roast Vegetables

Serves 4

10½ oz carrots (use red or purple if you can find them)

10½ oz parsnips (halved if they are thick)

10½ oz rutabaga, cut into chunks (unpeeled)

10½ oz turnips, halved, or quartered if large

¼ cup olive oil

2 large garlic cloves, grated

1 tsp dried oregano

1½ lemons, ½ juiced, the whole lemon quartered

½ oz thyme sprigs

1 oz raw hazelnuts, lightly crushed

sea salt and freshly ground black pepper

I love serving a big batch of these vegetables to complement my nut roast on page 195 or even as a lunchbox filler. The thyme and hazelnut combination works really well and hasselbacking them allows the marinade to penetrate the vegetables. It's a great way of using up vegetables (you can use any root vegetables) and it's my go-to dish when I know a few people are coming round and I want to prepare something easy and stress free.

Preheat the oven to 375°F and line a baking tray with baking parchment.

To hasselback the vegetables, slice them at ⅛-inch intervals, cutting only three-quarters of the way through their depth (using 2 wooden spoons as a guard and placing the vegetables in between them helps to achieve this without cutting the whole way through the vegetables). Try to keep the vegetables roughly the same thickness so they cook evenly.

Prepare the marinade by mixing together the oil, garlic, oregano, lemon juice, and thyme, along with some salt and pepper, in a bowl.

Smother the vegetables in the marinade, and place them on the lined baking tray. Cook for 30 minutes, tossing them once, then add the quartered lemons and cook for another 20–30 minutes (or more if needed), adding the hazelnuts for the final 7 minutes.

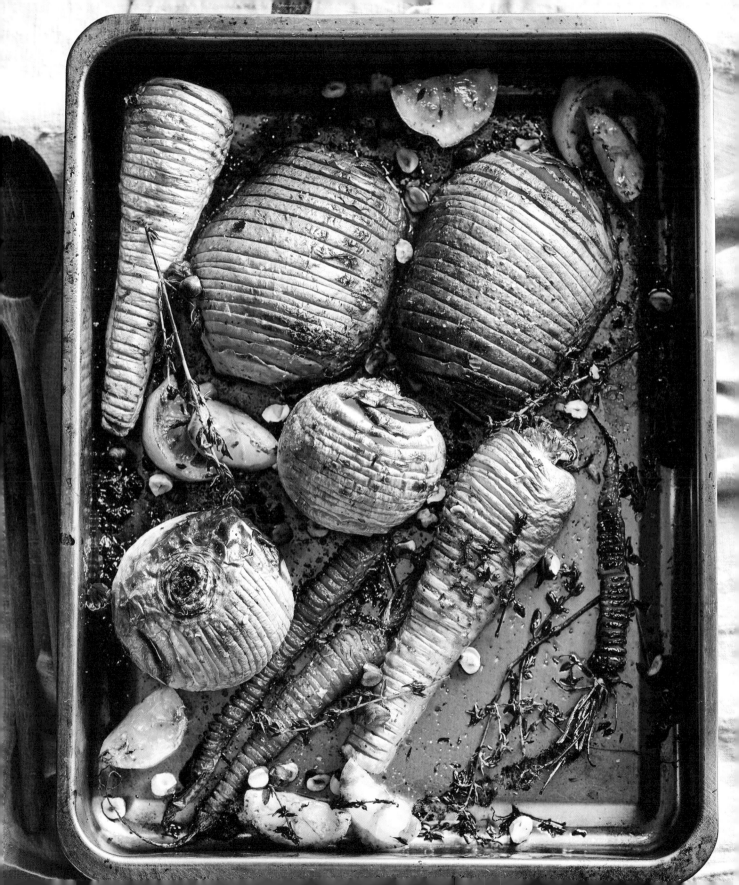

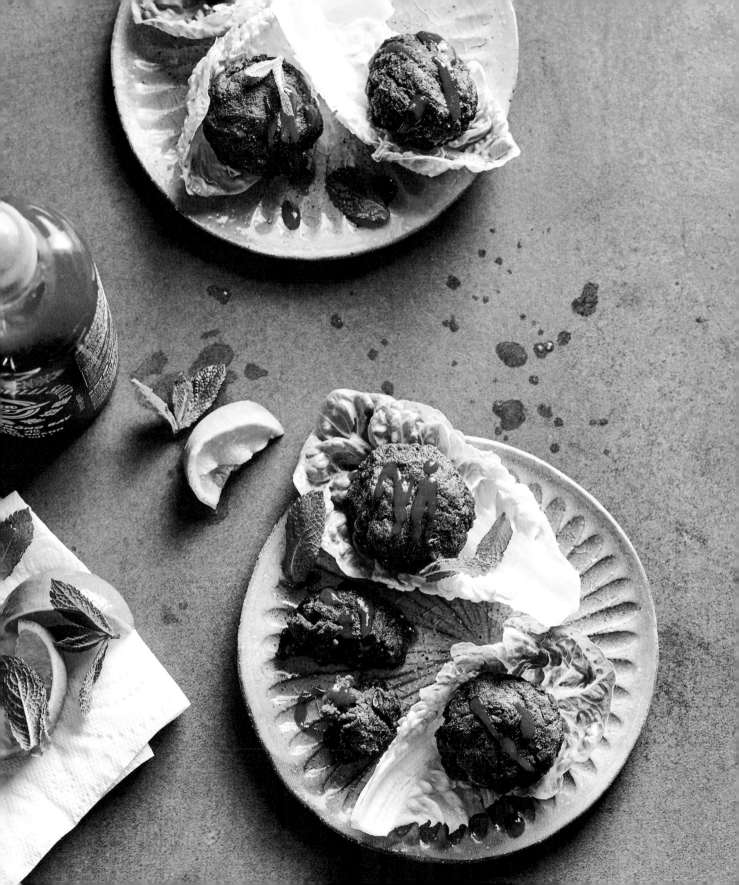

Cajun Corn Bites

I tend to make these in big batches so I can pair them up with salads and colorful vegetable platters for my work lunches. Black beans are a fantastic source of fiber and protein, and I always have a can in the cupboard so I can quickly whip up this recipe. The corn balls keep for a few days in the fridge, and the heat from the spices works really well in a lettuce wrap, paired with some lime wedges and sriracha sauce for a quick, delicious snack when friends come round at the last minute.

Preheat the oven to 400°F and line a baking tray with some baking parchment.

Put all the ingredients in a food processor with some salt and pepper, and blitz. You may need to scrape the ingredients down the sides of the machine intermittently to get a consistent mixture. The mixture will be quite wet.

Lightly dust your hands with flour, then form the mixture into 12 balls (around the size of a golf ball). Place the balls on the lined baking tray, and drizzle with a little oil. Bake in the oven for 30–35 minutes until crisp on the outside and cooked through.

Arrange the balls in lettuce leaves and serve with sriracha, lime wedges, and mint leaves.

TIP

+ As a cheat, instead of using the individual spices, you could simply use 3 heaping teaspoons of a good-quality Cajun spice blend.

Makes 12 balls

7 oz sweet corn kernels (fresh or canned)

14 oz tin black beans, drained and rinsed

3½ oz buckwheat flour (or regular whole-wheat flour), plus extra for dusting

1 tbsp extra-virgin olive oil, plus extra for drizzling

1 tsp fennel seeds

1 tsp ground cumin

1 tsp English mustard powder

1 tsp sweet paprika

½ tsp chili powder (optional)

sea salt and freshly ground black pepper

To serve

lettuce leaves

sriracha

lime wedges and mint leaves

142

Citrus and Pineapple Asian Salad

Serves 2

¾ oz unsalted peanuts or cashews, roughly chopped

7 oz fresh pineapple, cut into 1¼-inch cubes

5½ oz bean sprouts

3½ oz red pepper (about 1 small pepper), halved, deseeded, and cut into thin strips

For the dressing

¾ oz fresh coriander, stalks and leaves finely chopped

¾ oz fresh mint, leaves picked and finely chopped

¼ cup sesame oil

grated zest and juice of 2 limes

2 tsp fish sauce or soy sauce

1 shallot, finely chopped

1 garlic clove, finely chopped

1 tsp Rendang Curry Paste (see page 246) or store-bought paste (or another curry paste)

I love the flavors of Vietnamese, Malaysian, and Thai food. You can use any pre-made curry paste from these cuisines to make this beautiful fresh salad, such as sambal olek or Thai red curry paste. I've used my favorite ingredient, bean sprouts, to add a fresh crunch to this speedy dish, but feel free to use any sort of sprouts: mung bean, adzuki, or even red lentil sprouts can work equally well.

Mix all the dressing ingredients together in a bowl.

Toast the peanuts in a dry frying pan over medium heat for a few minutes until aromatic and starting to color.

Toss the pineapple, bean sprouts and red pepper together in a bowl with the toasted nuts and dressing, then serve.

VARIATION

+ Try using different vegetables and fruits in the salad, such as carrots, cucumber, and zucchini, or orange segments and peaches.

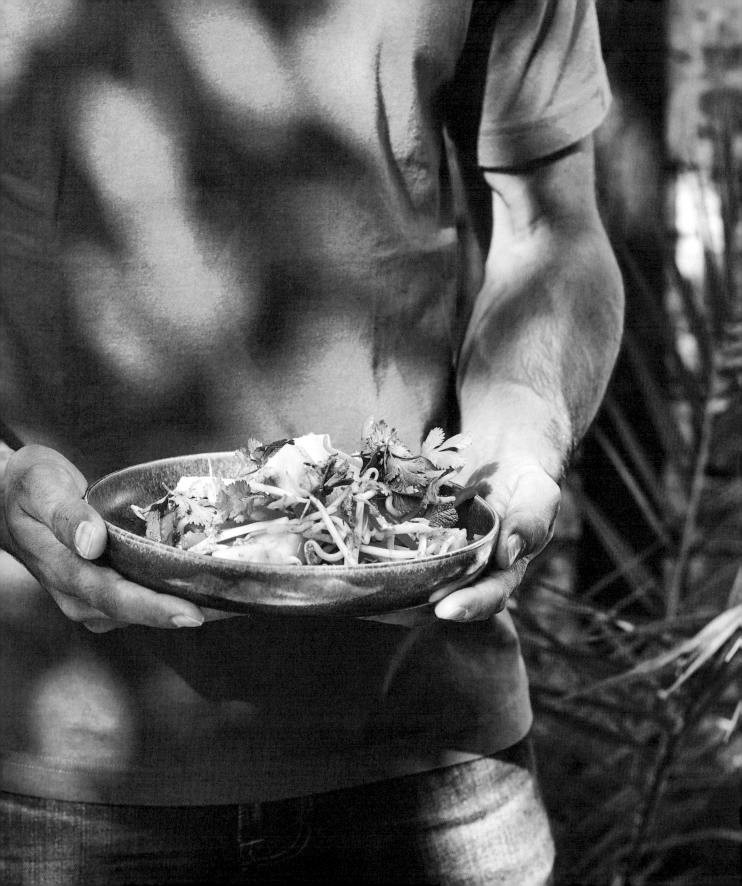

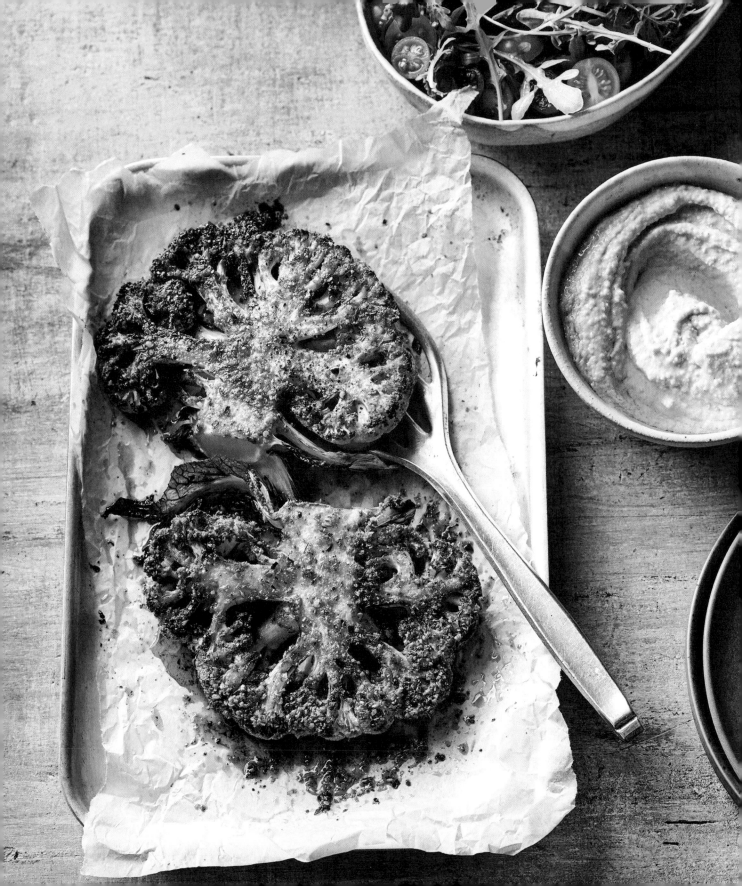

Herby Cauliflower Steaks

When I first came across "cauliflower steaks," I scoffed at the idea of cauliflower being passed off as a steak. But actually, aside from the fact that it is completely nutritionally different from an actual steak, it's a very satisfying dish to make. I am a fan of any innovative way of using brassica vegetables, like cauliflower, that delivers on taste and enjoyment. This simple recipe has incredible flavors and is perfect served as an accompaniment, or on its own as a light meal. Flaxseed makes an excellent crispy coating, but if you prefer you can also use whole-grain breadcrumbs or a little flour.

Serves 2

1 large cauliflower
3 tbsp extra-virgin olive oil
2 tsp dried tarragon
2 tsp dried thyme
½ tsp dried chili flakes
1 tsp sweet paprika
2 tbsp milled flaxseed
sea salt and freshly ground black pepper
1½ oz arugula, to serve
3½ oz cherry tomatoes, halved, to serve

For the white bean puree

14 oz canned white beans (cannellini beans or butter beans), drained and rinsed
2 garlic cloves
1 tbsp tahini
juice of ½ lemon
2 tbsp extra-virgin olive oil
5 tsp water

Preheat the oven to 400°F and line a baking sheet with some baking parchment.

Cut 1¼-inch-thick slices out of the cauliflower (you should get at least 2 proper steaks—the ends you can still roast in the spices or use in another dish).

Combine the oil with the tarragon, thyme, chili, paprika, flaxseed, and some salt and pepper in a bowl. Place the cauliflower steaks on the lined baking sheet, and brush them all over with the herb rub. Bake in the oven for 30–35 minutes until browned and soft.

Meanwhile, put the white bean puree ingredients in a food processor, and blitz to make a puree for the steaks to sit on.

Place the cauliflower steaks on a bed of bean puree, and dress each serving with arugula and tomatoes to serve.

TIP

+ Dry-toast ½ ounce shelled pistachios and roughly chop them to make a nice garnish for the steaks.

Fennel and Carrots with Star Anise

Serves 4 as a side

2 fennel bulbs, quartered

4 large carrots, quartered lengthways

3 star anise

2 tbsp extra-virgin olive oil

¾ oz raw hazelnuts

1 tsp butter

2 oz spinach, finely chopped

sea salt and freshly ground black pepper

Star anise is a beautiful match for carrots and fennel, and the combination of all three makes a fantastic quick side dish that you can serve with simple fish or even a roast dinner. Not many people use fennel, but it's a wonderful vegetable that contains a unique set of plant chemicals that have been shown to reduce inflammation.

Preheat your oven to 400°F.

Place the vegetables on a baking tray along with the star anise. Drizzle with the olive oil, season with salt and pepper, and bake for around 45 minutes until the vegetables are golden and tender, tossing them once halfway through.

Place the hazelnuts on a small baking tray and roast in the oven for the final 7 minutes of cooking time.

Remove the trays from the oven, and add the butter to the vegetables and fold in the spinach. Roughly chop the toasted hazelnuts, and garnish the dish with them before serving.

VARIATION

+ Add a teaspoon of garam masala if you want to pair this with an Indian dish, or perhaps Chinese 5-spice powder if you are making noodles.

Almond and Hazelnut Lentils with Capers

Serves 2

1¼ cups water

7 oz puy lentils, soaked in water for at least 20 minutes, then drained

grated zest and juice of 1 lemon

3 tbsp extra-virgin olive oil, plus extra for drizzling

1 oz raw hazelnuts

1 oz raw almonds

2 tbsp capers, drained and rinsed

1 spring onion, trimmed and finely chopped

½ oz fresh tarragon leaves, finely chopped

½ tsp dried chili flakes, plus extra to serve

3½ oz cherry tomatoes, halved

Puy lentils are cheap and super easy to prepare from scratch, but if you're really short of time there are many good-quality ready-cooked options. This is a simple, quick dish that I make with fridge and pantry staples. The sharp, salty taste of the capers is a great match for lentils and sweet tomatoes, and the dish is a fantastic lunchbox filler.

Bring the water to a boil in a pan, add the drained lentils and a little of the lemon zest and a drizzle of olive oil, and simmer for 15 minutes until cooked (they will still have a soft bite to them when ready).

Meanwhile, toast the hazelnuts and almonds in a dry pan over medium heat for 2–3 minutes until lightly colored. Remove, roughly chop, and set aside to cool.

Combine the capers, oil, lemon juice, spring onion, tarragon, toasted nuts, and chili in a bowl. Scatter the lentils and cherry tomatoes into a large, flat bowl and fold in the lemon caper dressing. Garnish with the remaining lemon zest and some extra chili flakes.

VARIATIONS

+ This dish works well with some smoked salmon slices.
+ Add watercress or arugula to bulk up the dish and add even more nutrients.

Radicchio, Peach, and Fennel Salad with Balsamic Croutons

Serves 4

7 oz radicchio, leaves separated and hand-torn

10½ oz fennel bulb, thinly sliced (use a mandoline if you have one)

2½ oz arugula

grated zest and juice of 1 lime

3 tbsp extra-virgin olive oil

2 ripe peaches, stones removed and flesh cut into wedges

2 slices of sourdough, cut into chunky cubes

1 tbsp balsamic vinegar

sea salt and freshly ground black pepper

I absolutely love using strong contrasting flavors and colors in small plates like these. The bitter notes of radicchio are a delicious accompaniment to sweet stone fruit and aromatic fennel. The inviting beauty of this dish will encourage you to enjoy the wealth of nutrition contained within these plants. The strong flavor of fennel and radicchio leaves are testament to the rich concentration of polyphenols and vitamins that neutralize free radicals in the body as well as help protect against eye disease. The crunchy balsamic croutons are worth the extra effort, too!

Combine the radicchio, fennel, and arugula with the lime zest and juice and 2 tablespoons of the oil in a large bowl, and season with salt and pepper.

Heat a griddle pan over high heat. When hot, add the peach wedges and sear on the cut sides for about 1 minute to leave brown marks on the fruit, then scatter them over the leaves.

Toast the sourdough cubes in the remaining tablespoon of olive oil in the griddle pan over medium heat for 2–3 minutes until the bread begins to lightly brown, then add the balsamic vinegar to the pan and stir the cubes to coat them in the oil and vinegar. After 2–3 minutes, when they become crisp, remove from the pan and scatter them over the salad.

VARIATION

+ Try using different leaf and stone fruit combinations, such as plum and Swiss chard or even bok choy and apricot.

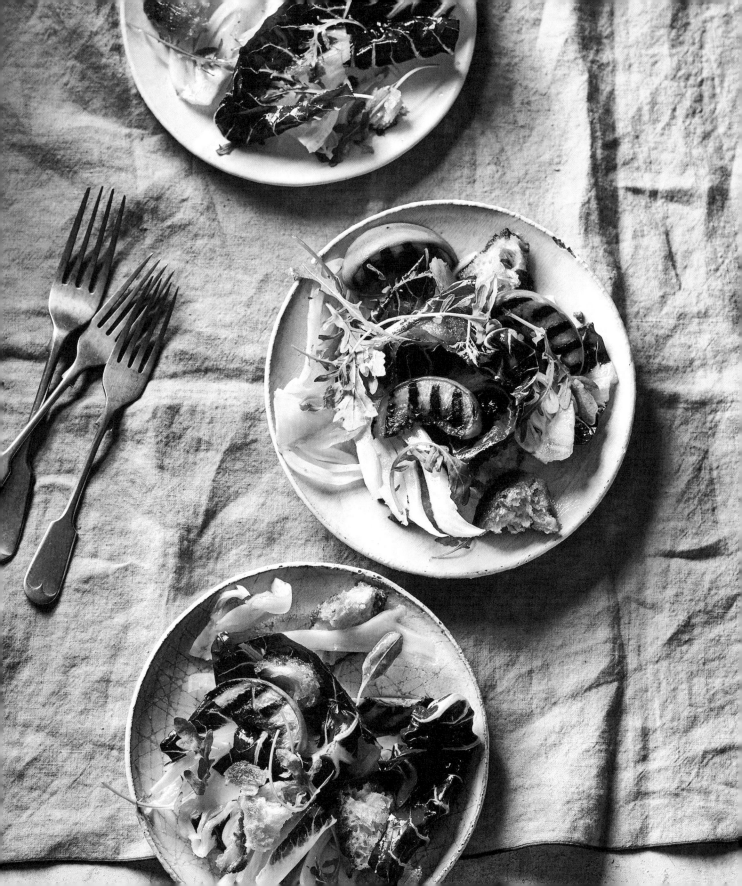

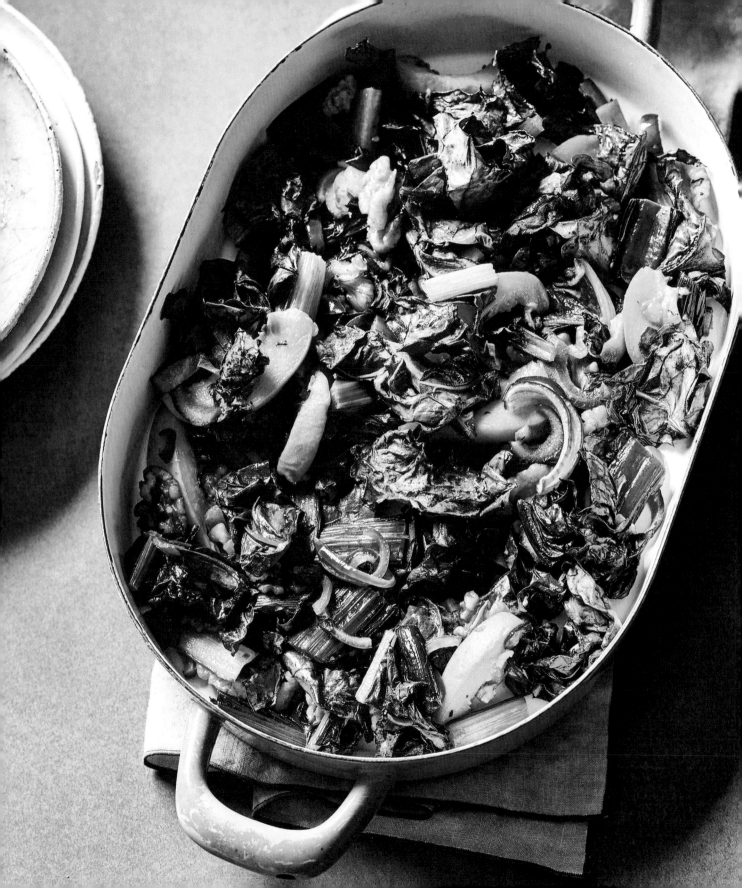

Baked Rainbow Chard with Apricot and Walnuts

Serves 2

1½ oz walnuts, whole or halved

1 red onion, halved and thinly sliced

7 oz Swiss chard, roughly sliced into ¾-inch-thick strips, stem included

1 fresh apricot, stoned and sliced into thin segments

2 tbsp extra-virgin olive oil, plus extra for drizzling

sea salt and freshly ground black pepper

Whenever I see beautiful rainbow chard on the shelves, I pick up a bunch. It is packed with vitamin K and magnesium, which are both essential for bone health, as well as antioxidant-rich phytochemicals like betalain. This dish marries the sweet flavor of stone fruit and chard's bitter compounds perfectly. The walnuts add texture as well as providing a source of fats that enable better absorption of the vitamins in chard.

Preheat the oven to 400°F.

Toss all the ingredients into a large roasting dish with plenty of salt and pepper. Bake in the oven for 18–20 minutes until the chard has slightly crisped up, then remove from the oven and serve with a drizzle of extra oil if needed.

VARIATION

+ I enjoy this with poached eggs as a breakfast meal, but it works equally well with pan-fried or poached white fish like bream or sea bass.

Fennel, Cumin, and Mackerel Salad

Serves 2

2 oz black olives, pitted

2 tomatoes, roughly chopped

1 red onion, thinly sliced

¾ oz fresh flat-leaf parsley, leaves and stalks roughly chopped

2 slices of rye bread, cut into ¾-inch cubes

2 tbsp olive oil

4 fresh mackerel fillets, skin on

3 tbsp labneh (or full-fat Greek yogurt)

For the dressing

2 tsp red wine vinegar

4 tsp olive oil

1 tsp pomegranate molasses (or maple syrup or honey)

1 tsp tomato puree

½ tsp chili powder

For the spice rub

1 tsp fennel seeds

1 tsp cumin seeds

1 tsp sumac

This salad reminds me of my travels to the Middle East where I first came across sumac. This wonderful spice has a unique sour lemon flavor and an exceptionally high antioxidant value. I love the freshness of this dish, and the spiced mackerel complements the strong flavors of the herbs and dressing. Labneh is a thick yogurt that contains a good amount of protein and typically also contains lactobacillus, which is great for gut health.

Mix all the dressing ingredients together in a bowl.

Place the olives, tomatoes, onion, and parsley in a bowl and toss together.

Heat a large frying pan over medium heat, add the rye bread cubes and toast for about 4 minutes until the edges begin to color, then add 1 tablespoon of the olive oil and gently fry for 2 minutes until the croutons become golden and firm. Transfer the croutons to a plate and set aside.

Grind the fennel seeds and cumin seeds using a pestle and mortar and combine with the sumac in a bowl, then spread out on a plate.

Press the mackerel fillets flesh side down in the spices, but leave the skin side uncovered.

Put the frying pan back over medium heat and add the remaining oil. Place the mackerel skin side down in the pan and cook for 3–4 minutes, pressing the fillets so the skin crisps up evenly. Remove from the heat and turn the fillets over so they are flesh side down. The residual heat will cook them through in about 1 minute.

Bring the salad together on a platter with the labneh in dollops, mackerel fillets and the dressing.

VARIATIONS

+ To make this salad plant-based, use slices of tempeh instead of mackerel fillets, dusted in the spices and cooked exactly the same way.
+ Swap the rye bread for any other type of bread, or add toasted hazelnuts for a bit of crunch.

Polenta and Greens

Serves 2

3½ oz polenta (white or yellow)

2 tbsp extra-virgin olive oil, plus extra for drizzling

2 spring onions, trimmed and roughly chopped

½ oz fresh flat-leaf parsley, leaves and stalks finely chopped

¾ oz sun-dried tomatoes (dry or in oil), roughly chopped

3½ oz peas (fresh or thawed)

3½ oz cavolo nero (or spring greens or cabbage), stems removed and leaves finely chopped

2 cups vegetable stock or boiling water

2 tbsp grated Parmesan cheese (or nutritional yeast flakes) (optional)

sea salt and freshly ground black pepper

I love using polenta to add fiber to dishes, and the quick-cook whole grain takes on the flavor of herbs and spices exceptionally well. Increasing the amount of fiber in our diets may help improve our immune response by giving our microbes a boost. Toasting the polenta in a pan really brings out the flavor of this nutty grain—this is a delicious side dish! I sometimes serve it with white fish that has been baked in the oven with a bit of lemon and oil.

Heat a dry saucepan over medium heat, add the polenta and toast it for about 2 minutes.

Add the olive oil, spring onions, parsley, sun-dried tomatoes, peas, and greens, season with salt and pepper and cook, stirring, for 2 minutes. Add the vegetable stock or boiling water and simmer for 8–9 minutes until the polenta is cooked and the greens have wilted. If the mixture is too dry, simply add a splash of boiling water, cover and cook for a minute longer.

Remove from the heat and divide between bowls. Sprinkle with the Parmesan (if using), drizzle with oil and serve.

VARIATION

+ Use any greens you like, such as spinach, chopped broccoli, or savoy cabbage.

Greek-Style Giant Beans

This is an incredible hearty Greek baked bean dish that I often make in big batches for work. I love the earthy herbs and spinach (Swiss chard or spring greens also work beautifully), and the sweetness from the honey and cinnamon brings a soothing homely element to the meal. The flavors develop even more when left to mingle and eaten the next day.

Serves 4

2 tbsp olive oil

½ red onion, thinly sliced

5½ oz chard, spinach, or spring greens, finely chopped

14 oz canned butter beans, drained and rinsed (or 9 oz dried beans cooked from scratch)

14 oz canned chopped tomatoes

1 tbsp runny honey

1 small red chili, deseeded and finely chopped

1 tsp ground cinnamon

1 tsp dried oregano

½ oz fresh flat-leaf parsley, leaves and stalks finely chopped

sea salt and freshly ground black pepper

Preheat the oven to 400°F.

Heat the oil in a large ovenproof frying pan over medium heat. Add the onion with plenty of salt and pepper and cook for 2–3 minutes until softened. Toss in the greens and cook for another 3–4 minutes, then add the beans, tomatoes, honey, spices, and oregano and stir to combine. Bring to a simmer then transfer to the oven and bake for 20 minutes until the edges brown and the flavors intensify (if you don't have an ovenproof frying pan, just transfer the mixture to a baking dish).

Remove from the oven, top with the parsley, and serve.

TIPS

+ Try serving this with some simple baked or pan-fried white fish.
+ Add an anchovy fillet to the pan with the onions for extra umami and saltiness.

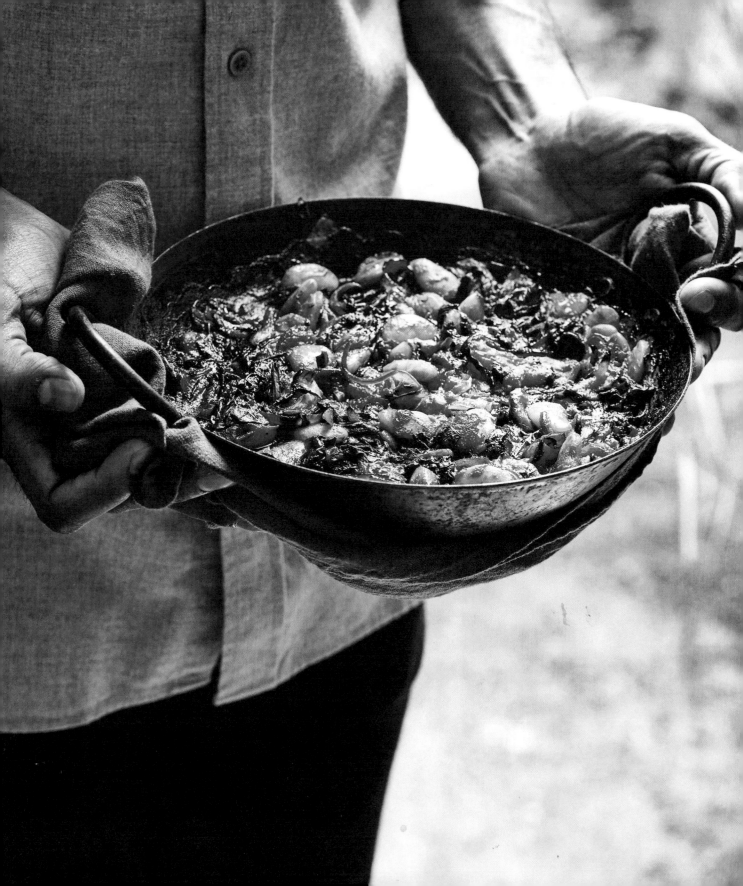

These are quick, foolproof recipes that generally take less than 30 minutes and leave your kitchen in a tidy state. Having these meals up your sleeve will prevent you from relying on convenience foods and give you more kitchen confidence. You'll be making speedy healthy meals in no time.

Rapid meals

Carrot and Zucchini Laksa

Making the paste for this delicious meal from scratch is so simple and totally worth the effort (see page 246), but you could use a ready-made Malaysian-style red curry (laksa) paste if you prefer—in fact, most southeast Asian pastes will work in this dish. Curries are a fantastic vehicle for nutrient-rich vegetables. Carrots are a rich and widely available source of beta-carotene, but you could easily use grated sweet potato or butternut squash for similar nutrient and health properties. The grated apple brings a touch of sweetness to the final dish that mellows the heat of the paste.

Serves 4 (with leftovers)

2½ cups water

1 vegetable stock cube

5½ oz Malaysian Laksa Paste (see page 246 or use 4 tbsp store-bought paste)

1¾ cups canned coconut milk

7 oz brown rice noodles

7 oz carrots, grated

10½ zucchini, grated

7 oz green beans, roughly chopped

½ red chili, finely chopped

a little chopped fresh coriander, to serve

½ red apple

1 lime, halved

Bring the water to a boil in a large saucepan and dissolve the stock cube in the water. Add the laksa paste and coconut milk and bring to a simmer.

Add the noodles and stir for 2–3 minutes, then add all the vegetables. Bring to a simmer and allow the flavors to marry for a few minutes before dividing among large bowls.

Scatter the chili over each serving along with a little chopped coriander. Grate some apple over each serving and finish with a squeeze of fresh lime juice.

VARIATIONS

+ Swap the brown rice noodles for white rice noodles or other noodles you have on hand (bearing in mind that they might take less or more time to cook).
+ Try grating other vegetables like celeriac, parsnip, or even beet for a delicious earthy twist.

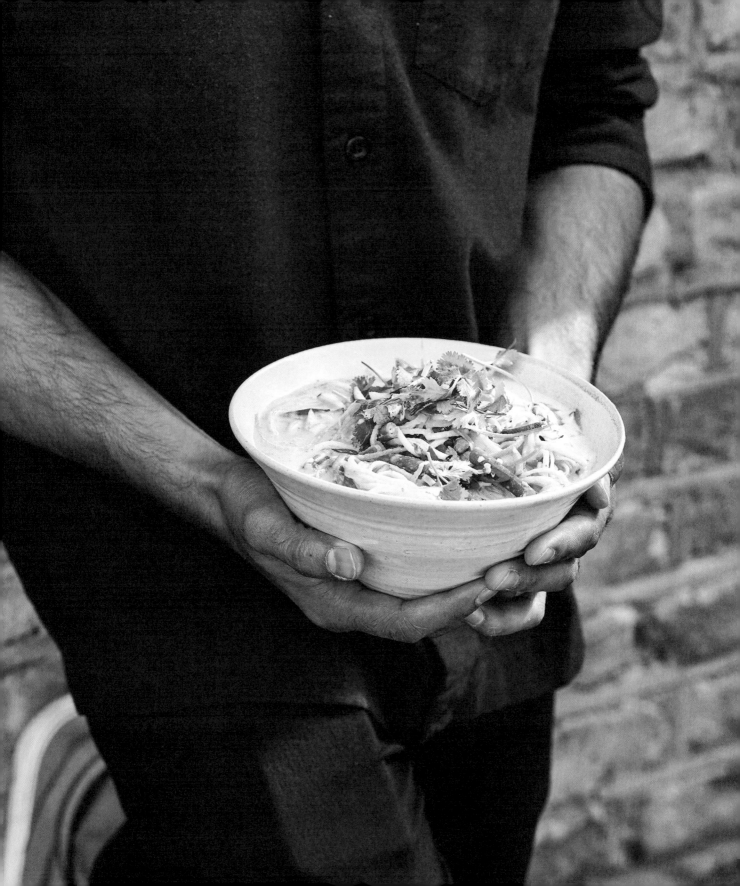

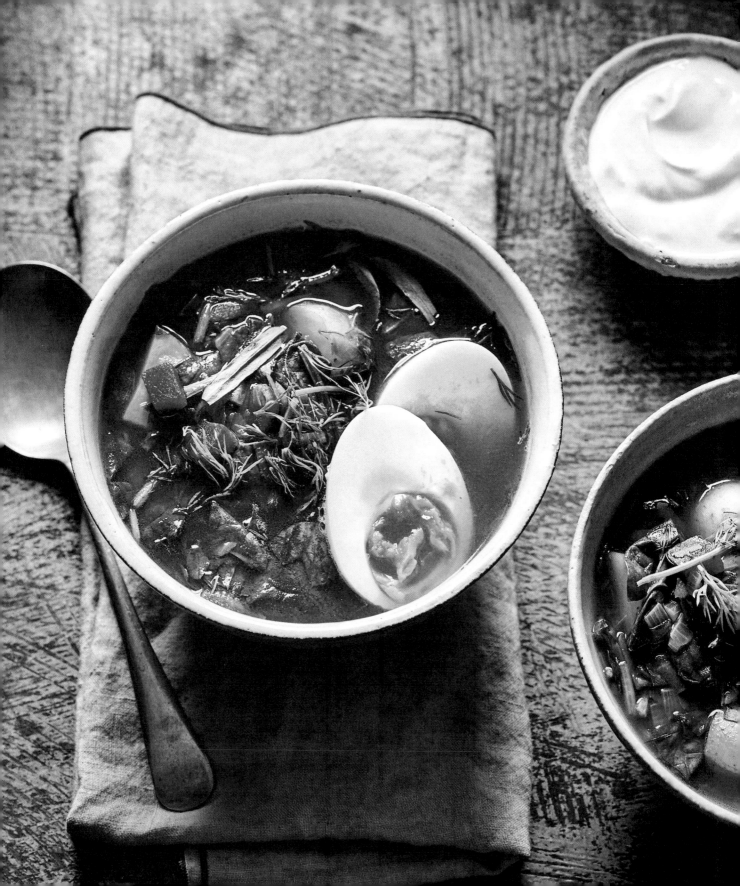

Spinach and Sorrel Borscht

Sorrel is a bit of an unusual vegetable and can be hard to get hold of, but many grocers now stock it. If you see it on the shelves, buy some! It's packed with nutrients and is particularly high in immune system–boosting micronutrients including vitamins A and C, plus it has a delightful lemon flavor that goes well with the spinach in this soup. Because of cultural integration in the US we've inherited incredibly varied culinary influences, which I love to incorporate into my food. Borscht is a typical Eastern European soup dish that I've put a vegetarian twist on, but you can make this with chicken stock, too. This is perfect food for when you need a boost or a comfort meal.

Serves 2

2 eggs (optional)
1 tsp butter
2 tbsp extra-virgin olive oil
3 garlic cloves, grated
1 shallot, finely diced
1 carrot, grated
2½ cups fresh vegetable stock (or 1 vegetable stock cube dissolved in 2½ cups boiling water)
2 bay leaves
3½ oz new potatoes, quartered
3½ oz sorrel, finely chopped
3½ oz spinach, finely chopped
3½ oz cooked beet, diced
½ oz fresh dill, finely chopped
½ oz fresh tarragon leaves, finely chopped
2 oz soured cream
½ tsp dried chili flakes
sea salt and freshly ground black pepper

If you want to serve your borscht with eggs, boil them for 7 minutes then set aside in cool water.

Melt the butter with the oil in a large saucepan over medium heat then add the garlic, shallot, and carrot and sauté for 2–3 minutes until softened. Season with salt and pepper, add the vegetable stock and bay leaves, bring to a simmer, add the potatoes and cook for 8 minutes. Stir in the chopped sorrel, spinach, and beet and simmer for a further 2 minutes. Take the pan off the heat and add the herbs, which will gently wilt in the residual heat.

Serve in bowls topped with sour cream, chili flakes, and the boiled eggs, peeled and cut in half (if using).

TIP

+ If you can't get hold of sorrel, use the same quantity of arugula or parsley, adding the juice of half a lemon to mimic sorrel's tangy flavor.

Rendang Stir-Fry

Serves 2

5½ oz brown rice noodles

2 tbsp sesame oil

½ oz gingerroot, peeled and grated

4-inch piece of lemongrass, tender base grated

7 oz tempeh (or chicken breast), cut into 2cm chunks at an angle

3½ oz savoy cabbage, thinly sliced

3½ oz Tenderstem broccoli, trimmed

3 tsp Rendang Curry Paste (see page 246) or store-bought paste

1 carrot, peeled into long strips with a vegetable peeler

¾ oz unsalted peanuts, toasted and crushed

1 spring onion, trimmed and finely chopped

sea salt

There's nothing I love more than a quick and easy stir-fry after work. It can be on the table in less than 15 minutes, requires minimal cleanup, and offers maximal nutrient value. I've used tempeh (a fermented soy bean product) in this colorful and flavorful stir-fry, but you could easily use chicken or marinated firm tofu instead. "Anti-inflammation" recipes always seem complicated and tend to include expensive ingredients: this totally bucks that trend and is one of the best meals to improve the balance of inflammation in your body.

Boil the noodles for 4 minutes (or according to the packet instructions), rinse well and leave to drain in a sieve.

Heat the sesame oil in a wok or large frying pan over medium heat. Add the grated ginger and lemongrass and sauté for 2–3 minutes, then add the tempeh and cook for 2 minutes (if using chicken make sure to cook until the juices run clear and there is no pink meat). Add the cabbage and broccoli and cook for a further 3 minutes, then add the paste and a pinch of salt and stir-fry for another 2–3 minutes. Add the noodles to the pan with the carrot strips and toss for about 1 minute before transferring to plates or bowls.

Garnish with the peanuts and spring onion.

VARIATION

+ Try this with other pastes like sambal olek or green or red Thai curry paste.

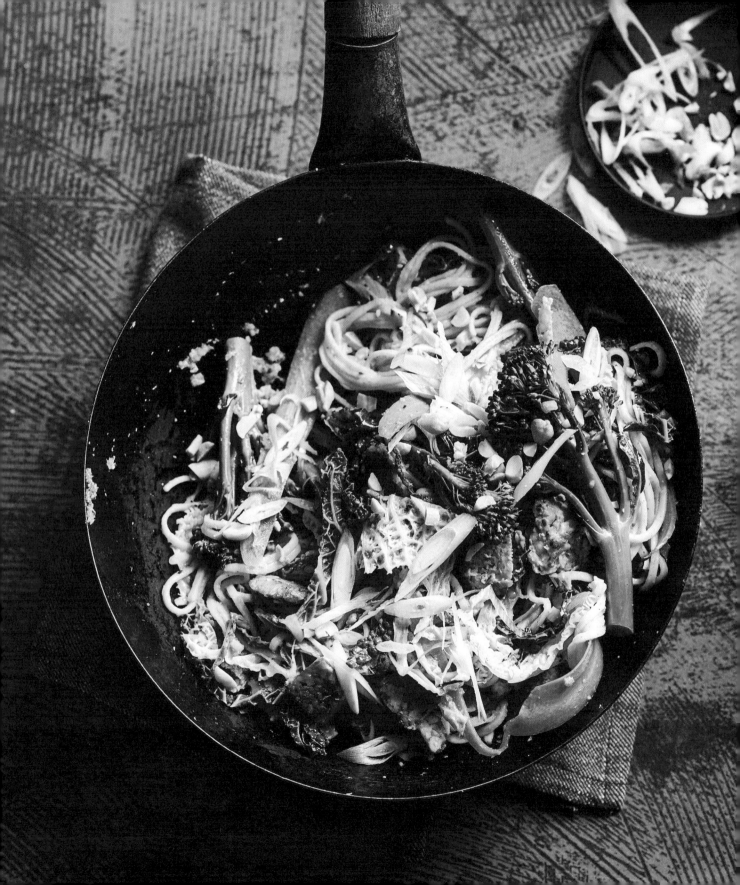

Harissa Beans and Greens

Serves 2

2 tbsp extra-virgin olive oil

7 oz Tenderstem broccoli

7 oz sugar snap peas

3 tbsp water

3 garlic cloves, finely chopped

½ oz fresh thyme, leaves stripped

14 oz canned butter beans, drained and rinsed

1 tbsp harissa paste, or more (to taste)

grated zest and juice of 1 lemon

sea salt and freshly ground black pepper

Harissa pastes contain such wonderful flavors, but you can make simple store-bought pastes taste even better with the addition of fresh garlic and herbs to heighten the flavors and nutrient density of the dish. The white beans take on spice really well, and this meal contains plenty of plant-based protein from the pea sources, too. This is an easy dish to knock together in 15 minutes or less. Experiment with different bean varieties and, of course, greens!

Heat 1 tablespoon of the oil in a large, lidded frying pan over medium heat. Add the broccoli and sugar snap peas and fry for a minute then add 4 teaspoons of the water, cover and cook for 5 minutes, tossing occasionally. When cooked, remove the broccoli and sugar snap peas from the pan and set aside.

Return the pan to the heat and add the remaining oil. Add the garlic and thyme leaves, and sauté for 30 seconds, then add the beans and the harissa paste, half the lemon juice, and the rest of the water. Stir for 2 minutes until heated through, then add the broccoli and sugar snap peas. Toss to combine. Top with lemon zest and season with salt and pepper. Add more lemon juice, if desired, to taste.

Butter Beans, Butternut Squash, and Spicy Couscous

Serves 2

7 oz butternut squash, peeled and cut into ¾-inch cubes

2 tbsp extra-virgin olive oil

2 tsp barbecue spice blend

14 oz canned butter beans, drained and rinsed

5½ oz couscous

2 oz sun-dried tomatoes (dried or in oil)

2½ oz frozen peas

¼ tsp sweet paprika

¾ cup boiling water

The issue with working in clinical medicine is that no day is the same, and it's rarely the case that you finish on time. Like the majority of people, we can also slip into the unhealthy habit of ordering a takeout and turning to comfort food more regularly than we should. This is one of those meals I made up from random bits in the fridge after coming back late from work. The beans and butternut squash are so satisfying in the spice mix, plus the couscous is incredibly easily to prepare. This is barely cooking. It's simply prepping a few things and turning the oven on, which allows you to focus on winding down after a hard day.

Preheat the oven to 400°F.

Scatter the squash on a baking tray and combine with the oil and barbecue spice blend. Bake for 15 minutes, then add the butter beans and bake for a further 10–15 minutes until the squash cubes soften and cook through.

While the beans and squash are baking, mix the couscous, tomatoes, peas, and paprika in a medium heatproof bowl and pour over the boiling water. Cover with a plate or large dish and set aside for 5 minutes. Once all the water has been absorbed, fluff up the grains with a fork.

Serve the meal in bowls with the beans and squash on top of the couscous.

TIP

+ Pre-mixed barbecue spice blends can easily be store-bought, or you can make your own: combine equal quantities of cayenne pepper, onion powder, ground cumin, crushed coriander seeds, mustard powder, and dried oregano, and add a good pinch of salt and pepper.

Creole Couscous with White Beans and Parsley

Serves 2

3 tbsp olive oil

1 red onion, cut into thin strips

3 tsp Creole Spice Blend (see page 245) or store-bought blend

1 red pepper, halved, deseeded, and cut into thin strips

3½ oz colored Swiss chard, leaves and stems chopped (stem bases removed)

7 oz couscous

1¼ cups water

1¾ cups canned cannellini beans, drained and rinsed

1½ oz fresh flat-leaf parsley, leaves and stalks finely chopped

3½ oz arugula

When I visited Tulane medical school in New Orleans to discuss how to start a culinary medicine program in the UK, I got to experience authentic Louisiana Creole cuisine. It's an incredible blend of flavors that includes Haitian, French, West African, and Spanish influences. Jambalaya and gumbo are some of the most well known dishes, but unfortunately they're far from healthy! I was determined to weave similar beautiful spices into recipes that could be enjoyed more regularly without losing that authentic Creole flavor.

Heat 1 tablespoon of the olive oil in a large saucepan over medium heat and add the onion, Creole Spice Blend and red pepper strips. Sauté for 5–6 minutes until the onions soften, then add the Swiss chard leaves and cook for a further 2–3 minutes to gently wilt them.

Put the couscous in a heatproof bowl. Bring the water to a boil and pour it over the couscous, add the remaining oil, beans, and parsley and mix thoroughly. Cover and leave for 5 minutes, then scatter the cooked couscous and white beans over the vegetables in the pan to combine the flavors.

Serve on a bed of arugula.

VARIATION

+ Try swapping the cannellini beans for different beans or legumes such as red kidney beans or black-eyed peas.

TIP

+ Use a store-bought Creole spice blend to save time.

Black Bean Goulash

Serves 4

2 tsp butter
2 tbsp extra-virgin olive oil
2 tsp caraway seeds
2 tsp sweet smoked paprika
1 tsp English mustard powder
1 tsp freshly ground black pepper
1 tsp salt
3 garlic cloves, finely chopped
5½ oz red onion, diced
1 red pepper, halved, deseeded, and diced
7 oz fennel, diced
7 oz carrots, diced
7 oz leeks, diced
2 tsp tomato puree
14 oz canned chopped tomatoes
1 cup vegetable stock
28 oz canned black beans, drained and rinsed

To serve

3½ oz probiotic yogurt (or dairy-free equivalent)
½ oz fresh flat-leaf parsley, leaves and stalks roughly chopped
4 slices of toasted rye bread

This is healthy comfort food at its best. Goulash is usually considered heavy, but this version makes a light yet satisfying meal. The flavors are incredibly warming. The paprika and caraway I've used to give the dish that authentic Hungarian flavor also contain vitamin C and phytochemicals that ease digestion. A goulash like this is a fantastic way to get fiber and a complete rainbow of vegetables into your diet. The tangy, sharp flavor of the probiotic yogurt cuts through the heat of the spices, but you could just use a hint of lemon juice instead.

Heat the butter with the oil in a large saucepan over medium heat. Add the caraway seeds, spices, and salt, along with the garlic and onion, and cook for 5 minutes, stirring occasionally, until starting to soften.

Add the pepper, fennel, carrots, and leeks and sauté for 15 minutes until softened, stirring occasionally. Add the tomato puree, canned tomatoes, vegetable stock, and black beans, bring to a simmer and cook for 10–15 minutes, or until the vegetables are soft.

Serve in large bowls topped with the yogurt, parsley, and a slice of toasted rye bread.

VARIATION

+ Try using different vegetables such as parsnips or whole new potatoes.

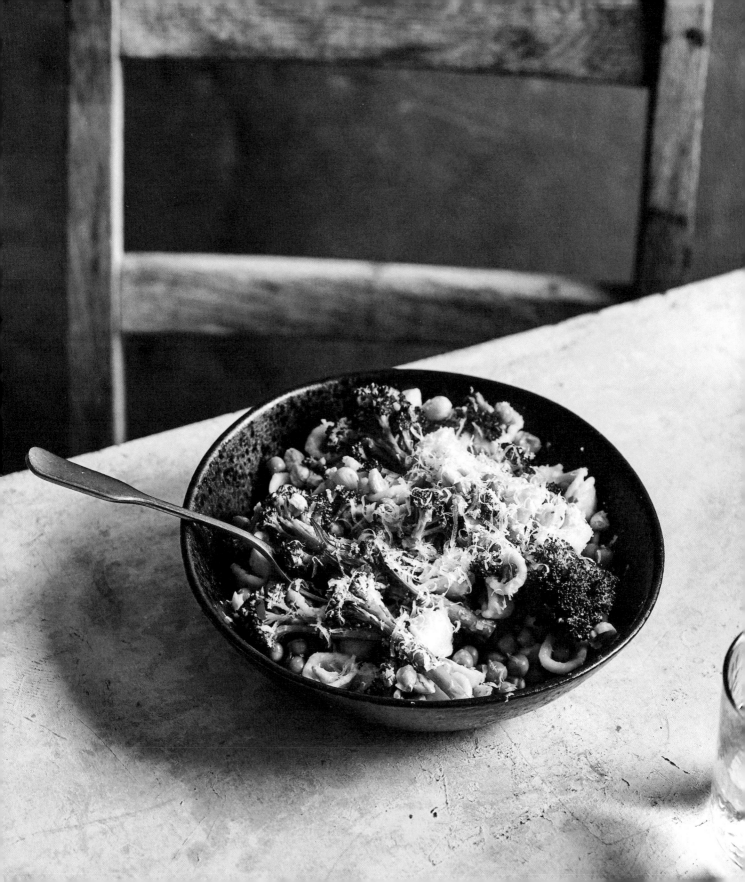

Pea Orecchiette with Purple Sprouting Broccoli and Hazelnuts

Serves 2

5½ oz whole-wheat orecchiette (or whole-wheat pasta of your choice)

3 tbsp extra-virgin olive oil

4 small garlic cloves, finely chopped

1 small red chili, deseeded and finely chopped

7 oz purple sprouting broccoli (or Tenderstem)

7 oz garden peas (fresh or frozen)

grated zest of ½ lemon

½ oz Parmesan cheese, grated (optional)

¾ oz raw hazelnuts

sea salt and freshly ground black pepper

Pasta is one of my favorite foods. Over the last few years, "carb bashing" has demonized pasta, so it's no longer thought of as a healthy option, but I believe it's about balance. Whole-wheat pastas are good higher-fiber options, but even white pasta on occasion is something to enjoy. The focus in this recipe is on delicious greens that accompany the pasta; the protein-packed peas and vibrant purple broccoli pair really well with the salty Parmesan and sharp lemon zest.

Bring a saucepan of salted water to the boil. Add the pasta and cook it for 2 minutes less than the package instructions advise.

Meanwhile, heat the olive oil in a large frying pan over medium heat, add the garlic and sauté for a minute, then add the chili, broccoli, and some salt and pepper, cover, and cook for 4–5 minutes.

Drain the pasta, reserving ¼ cup of the pasta cooking water, and add the pasta and water to the pan of broccoli, along with the peas. Cook for a further 2–3 minutes, then add the lemon zest and Parmesan (if using) and remove from the heat.

Lightly toast the hazelnuts in a separate dry frying pan over medium heat for 1–2 minutes, then roughly chop and scatter them over the pasta at the table.

TIPS

+ You can use any whole-wheat (or even gluten-free) pasta for this dish. I love using whole-wheat fusilli or penne made from red lentils.
+ To make the dish vegan, swap the Parmesan for nutritional yeast flakes, which will give the dish a similar umami taste without the dairy.

Spanish Chickpea Stew with Roasted Peppers

Serves 2 (with leftovers)

3 tbsp extra-virgin olive oil, plus extra for drizzling

4 garlic cloves, finely chopped

2 anchovy fillets in oil, finely chopped (optional)

½ small red onion, finely diced

2 tsp sweet paprika

½–1 tsp dried chili flakes (according to taste)

5½ oz roasted red peppers from a jar, finely chopped

5½ oz celery stalks, thinly sliced

14 oz canned chickpeas, drained and rinsed

7 oz plum tomatoes, chopped

¾ cup vegetable stock

sea salt and freshly ground black pepper

2 tbsp full-fat Greek yogurt (optional), to serve

½ oz basil leaves, roughly torn, to serve

I love making a stew using the beautiful flavors of Spain. The heavenly combination of paprika and roasted peppers provides gorgeous color as well as anti-inflammatory phytochemicals. The dish also contains high amounts of the antioxidant lycopene, which is released from the tomatoes with longer cooking. This simple, quick dish takes very little effort and delivers nutrition in every mouthful. Serve the stew with some sourdough, if you wish, to soak up the juices.

Heat the oil in a large saucepan over medium heat, add the garlic, anchovies (if using), and onion and sauté for 2 minutes until softened, then add the paprika, chili, red peppers, and celery. Cook for another 5 minutes before adding the chickpeas, tomatoes, and vegetable stock. Season with salt and pepper, bring to a boil, cover and simmer for 10 minutes.

Divide the stew between large bowls and serve with a dollop of yogurt, a drizzle of oil, and some torn basil leaves.

VARIATION

+ Adding 1 ounce thinly sliced chorizo to the pan with the garlic and onions is an amazing way to introduce spicy, deep, earthy flavors without using too much meat (chorizo is a processed meat, but there are good-quality chorizo producers that do not use potassium nitrate or other preservatives—I always opt for those).

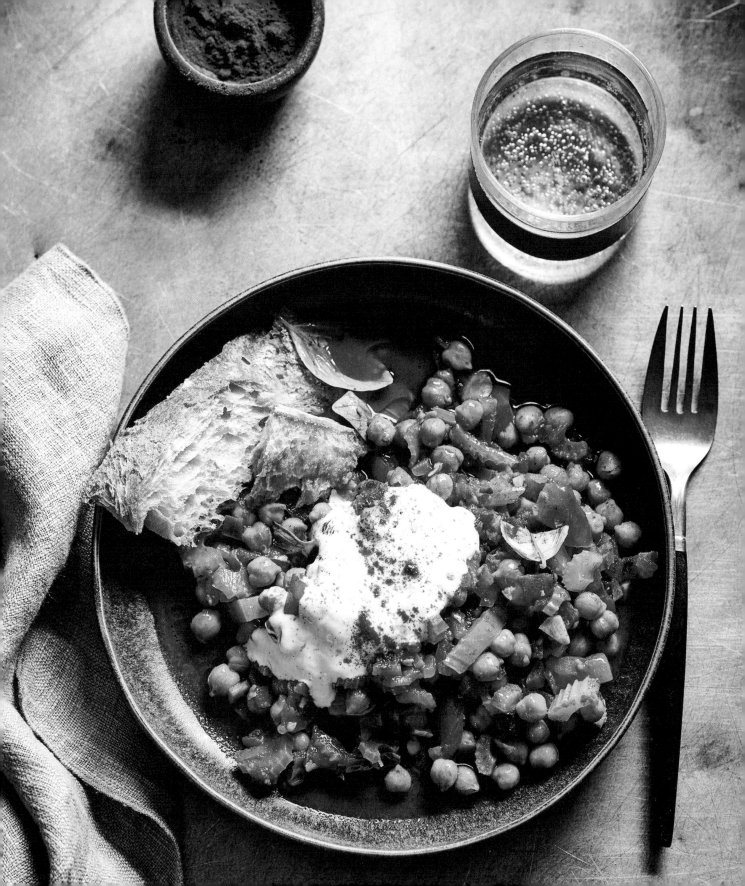

Spicy Peanut and Lime Stir-Fry

Serves 2

2 tbsp sesame oil (or coconut oil)

2-inch piece of gingerroot, peeled and grated

3½ oz red or brown rice, cooked and cooled

5½ oz bean sprouts

3½ oz spinach, roughly chopped

3½ oz carrot, peeled into thin strips with a vegetable peeler

3½ oz snow peas, roughly chopped

1½ tsp sesame seeds

juice of 1 lime (use the lime from the dressing)

For the peanut dressing

2 tbsp smooth peanut butter

½ tsp dried chili flakes

2 tbsp soy sauce (or tamari)

⅓ cup hot water

grated zest of 1 lime

One of the common misconceptions driven by the low-fat foods industry is that all fat should be avoided. A key component of a healthy lifestyle is consuming good sources of quality wholesome fats, and we can get these from nuts and seeds. This recipe makes great use of delicious smooth nut butter, which also helps absorption of micronutrients found in the greens. It's the quality dressing that transforms a rapid stir-fry into a wholesome comfort food that is as delicious as it is healthy.

Put all the dressing ingredients in a bowl and stir with a spoon.

Heat the sesame oil in a wok over medium heat, add the ginger and sauté for 2 minutes until slightly colored, then add the cooked rice and bean sprouts and stir-fry for 2–3 minutes so they take on the flavor of the oil.

Throw in the chopped spinach, carrot, and snow peas and stir-fry for another minute then remove the pan from the heat and add the dressing (hold back a little dressing to serve).

Toast the sesame seeds in a dry frying pan then scatter them over the dish before serving drizzled with the lime juice and the rest of the peanut dressing.

Sunflower Sprouts with Caraway and Porcini Mushrooms

Serves 2

2 tbsp olive oil, plus extra for drizzling

4 garlic cloves, finely chopped

2 tsp caraway seeds

2 tsp dried oregano (or 5g fresh leaves)

3½ oz porcini mushrooms (or 1 oz dried porcini mushrooms, rehydrated in warm water for 10 minutes then drained)

7 oz sunflower sprouts (see Tip)

5½ oz peas (fresh or thawed)

2 slices of whole-grain bread (or a gluten-free equivalent), cut into small squares

salt

5½ oz lamb's lettuce, arugula, or pea shoots, to serve

Dried beans and seeds are some of the cheapest ingredients in the supermarket and are packed full of protein as well as antioxidants, micronutrients, and enzymes that are wonderful for overall health. They're very easy to sprout at home, and this is a fantastic way to release their nutritional content. The aromatic caraway works well with earthy porcini mushrooms, but feel free to use any mushrooms you can get hold of.

Heat the oil in a large frying pan over medium heat, add the garlic, caraway and oregano, and sauté for 1 minute until aromatic, then add the porcini mushrooms. Cook for 2–3 minutes before tossing in the sunflower sprouts and peas and cooking for a further 2–3 minutes. The sprouts should soften but still maintain some crunch.

Prepare the croutons by tossing the bread in a dry frying pan over high heat. Once the bread begins to toast, drizzle a little oil in the pan with a pinch of salt. Allow to crisp up and remove from the heat.

Serve the mushrooms and sprouts on a bed of lamb's lettuce, arugula, or pea shoots, topped with the croutons.

TIP

+ For information on how to sprout, check out my website: www.thedoctorskitchen.com.

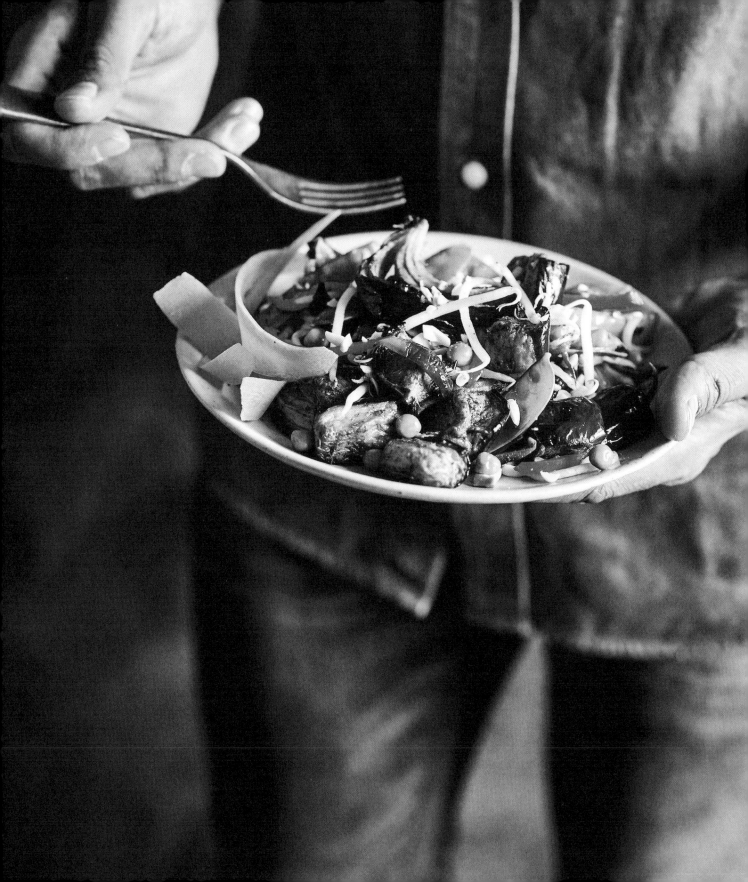

5-Spice Sticky Eggplant Bake

Serves 2 (with leftovers)

10½ oz eggplant, cut into 1¼-inch chunks

1 red onion, thinly sliced

5½ oz peas (fresh or thawed)

3½ oz snow peas, roughly sliced

1 red pepper, halved, deseeded, and thinly sliced

3½ oz beansprouts

1 small carrot, peeled into long strips with a vegetable peeler

1 oz unsalted cashews, roughly chopped

For the marinade

2 tsp Chinese 5-spice powder

¾ oz gingerroot, peeled

2 tbsp coconut oil

1 tbsp soy sauce

1 tbsp maple syrup

juice of 1 lime

I love making simple savory bakes from scratch. Here, the Chinese 5-spice marinade takes roasted vegetables to another level—this quick dish is "health" food at its most flavorful. It contains seven sources of plant nutrients, the vegetables provide a healthy dose of fiber and antioxidants, and all of the spices are anti-inflammatory. Serve this bake as it is or with steaming bowls of brown rice.

Preheat the oven to 400°F.

Put the marinade ingredients in a small blender or food processor and blitz until smooth.

Put the eggplant and red onion into a baking tray, add the marinade and rub it all over the vegetables. Bake in the oven for 25–30 minutes until golden and crispy.

Put the peas and snow peas in a saucepan over a medium heat. Pour in a splash of water (about 2 tablespoons), cover, and cook for 2–3 minutes, adding more water if needed.

Stir in the red pepper and bean sprouts, cover again and cook for a further 3 minutes.

Once the eggplant and onions are golden and tender, remove the tray from the oven. Tip the greens and bean sprouts into the oven tray and mix them with the eggplant and onion, adding 2 tablespoons of hot water to the mixture.

Divide between two bowls and garnish with the carrot strips and cashews.

Cod Bites with Lemon and Seaweed

This is a kind of posh take on fish and chips, using ingredients we definitely need more of in our diets: sea vegetables. The micronutrient value of seaweed is incredible, plus it's cheap if you buy it from fishmongers and grows on our coasts during the summer months. There are different varieties of sea vegetables available, including dulse and kelp, and many supermarkets have started stocking marine plants. There are dehydrated versions of seaweed, too. These cod bites are breaded in a spiced flaxseed mix, which gives them a crispy delicious crust.

Serves 2

14 oz cod cheeks, cut into 2-inch chunks (white fish fillets such as cod, hake, and pollock also work well if you can't find cod cheeks)

4 tbsp olive oil

5½ oz skin-on new potatoes, quartered

3½ oz seaweed

7 oz arugula

2 oz pickled red cabbage (sauerkraut)

1 lemon, cut into wedges

sea salt and freshly ground black pepper

For the spiced flaxseed mix

2 oz milled flaxseed

2 tsp sweet paprika

1 tsp ground cumin

1 tsp dried thyme

1 tsp cayenne pepper

Preheat the oven to 425°F and line a baking tray with baking parchment.

Mix the flaxseed and spices in a bowl. Coat the fish chunks with half of the oil, then thoroughly coat with the spice mix, sprinkle with a little salt and pepper and lay them out on the lined baking tray. Bake for 12–14 minutes until the chunks become golden and are cooked through.

Meanwhile, bring a pan of unsalted water to a boil, add the potatoes and parboil them for 6 minutes, then drain and set aside.

Add the rest of the oil to a frying pan over medium heat and add the new potatoes without seasoning (the seaweed is salty enough). Sauté them for a few minutes until they form a light golden brown crust. Toss the seaweed into the pan with the potatoes for 1–2 minutes, to cook it just lightly, then plate onto dishes with the arugula. Serve with the pickled red cabbage, lemon wedges and baked cod bites on top.

VARIATION

+ You can use a piece of whole-wheat bread blitzed in a food processor to make crumbs if you can't find flaxseed.

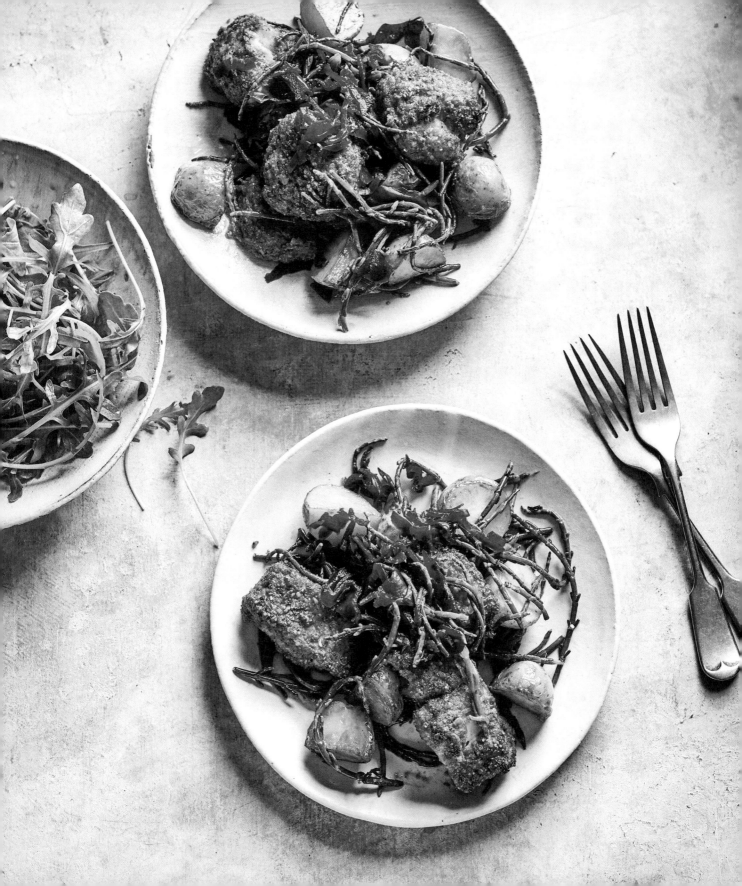

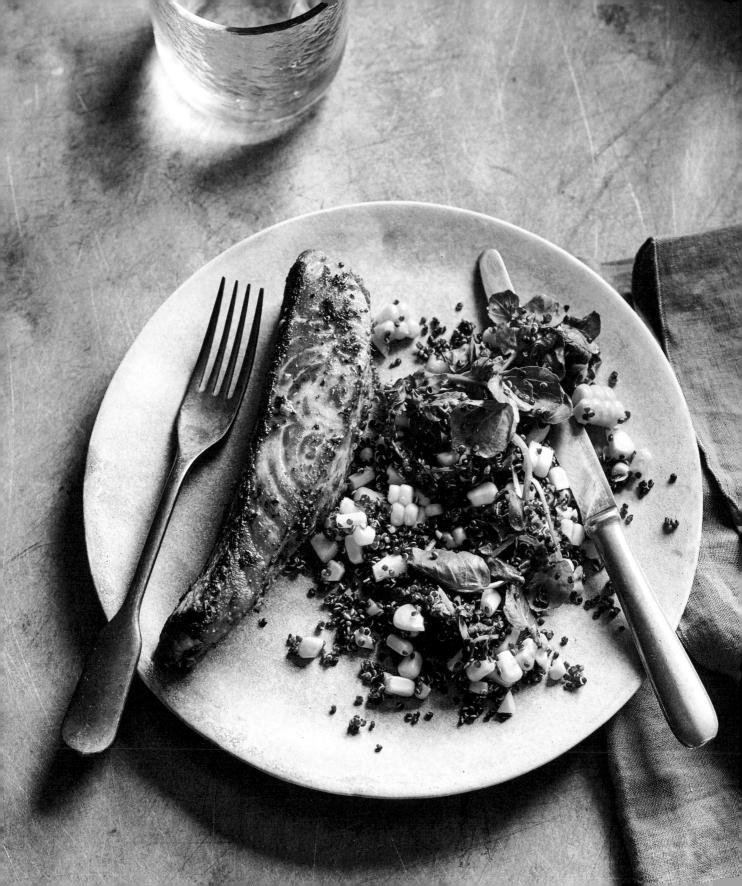

Sweet Cajun Salmon

Salmon is a fantastic oily fish that contains essential fatty acids to support brain and heart health. Combined with quinoa, watercress, and sweet corn, it's a delicious satisfying meal. The hot Cajun spices contrast well with a small amount of sweetness from brown sugar.

Serves 2

2 x 7 oz salmon fillets (preferably wild, line-caught)

7 oz quinoa

2 cups water

1 tsp sweet paprika

5½ oz sweet corn, sliced off the cob (or frozen kernels)

sea salt and freshly ground black pepper

5½ oz watercress, roughly chopped, to serve

For the Cajun marinade

2 tbsp milled flaxseed (or whole-wheat breadcrumbs will work)

2 tsp Cajun spice blend

grated zest and juice of 1 lime

1 tsp brown sugar or coconut sugar

2 tbsp coconut oil, melted

Mix the marinade ingredients together in a bowl. Add the salmon fillets and leave to marinate for 20 minutes. While the salmon is marinating, soak the quinoa in a bowl of water for the same amount of time.

Add the quinoa to a dry saucepan over medium heat and toast the grains for a few minutes. Boil the 2 cups water, then add it to the pan of quinoa along with the paprika, sweet corn, and some salt and pepper. Simmer for 15 minutes, then plate up with the watercress.

Heat a frying pan over medium-low heat and place the marinated fillets in the pan skin side down, pressing them gently for the first 30 seconds. Cook for about 6 minutes until the top side begins to turn opaque, then flip the fillets over and cook on the other side for a further 3–4 minutes until cooked through.

Place the salmon on top of the quinoa and watercress and enjoy.

Fennel Sardines with Pine Nuts

**Serves 2 as a main
or 4 as a side**

5½ oz skin-on new potatoes,
  quartered

2 tbsp extra-virgin olive oil

1 white onion, thinly sliced

1 fennel bulb, thinly shaved,
  fronds reserved and chopped

1 tsp fennel seeds

½ tsp dried chili flakes

7 oz fresh sardines (or unsalted
  canned sardines in oil, drained)

3½ oz spinach, finely chopped

grated zest and juice of 1 lemon

1 oz toasted pine nuts

sea salt and freshly ground black
  pepper

Sardines are fantastic—they are cheap and a good source of long-chain Omega-3 fatty acids that are excellent for brain health. You can use other oily fish, but this is my favorite. They're a staple in the Mediterranean and MIND diets (for more information, see page 14), which have been shown to reduce the likelihood of cognitive decline. Adding herbs and greens to the dish creates a nutrient-dense inflammation-lowering and delicious recipe.

Put the quartered new potatoes in cold salted water, bring to a boil, and simmer for 7–8 minutes until tender, then drain and set aside.

Heat the olive oil in a large frying pan over medium heat, add the onion and shaved fennel and sauté for 4–5 minutes until softened, then add the fennel seeds and chili and cook for 1 minute. Finally, move the vegetables to the edges and add the fish (skin side down) seasoned with salt and pepper to the center of the pan and cook for 3–4 minutes.

Add the spinach and potatoes to the same pan and stir through the vegetables to coat in the spices, flipping the fish to cook on the other side for 1 minute. Finish with the lemon juice and zest, pine nuts, and chopped fennel fronds.

VARIATION

+ To make a plant-based version of this dish, swap the sardines for cannellini beans.

Chili and Lime Fish Skewers with Mint and Red Cabbage Salad

Serves 2

For the fish skewers

7 oz monkfish (or skin-on salmon), cut into 1½-inch chunks

For the marinade

1 tbsp extra-virgin olive oil

½ tsp chili powder

1 tsp sweet paprika

grated zest and juice of 1 lime

2 tsp honey or maple syrup

For the salad

5½ oz shredded red cabbage

½ oz fresh mint leaves, finely chopped

juice of 4 limes and grated zest of 1

1 tsp dried chili flakes

½ oz fresh coriander, leaves and stalks finely chopped

1 tbsp apple cider vinegar

1 ripe avocado, stoned, peeled, and cut into ¾-inch chunks

2 oz cherry tomatoes, quartered

sea salt and freshly ground black pepper

To serve

1 avocado, stoned, peeled, and cut into ¾-inch chunks

2 oz cherry tomatoes

2 tbsp extra-virgin olive oil, for drizzling

For a delicious and easy summer recipe, I love making fish skewers with a simple salad on the side. The skewers can be cooked on the barbecue, but they also come out really well on the grill. It's a delicious way of getting bags of color onto your plate from one of the cheapest yet most nutrient-dense vegetables on the shelves, the humble red cabbage. Marinating it in the fridge softens the crisp cabbage and infuses it with flavor, and you can marinate it for longer if you want to make it in advance.

Mix the marinade ingredients in a bowl with some salt and pepper and stir in the fish chunks. Cover and leave to marinate for at least 20 minutes (ideally overnight in the fridge). Preheat the grill to medium-high.

Mix all the salad ingredients together in a bowl, season well with salt and pepper, and place in the fridge for at least 30 minutes. If using bamboo or wooden skewers, soak them in water for 20 minutes to prevent them burning on the grill.

Push the marinated fish chunks onto the skewers and place them on a baking tray. Grill for 20 minutes, turning the skewers halfway through the cooking time (you can also cook them on the barbecue).

Serve the skewers with the salad and an extra helping of diced avocado and cherry tomatoes drizzled in oil.

Heirloom Tomatoes, Horta, and Mackerel

Serves 4

2 liters water

1 tbsp apple cider vinegar

28 oz mixed greens (a combination of any of the following: dandelion greens, nettles, kale, collard greens, English spinach, Swiss chard), woody stems removed

5 tbsp extra-virgin olive oil

juice of 1 lemon

18 oz heirloom tomatoes (a variety of colors and sizes), sliced into ½-inch-thick rounds

1 tsp dried oregano

8 mackerel fillets, deboned (you can ask your grocery store to do this)

pinch of chili powder

sea salt and freshly ground black pepper

sourdough bread or whole-grain flatbreads, to serve

I tend to use simple recipes like this when I've had an opportunity to visit a farmers' market and grab some fresh produce that I don't want to mess around with too much—when the ingredients are of such high quality, less is more. Keeping things simple helps preserve the nutrient value of the ingredients, but also makes them taste more gratifying. Every Greek household has their version of horta, which is simply boiled greens with good-quality olive oil. This is a testament to how healthy cooking can be enjoyable and almost no work at all!

Bring the water to a boil in a large saucepan with a good pinch of salt and the apple cider vinegar. Plunge the greens into the water, cover, and simmer for 6–8 minutes until tender. Drain and place in a large bowl, drizzle with 3 tablespoons of the oil and the lemon juice and season with plenty of salt.

Dress the tomatoes in another bowl with the oregano and 1 tablespoon of the olive oil and season with salt and pepper.

Heat the remaining oil in a frying pan over high heat. Season the fish and cook the mackerel fillets in batches, placing the fish skin side down in the pan and cooking for 3–4 minutes until the skin has browned, then flipping the fillets over and cooking for a further 1–2 minutes. Set the fish aside on a plate and dust with the chili powder.

Serve the greens, fish, and tomatoes with sourdough or whole-grain flatbreads.

TIP

+ You can use any greens, but I love using nettles and dandelion. The cooking process is a great way of mellowing their natural bitterness, and these particular greens have fantastic nutrient value.

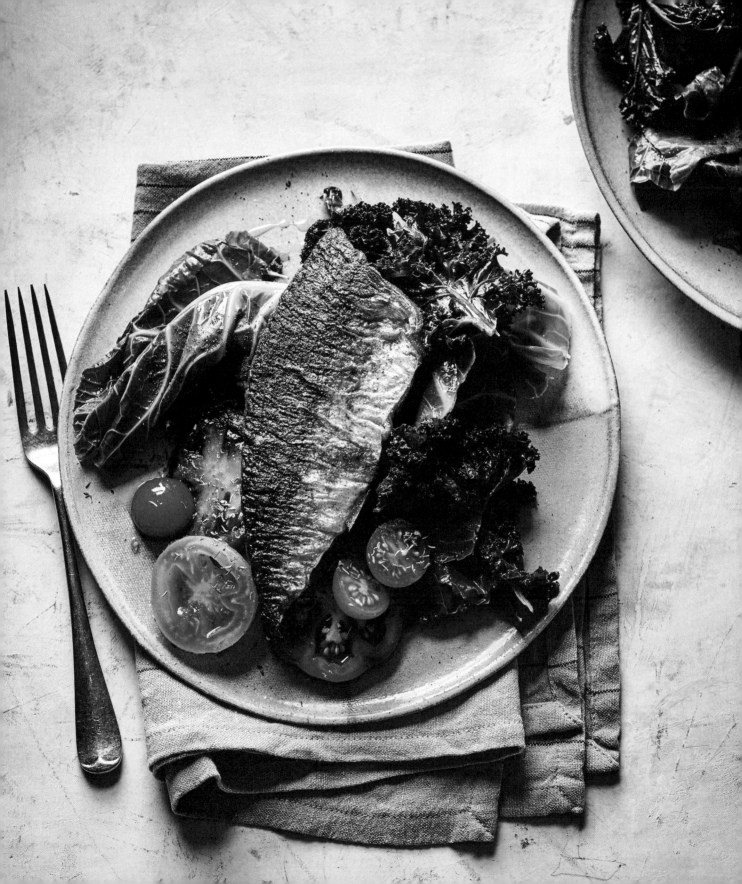

Every meal I create, I think about the science behind the ingredients I'm using and how I can incorporate flavors from around the world to make food that is visually beautiful as well as delicious. These meals are formulated with this exciting nutritional science in mind and have both culinary techniques and flavors from across the globe woven into them. There's no better way to eat to beat illness.

Main meals

Serves 4

2 tbsp olive oil

1 red onion, finely diced

3 carrots, finely diced

4 celery stalks, finely diced

10½ oz fennel bulb, finely diced

7 oz zucchini, finely diced

3½ cups water

10½ oz podded broad beans
(fresh, canned or frozen)

2 large tomatoes, cut into 1¼-inch
cubes

sea salt and freshly ground black
pepper

½ oz Parmesan cheese, grated
(or nutritional yeast flakes if you
prefer a plant-based soup), to
serve

For the red pesto

1 oz fresh basil leaves

¼ cup olive oil

3½ oz sun-dried tomatoes in oil,
drained

3½ oz roasted red peppers from
a jar

2 garlic cloves

Seasonal Soup with Red Pesto

The simplest meals are often the most satisfying. Instead of having to remember complicated cooking steps and intricate techniques, you can focus on what's important—flavor! This dish is incredibly versatile and straightforward, it delivers so much in the way of nutrition, it's exceptionally pleasing to the eye, and it's a perfect dish for the family. You can mix up the vegetables to suit your taste or depending on what's in season. You'll be eating the rainbow in no time.

Heat the olive oil in a large saucepan over medium-high heat and add all the vegetables, apart from the broad beans and tomatoes. Season with salt and pepper and sauté for 20–25 minutes, stirring occasionally, until the vegetables have slightly caramelized. Boil the water and add it to the saucepan along with the broad beans (you can add frozen ones as they are—no need to defrost first) and simmer for another 6–8 minutes until the vegetables are soft but not mushy. Add the tomatoes and cook for a further minute, then take off the heat.

Put all the red pesto ingredients into a blender or food processor and blitz until nice and smooth.

Pour the soup into bowls, swirl the pesto into the soup, and sprinkle with a dusting of Parmesan for umami flavor.

VARIATION

+ Swap the broad beans for canned cannellini beans or borlotti beans
if you like.

TIP

+ Jarred red peppers and sun-dried tomatoes tend to have added salt,
so be mindful of this when seasoning during the cooking process.

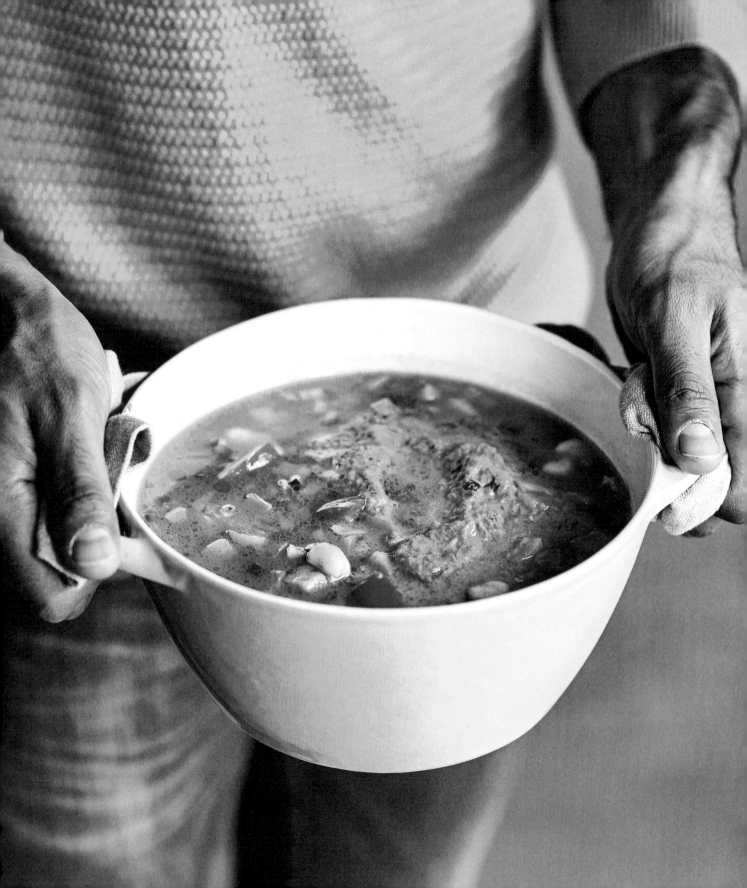

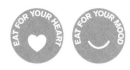

Roast Walnut and Squash Medley with Persillade

Serves 2 (with leftovers)

1 red onion, thickly sliced

10½ oz peeled winter squash, cut into 1½-inch cubes

7 oz chicory, roughly chopped (about 2 heads)

7 oz portobello mushrooms, thickly sliced

7 oz red peppers, halved, deseeded, and roughly chopped

2 oz walnuts, halved

2 oz cooked chestnuts, halved

2 tbsp olive oil

sea salt and freshly ground black pepper

For the persillade

4 tbsp extra-virgin olive oil

1 oz fresh flat-leaf parsley, leaves and stalks finely chopped

½ oz fresh tarragon leaves, finely chopped

½ oz fresh dill, finely chopped (chervil, fennel fronds, or chives will also work)

½ shallot, finely chopped

1 garlic clove, finely chopped

Think of all the activities that your microbes do for you, from releasing vitamins to creating fatty acids and hormones that impact your mood and inflammation. This dish—a one-tray vegetable bake with a little French flair—contains a variety of different sources of fiber and colors to help gut microbes bloom and shows how supporting your gut health can be easy, with no compromise on flavor. Persillade is an herby sauce, a little like a French pesto, made with ingredients we have an abundance of in the US.

Preheat the oven to 400°F.

Arrange the vegetables and nuts on a large baking tray, drizzle with the olive oil, season with salt and pepper, and toss to coat. Bake in the oven for 45 minutes, tossing everything halfway through so the ingredients cook evenly, until the vegetables are tender and the nuts are toasted.

Combine the persillade ingredients in a bowl with some salt and pepper.

Remove the roasted vegetables and nuts from the oven, transfer to serving bowls, and dollop the persillade over the top.

TIP

+ Serve this dish with a little brown rice or red quinoa to turn it into a more substantial meal.

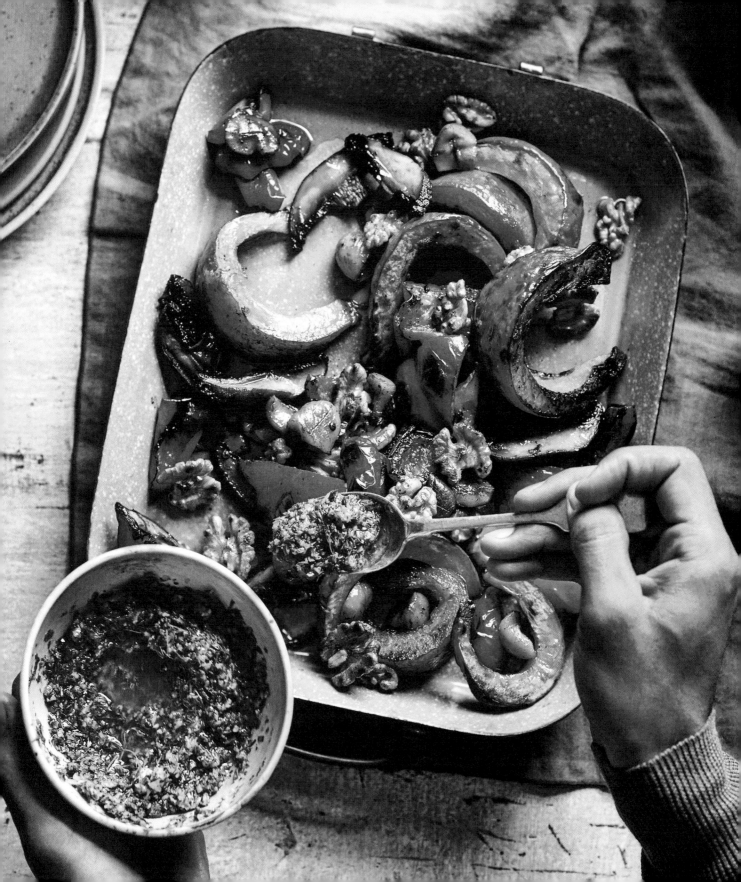

Chicken Thighs with Red Onion, Apple, and Chestnuts

Serves 2

2 tbsp olive oil

14 oz bone-in, skin-on chicken thighs (2 or 3 pieces)

½ red onion, thinly sliced

½ red apple, thinly sliced

1 oz cooked chestnuts, roughly chopped (or use unsalted walnuts or hazelnuts)

3½ oz savoy cabbage, finely chopped

½ oz fresh sage leaves, roughly chopped

For the sauce

1 tsp yeast extract (e.g., Marmite)

1 tsp tomato paste

½ vegetable stock cube

½ cup hot water

I made this sauce when trying to make a vegetarian stock that mimics the deep flavor of a red wine and beef reduction. The tanginess of yeast extract and the sweetness of the tomato give the vegetables and fruit in this dish a beautiful sticky, umami finish, and the punchy flavors help counter the bitterness of the greens. The classic pairing of apple and sage works quite well with dark greens that are chock-full of vitamin C and folate—you could also use kale, chard, or spring greens instead of savoy cabbage if you prefer.

Preheat the oven to 400°F.

Heat the oil in a large ovenproof frying pan over medium heat. Lay the chicken thighs in the pan skin side down and sauté gently for 6 minutes until the skin browns, then flip them over to cook on the other side. Drain off any excess fat, add the red onion, apple, and chestnuts and cook, stirring, for 2–3 minutes.

Combine the sauce ingredients in a bowl. Add the cabbage, sage, and sauce to the frying pan and transfer to the oven for 15 minutes, or until the chicken is cooked through (if you don't have an ovenproof frying pan, just transfer the contents of the pan to a baking tray). Remove from the oven and allow to cool a little before serving.

VARIATIONS

+ Add 3½ ounces fresh or frozen peas to the dish with the sage before putting in the oven.
+ To increase the fiber content of the meal, add 5½ ounces cooked puy lentils or butter beans to the pan before putting in the oven.

TIP

+ Deglaze the pan with a little red wine, after plating the chicken and vegetables, to make a jus to dress the chicken.

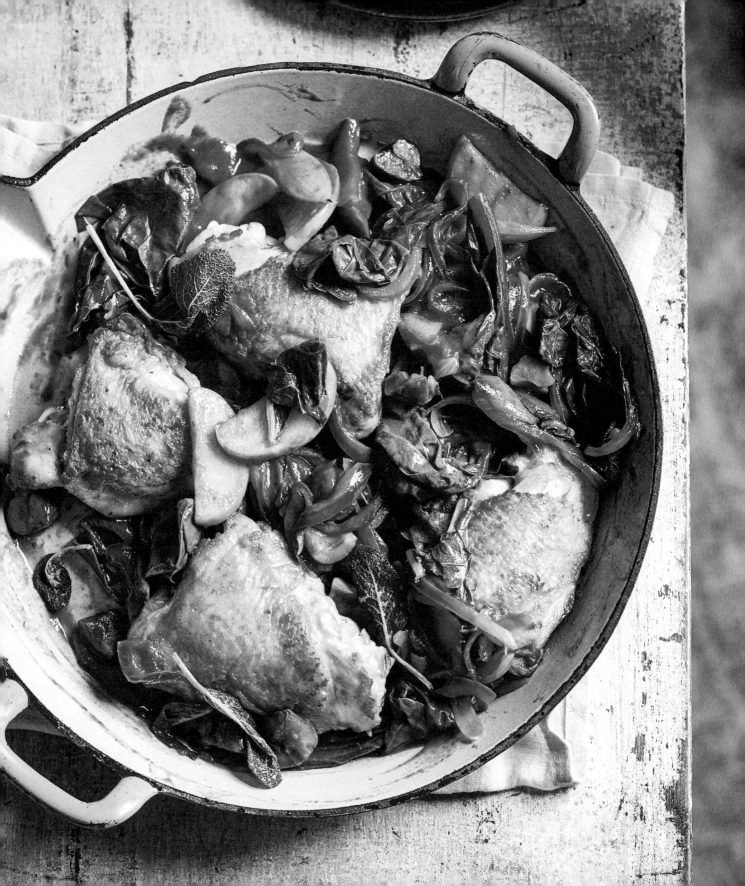

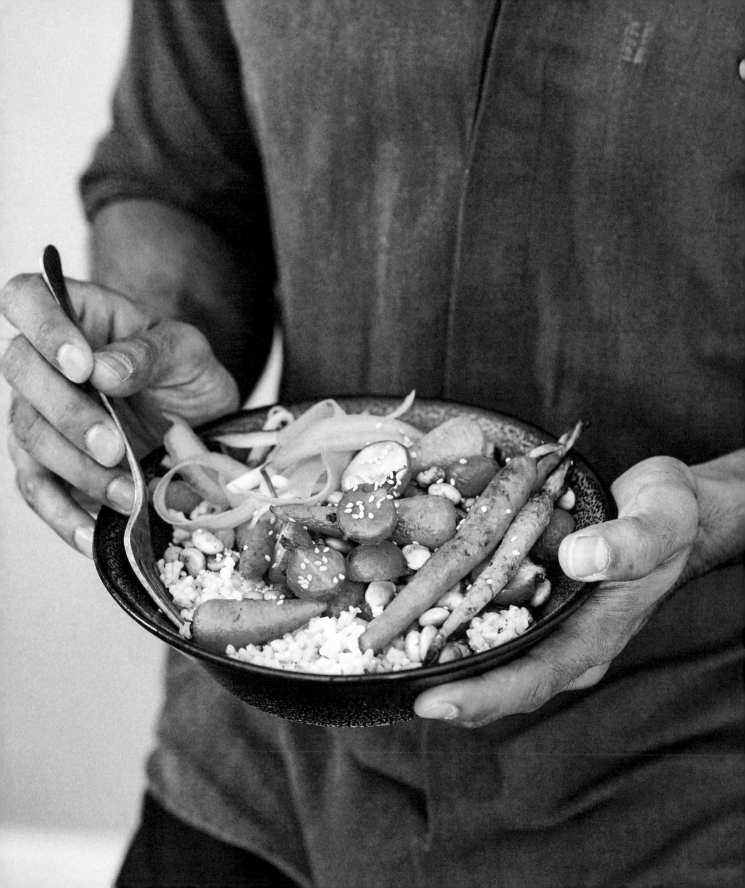

Glazed Asian Vegetable Rice Bowls

Serves 2

5½ oz brown rice, soaked in water for at least 20 minutes, then drained

7 oz baby carrots (or regular carrots quartered lengthways)

5½ oz radishes, halved

5½ oz edamame beans (fresh or thawed)

2½ oz carrots, peeled into long strips with a vegetable peeler

3½ oz cucumber, cut into long, thin strips

1 tsp toasted sesame seeds

For the miso marinade

1 tsp white miso paste

5 tsp sesame oil

grated zest and juice of 1 lemon

1 tsp maple syrup

1 tsp dried chili flakes

For the quick pickle

½ cup water

¼ cup rice vinegar

5 tsp sweet rice wine

2 garlic cloves, crushed

½ oz roughly chopped gingerroot

I love the umami flavors in this comforting dish, and it's really worth making your own quick pickle. You can experiment with different flavors in the liquids (try cloves, black peppercorns, fennel, or coriander seeds), adjusting the sharp tastes to balance the sweetness of the glazed carrots. Edamame beans are a fantastic protein and fiber source, though you can use frozen or freshly podded broad beans if you prefer.

Preheat the oven to 425°F.

Put the rice in a saucepan of boiling water and cook for 20–25 minutes.

Meanwhile, combine the marinade ingredients in a medium bowl. Add the baby carrots, radishes, and edamame beans to the bowl and toss well. Spread onto a baking tray and bake for 20–25 minutes until golden and cooked, tossing once halfway through.

Make the quick pickle while the rice and marinated vegetables are cooking. Bring the water to a boil in a small saucepan, add the vinegar, sweet rice wine, garlic and ginger, and bring back to a boil, then reduce the heat and simmer for 5 minutes. Put the strips of carrot and cucumber in a heatproof bowl, pour the pickle liquor over them, and allow to cool.

Divide the baked vegetables and the miso marinade sauce between two bowls and add the toasted sesame seeds, pickled vegetables and a little of the pickling liquid. Serve with the drained rice.

Crispy Mushroom Bowl

Serves 2

3 tbsp milled flaxseed (or whole-grain breadcrumbs)

3 tsp Cajun spice blend

10½ oz oyster mushrooms

4 tbsp olive oil

7 oz broad beans, podded

14 oz canned chickpeas, drained and rinsed

2 tsp dried oregano

7 oz tomatoes, roughly diced

grated zest and juice of 1 lemon

sea salt and freshly ground black pepper

For the tapenade

2 oz pitted kalamata olives

1 tbsp capers

1 tbsp olive oil

1 tsp freshly ground black pepper

½ oz sun-dried tomatoes in oil

There's nothing more satisfying then tucking into a big bowl of delicious food that you know is going to nourish your body and satisfy your taste buds. Bowl food is my favorite kind of meal to prepare, and all the different elements in this dish bring a unique taste and nutritional quality to the table: the sharp olive tapenade is sweetened with sun-dried tomatoes and pairs beautifully with the fiber-rich beans; the oyster mushrooms contribute another source of protein and B vitamins and crisp up beautifully in the oven with the flaxseed; and the Cajun spice brings a welcome heat to the dish.

Preheat the oven to 425°F.

Mix the flaxseed in a bowl with the Cajun spice blend and season the mixture with salt and pepper.

Coat the mushrooms with 2 tablespoons of the olive oil, then dunk them into the spiced flaxseed mixture to coat. Lay them on a baking tray and bake in the oven for 20–25 minutes until browned and crispy.

Meanwhile, put the ingredients for the tapenade in a food processor and blitz until coarsely ground.

Cook the podded broad beans in a saucepan of boiling water for 8–9 minutes.

Drain the broad beans, return them to the pan, then add the remaining olive oil, along with the canned chickpeas, oregano, and some salt and pepper. Stir gently over a medium heat for a few minutes to warm everything through.

Divide the broad beans and chickpeas between two bowls and add the tomatoes, lemon juice and zest, and tapenade. Place the crispy mushrooms on top and enjoy.

VARIATION

+ Try swapping the oyster mushrooms for other large, fleshy mushrooms such as shiitake, wood ear, or even girolles.

Herby Walnut and Cashew Roast

Serves 4

¾ oz dried wild mushrooms, rehydrated for 10 minutes in warm water and drained (reserve the soaking water) (optional)

2 oz raw walnuts

2 oz raw cashews

3 oz oats

3 oz milled flaxseed

4 tsp herbes de Provence

1 vegetable stock cube

sea salt and freshly ground black pepper

As far as roasts go, this is perhaps the quickest to prepare. I usually throw this together and put it straight into the oven on a tray surrounded by whatever root vegetables I have. It's a nice way to put a twist on typically meat-heavy Sundays, without sacrificing the flavor or enjoyment of a traditional roast. Nut roasts are a great way to increase your intake of quality fats and seeds, plus you can enjoy the leftovers as lunchbox fillers or cubed and used as croutons to top steamed greens and salads.

Preheat the oven to 400°F.

Rinse and roughly chop the rehydrated mushrooms (if using). Pass the mushroom soaking water through a fine-mesh sieve into a measuring jug.

Put the walnuts, cashews, oats, flaxseed, and herbs in a food processor, season with salt and pepper and blitz to form a rough mixture.

Add boiling water to the measuring jug with the mushroom water to make up 1 cup and dissolve the stock cube in it. Add this stock to the nut and oat mixture.

Fold in the mushrooms (if using). Add more water if the texture seems too dry and crumbly, then transfer the nut roast mixture to a non-stick 30-ounce loaf pan. Allow the mixture to sit for 5 minutes, then bake in the oven for 45 minutes until brown and set.

Remove from the oven, let the roast cool for a few minutes, then remove it from the pan and serve.

VARIATION

+ Try using different spice blends such as simple dried oregano and fennel seeds or even a Cajun spice blend.

TIPS

+ If the texture of the roast is too wet before baking, add 2 ounces whole-grain breadcrumbs to the mixture.
+ Try serving this with simple steamed greens or even the Seasonal Soup with Red Pesto on page 186.

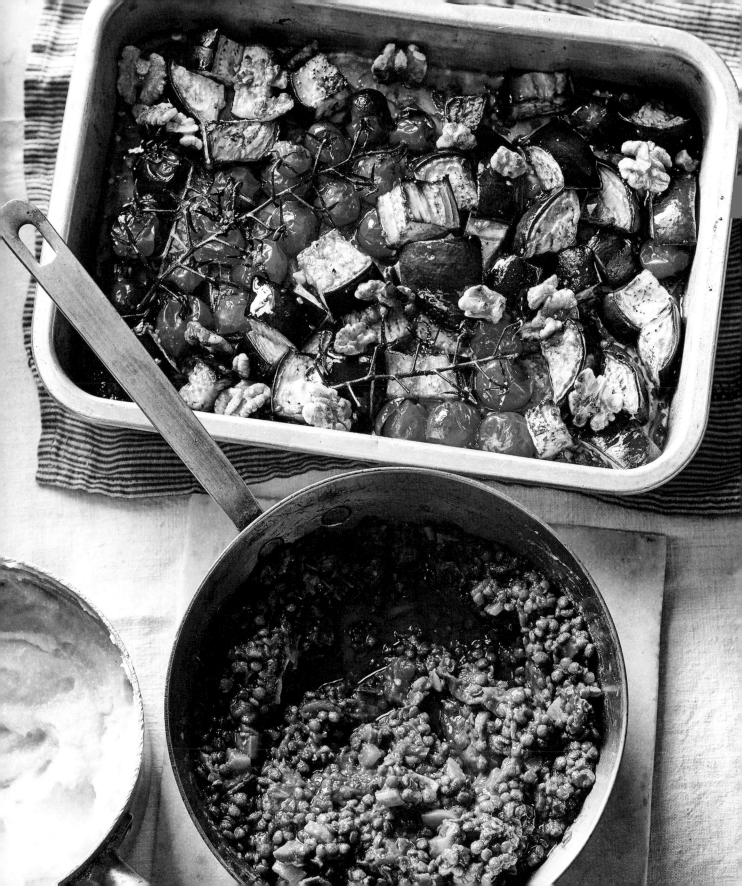

Eggplant and Walnut Ragu

Serves 6

7 oz cherry tomatoes

14 oz eggplants (about 2), cut into 1¼-inch chunks

2 oz walnuts, roughly chopped

2 tbsp olive oil

3½ oz celery, finely chopped

1 carrot, finely chopped

1 shallot, finely chopped

½ oz rosemary needles, finely chopped

2 anchovy fillets from a can, chopped (optional)

5½ oz puy lentils, soaked in water for at least 20 minutes, then drained

½ oz dried porcini mushrooms, rehydrated in warm water for 10 minutes, drained, and rinsed

14 oz canned chopped tomatoes

1¾ cups boiling water

5–6 sun-dried tomatoes, sliced

½ oz fresh flat-leaf parsley, finely chopped

½ oz Parmesan cheese, finely grated

sea salt and freshly ground black pepper

For the marinade

2 tbsp olive oil

4 tsp balsamic vinegar

6 garlic cloves, roughly chopped

1 tsp dried chili flakes

Italian food is one of my go-to cuisines when I'm making a meal for more than four people. The simplicity of ingredients and cooking methods makes it much less stressful in the kitchen, so you can focus on enjoying the company of your guests. Here, I've drastically reduced the amount of time it takes to make a traditional ragu and added nutrient-dense vegetables at every step. The nuts provide Omega-3 fats, plus lentils give the dish a good amount of fiber. In combination, these ingredients have a positive impact on your gut microbes, lower inflammation, and taste delicious. I usually serve this with a simple green salad as it's quite satisfying.

Preheat the oven to 425°F.

Mix the marinade ingredients in a bowl and season with salt and pepper.

Scatter the cherry tomatoes, eggplant chunks, and walnuts in an oven dish and pour over the marinade. Mix everything together well and bake in the oven for 30–35 minutes until the eggplant and tomatoes have softened and the walnuts have browned, tossing the mixture halfway through so it cooks evenly.

Meanwhile, heat the olive oil in a large saucepan over a medium heat, add the celery, carrot, shallot, and rosemary, season with salt and pepper, and sauté gently for 5 minutes until softened. Add the anchovy fillets (if using), lentils, and mushrooms and cook for a further 2 minutes to allow the flavors to infuse. Add the canned tomatoes, boiling water, and sun-dried tomatoes, bring to a simmer, and cook for 15 minutes until the liquid has reduced to a thicker sauce consistency. Add the roast eggplant, cherry tomatoes, and walnuts and simmer for 5 minutes until the puy lentils have cooked but still have a slight bite to them.

Sprinkle with the parsley and Parmesan and serve.

TIP

+ You could also use any pre-cooked lentils you like for added protein and fiber, or you can leave them out if you prefer a less substantial meal.

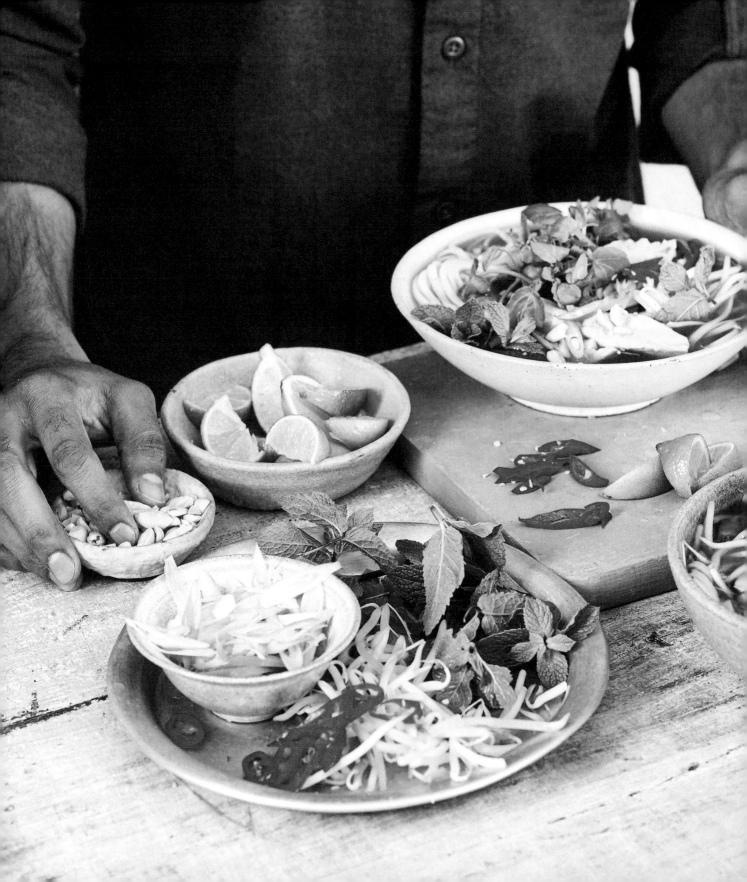

Aromatic Vietnamese Pho

Serves 2

For the broth

4 garlic cloves, bruised

1 red chili, thinly sliced

¾ oz piece of gingerroot, peeled and roughly chopped

1 stick of lemongrass, bruised

½ white onion

1 star anise

2 tsp fish sauce (optional)

1 vegetable stock cube

3 cups water

For the poached chicken and noodles

10½ oz skinless chicken breasts

½ oz piece of gingerroot, sliced

pared zest of ½ lime

3 oz rice noodles

sea salt and freshly ground black pepper

To serve

¾ oz mint leaves

2 oz bean sprouts

2 oz watercress

1 red chili, sliced

½ lime, cut into wedges

½ oz peanuts, crushed

1 spring onion, trimmed and thinly sliced

This is the most incredibly flavored dish in the book. It takes just minutes to prepare, and the number of senses it will hit makes the slightly longer ingredients list worthwhile. When I sip the clear broth, it instantly takes me back to my first pho (pronounced "fur"), which I had when I was traveling in Vietnam. The aromatic spices have incredible antioxidant value, and I like to prepare this meal for myself or others as a "pick-me-up." I've added watercress for its high nutrient value.

Put all the aromatics for the broth in a large saucepan with the fish sauce (if using) and vegetable stock cube. Boil the water and add it to the pan. Simmer over a medium heat for at least 15 minutes.

Put the chicken breasts in a separate small saucepan, cover with cold water and add the sliced ginger, a little salt and pepper, and the pared lime zest. Bring to a boil, then reduce the heat and simmer for 10–12 minutes until the chicken is cooked through—there should be no pink juices when you slice through it. Remove the chicken from the poaching water, set it aside, then add the rice noodles to the water and simmer for 3 minutes. Drain the noodles, picking out the aromatics (the ginger and lime zest), and slice the chicken.

Build your pho bowls with the cooked noodles, mint leaves, bean sprouts, watercress, and chicken slices. Pass the broth through a sieve into the bowls and garnish with sliced red chili, lime wedges, peanuts, and spring onion.

VARIATION

+ For a plant-based pho, replace the chicken with cubes or slices of firm organic tofu (there's no need to poach it).

Okra and Lentil Curry with Buckwheat Uttapam

Serves 4

For the coconut and mint chutney
2 oz desiccated coconut
2 tbsp water
juice of ½ lime
½ oz fresh coriander
½ oz fresh mint leaves
¼ oz peeled gingerroot, grated
1 green chili (optional)
sea salt and freshly ground black
  pepper

**For the buckwheat uttapam
(makes about 6)**
3 oz buckwheat flour
¾ cup almond milk
pinch of salt
1 tsp bicarbonate of soda
2 tsp garam masala
¾ oz spring onions, trimmed and
  finely chopped
3 tsp coconut oil

For the okra and lentil curry
¾ cup water
7 oz yellow lentils, soaked in water
  for at least 20 minutes, then
  drained
14 oz canned chopped tomatoes
1 tsp ground turmeric
1 tbsp tamarind paste
2 tbsp coconut cream
3½ oz spinach, finely chopped
1 tsp coconut oil
1 tsp black mustard seeds
1 red onion, thinly sliced
8 curry leaves (optional)
2 tsp garam masala
5½ oz okra, cut into ¾-inch-thick
  discs
sea salt and freshly ground black
  pepper

I find using delicious curry spices is a fantastic way of reducing inflammation and introducing antioxidants. I've included a recipe for my buckwheat version of uttapam (masala) pancakes, but the curry works equally well served with simple brown rice.

Put all the chutney ingredients into a small food processor or blender and blitz, adding the green chili if you like it hot. Season to taste with salt and pepper and set the chutney to one side.

Bring the water for the curry to a boil in a saucepan over medium heat. Add the lentils, reduce the heat and simmer for 12–14 minutes until the lentils are soft, then add the tomatoes, turmeric, tamarind paste, coconut cream, and some salt and pepper and simmer for a further 10 minutes. Remove from the heat and fold in the spinach.

While the curry is cooking, make the uttapam. Whisk together all the ingredients in a bowl or jug, except the spring onions and coconut oil, to form a batter that gently drops off the spoon, adding more flour or milk as needed.

Melt half a teaspoon of the coconut oil in a frying pan over medium heat. Add 2 teaspoons of mixture per uttapam (cook them one at a time) and fry for 2–3 minutes, scattering some of the chopped spring onions on the uncooked side, then flip the uttapam over and cook for a further 2 minutes until cooked through and the onions are browned. Set the uttapam aside and repeat with the remaining batter to make a stack of uttapam.

Heat the coconut oil in a frying pan over a medium heat. Add the mustard seeds, onion, curry leaves (if using), and garam masala and sauté for 3–4 minutes, then add the okra and cook for a further 4 minutes. Transfer the okra mixture to the lentils and gently stir through. Serve the curry with the uttapam, topped with the coconut and mint chutney.

VARIATION
+ Swap the okra for diced eggplant, zucchini, or even sliced French beans.

TIP
+ If you can't find tamarind paste, a teaspoon of maple syrup and some lemon juice will help bring a sweet tangy flavor to the curry.

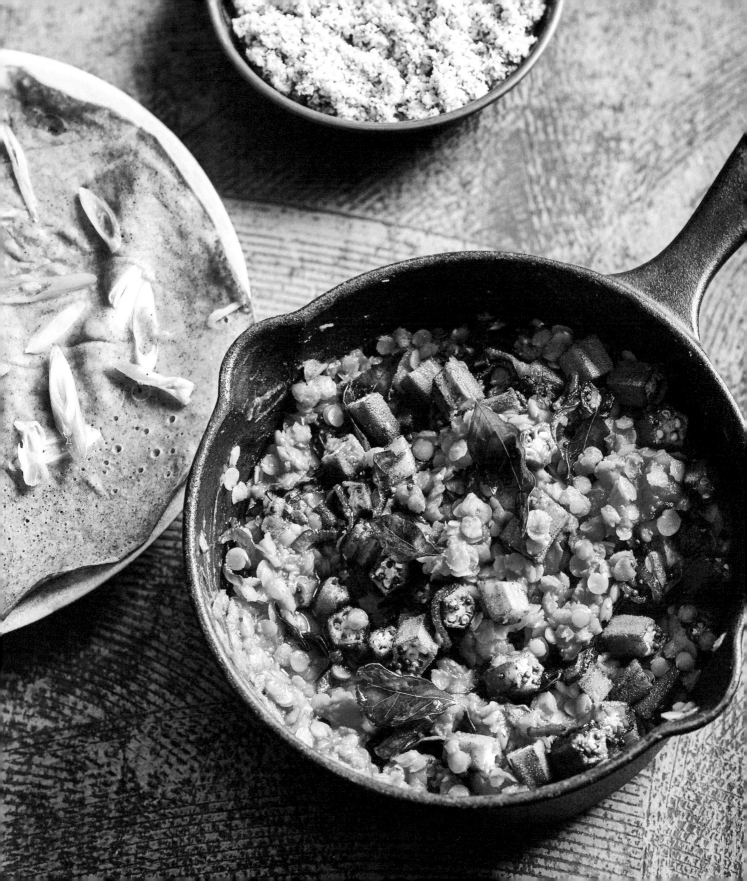

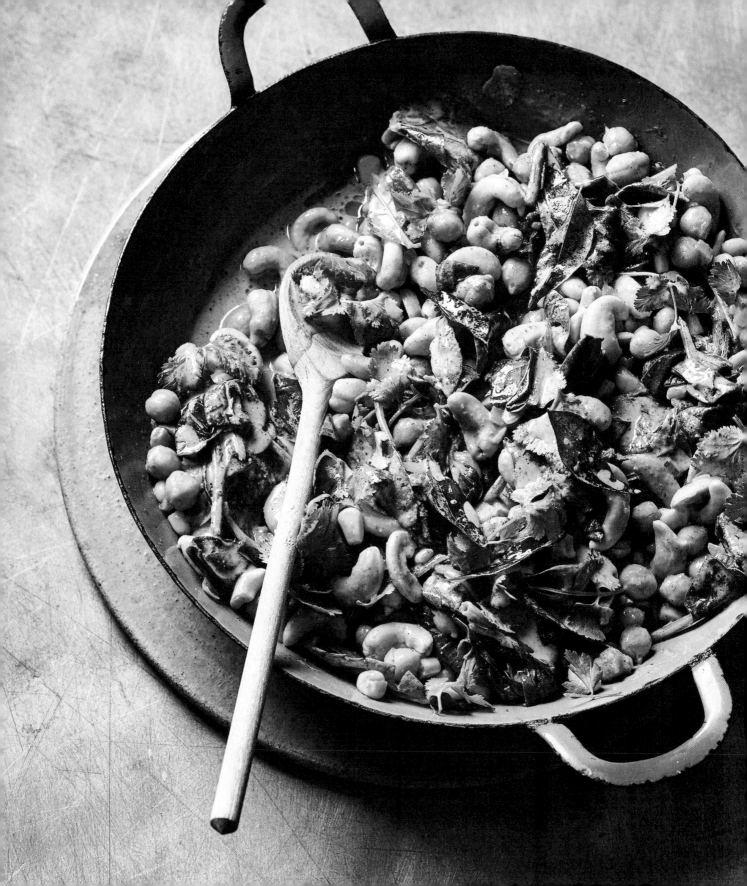

Sri Lankan Cashew Curry

I was lucky enough to travel to the beautiful and exotic country of Sri Lanka for the first time in 2018, but I'd fallen in love with the food long before, when my good friend introduced me to the cuisine while at medical school. One of the first dishes I tried was this gorgeous cashew curry. Rich in flavor, this bowl of goodness pairs beautifully with simple brown rice but also tastes fantastic on its own. Cashews are a great source of resistant starch that releases sugar into the bloodstream much more slowly than potatoes or other starchy foods, and helps boost our community of gut microbes.

Serves 4

2 tbsp coconut oil

½ oz gingerroot, peeled and grated

5 garlic cloves, grated or finely chopped

1 bay leaf

1 shallot, finely diced

8–10 curry leaves (optional)

2-inch piece of lemongrass (tender base only), thinly sliced (optional)

3 tsp curry powder (Sri Lankan or regular)

9 oz unsalted cashews, soaked in water for 20 minutes, then drained

14 oz canned coconut milk

½ cup hot water

14 oz canned chickpeas, drained and rinsed

3½ oz sweet corn kernels (frozen, fresh or canned)

2 oz baby spinach

½ oz fresh coriander, finely chopped

sea salt and freshly ground black pepper

Melt the coconut oil in a large saucepan over medium heat, then add the ginger, garlic, bay leaf, shallot, curry leaves, and lemongrass (if using), and sauté for 2–3 minutes until softened and lightly colored.

Add the curry powder and drained cashews, along with a pinch each of salt and pepper, and cook, stirring, for 2–3 minutes. Add the coconut milk, hot water, and chickpeas, bring to a simmer, cover, and cook for 20 minutes.

Add the sweet corn and spinach, re-cover, and cook for a further 2–3 minutes to gently cook the greens. Remove from the heat, stir in the coriander, and serve.

VARIATIONS
+ Try peas instead of sweet corn.
+ Green radish leaves, chard, or other leafy greens work well instead of spinach.

Jambalaya

This well spiced and incredibly flavorful dish is one of my favorite one-pan recipes. I like to describe it as Louisiana's take on a paella. It is packed with vegetables and completely plant-based but still has the authentic Creole flavor. Although it's great as it is, I sometimes serve it with simple grilled prawns, for extra flair, and a side of collard greens.

Serves 4

3 tbsp extra-virgin olive oil, plus extra for drizzling

2 red onions, thinly sliced

4 garlic cloves, finely chopped

3 tsp Creole Spice Blend (see page 245) or Cajun spice mix

½ oz fresh thyme leaves

1 bay leaf

3 celery stalks, finely chopped

5½ oz leeks, trimmed and finely chopped

1 yellow pepper, halved, deseeded, and cut into thin strips

3½ oz puy lentils, soaked in water for at least 20 minutes, then drained

7 oz red Camargue (or whole-grain) rice, soaked in water for at least 20 minutes, then drained

14 oz canned chopped tomatoes

1¼ cup vegetable stock (or 1 vegetable stock cube dissolved in 1¼ cup hot water)

¾ cup water

7 oz collard greens, roughly chopped (or use kale, cavolo nero, or spring greens)

sea salt and freshly ground black pepper

¾ oz fresh parsley, finely chopped, to serve

Heat the oil in a large frying pan over medium heat, add the onions and garlic, and sauté for 2–3 minutes. Add the spice mix, thyme, bay leaf, celery, leeks, and yellow pepper, stir, and cook for a further 3 minutes.

Add the lentils and rice to the pan with a good amount of salt and pepper. Stir to coat them in the spices, and cook for about 3 minutes, then add the canned tomatoes and vegetable stock. Cover and simmer for 22–25 minutes until the water has been absorbed and the ingredients are cooked.

Meanwhile, bring the water to a boil in a small saucepan, add the collard greens, cover, and cook for 6 minutes until the leaves wilt (most of the water will evaporate). Drain and drizzle with olive oil.

Garnish the jambalaya with parsley, and serve with the cooked greens.

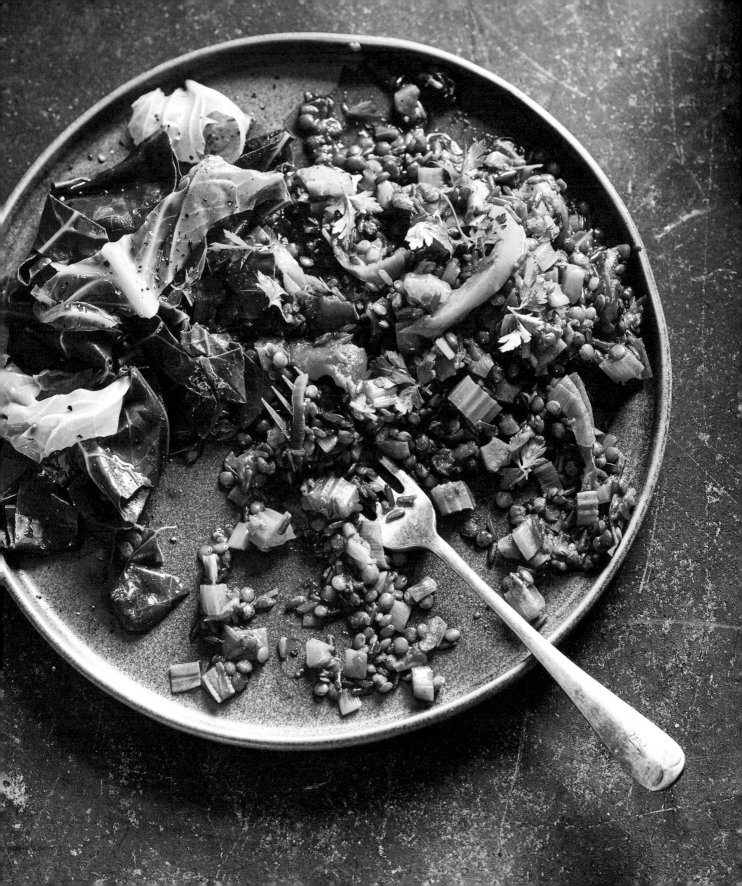

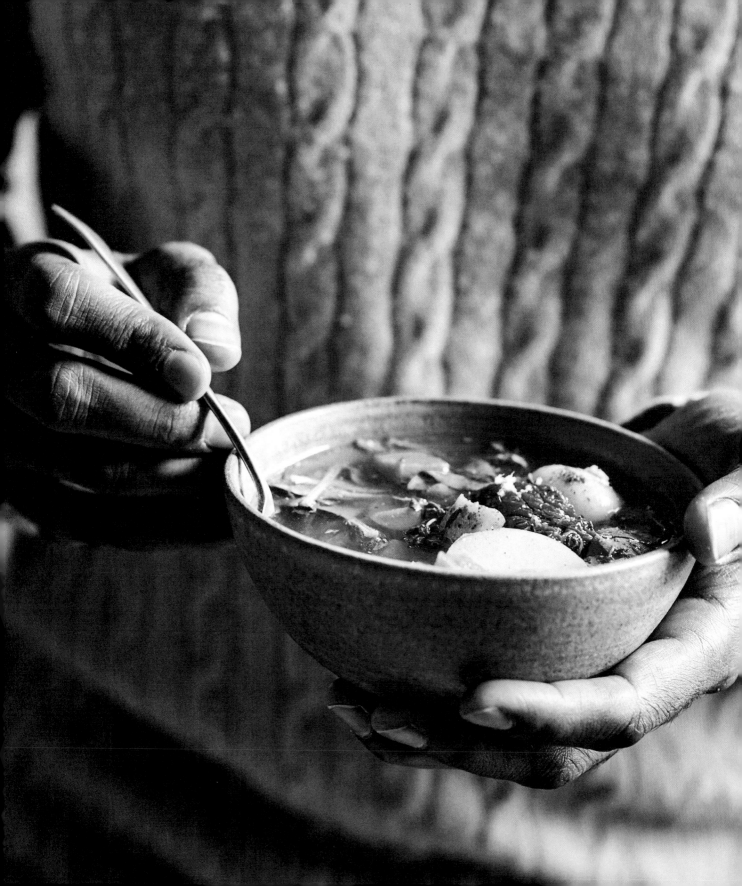

Thyme and Ginger Comfort Soup

Serves 4

2 tbsp coconut oil

6 garlic cloves, peeled

4-inch piece of gingerroot, peeled and grated, plus extra to serve

2 tsp ras el hanout spice blend (see page 245) or store-bought blend, plus extra to serve

7 oz new potatoes, scrubbed

7 oz carrots, scrubbed and roughly chopped

3½ oz dry sun-dried tomatoes (not in oil)

1 oz thyme stalks, tied together with string, plus extra leaves to serve

1 bay leaf

5 cups boiling water

3½ oz spinach, roughly chopped

I always recommend broths and soups for patients and colleagues during a viral illness such as the flu. Soups are a great way to introduce micronutrients to support your body's defenses when you're not feeling strong enough to make a complicated meal or you lack appetite. My inclination is always to make a turmeric and chili "medicinal broth" like the one in my first book, but it's not always to everyone's taste. This is a more lightly spiced version, with thyme and ginger as the central antiviral ingredients. You'll love the mellow flavors in this, and it's sure to comfort when you're feeling poorly.

Melt the coconut oil in a large saucepan over medium heat. Add the garlic and ginger, and sauté for 2 minutes until lightly browned, then add the spice blend, potatoes, carrots, sun-dried tomatoes, bunch of thyme, and bay leaf, stirring for a few minutes to marry the flavors in the oil.

Pour in 4¼ cups of the boiling water, cover, and simmer for 20 minutes until the potatoes and carrots are soft. Take off the heat, remove the thyme bunch and bay leaf, and add the spinach and the remaining ¾ cup water. Cover and cook for a further 2 minutes to wilt the greens.

Serve the soup as a consommé, or blend the ingredients with a stick blender until the soup has a smooth consistency.

Divide the soup among the bowls, and garnish with a dash of the ras el hanout spice, some freshly grated ginger, and extra thyme leaves.

VARIATION

+ Swap the carrots and potatoes for peeled butternut squash, parsnips, or rutabaga, or a combination.

TIPS

+ Avoid seasoning the dish, as the dry sun-dried tomatoes tend to be quite salty.

+ If you can't source dry sun-dried tomatoes, use fresh tomatoes instead.

+ Ras el hanout is easy to find in most supermarkets. It's a wonderful North African spice blend made with cinnamon, cardamom, and coriander.

Serves 4

10½ oz butternut squash, peeled and cut into rough ¾-inch cubes

18 oz parsnips, cut into rough ¾-inch cubes

3 tbsp extra-virgin olive oil, plus extra for drizzling

1 tsp fennel seeds, ground

1 tsp cumin seeds, ground

1 tsp ground turmeric

1 tsp freshly ground black pepper

3½ oz sprouted lentils (store-bought or sprouted at home)

3½ oz arugula

2 oz full-fat Greek yogurt, to serve (optional)

For the flatbreads

5½ oz spelt flour, plus extra for dusting

⅓ cup tepid water

1 tbsp olive oil

generous pinch of salt and pepper

¼ tsp ground coriander

Parsnip and Butternut Squash with Flatbreads

Some of the easiest meals I prepare are those made from simple roast vegetables. It's no fuss, there's minimal cleanup, and it is exactly what I need after a long day in the clinic. Root vegetables are wonderful sources of nutrients and are largely forgotten over their green, leafy counterparts. Parsnips contain potassium and magnesium—critical minerals for heart health. Keeping their delicious skins on means you will benefit from a lot of their chemical compounds, which are concentrated in these layers, not to mention plenty of fiber. I love making my own flatbreads, but to save time you can simply use thin store-bought ones.

Preheat the oven to 400°F.

Put the cubed butternut squash and parsnips in a baking tray, drizzle with the oil, and scatter the spices on top, tossing to thoroughly coat the vegetables in the spiced oil. Bake in the oven for 35 minutes, tossing them once halfway through and adding the sprouted lentils after 15 minutes, until the vegetables are golden.

In the meantime, make the flatbreads. Mix the flour with the water, oil, and spices in a bowl. Knead until the dough comes together and is smooth and not sticky, adding more water if necessary, then separate the dough into 4 small balls.

Dust the work surface with flour, and roll out the balls of dough using a floured rolling pin (or wine bottle) until you have breads about 8 inches in diameter.

Heat a large, dry frying pan over high heat, then cook each flatbread for 1–2 minutes on each side until lightly browned.

When the vegetables are cooked, remove the tray from the oven, and fold the arugula into the root vegetables. This will gently wilt the leaves.

Build your flatbreads, drizzling with a little olive oil or yogurt on top if you like.

TIP

+ If you can't source sprouted lentils, pre-cooked puy lentils or canned butter beans work well, too.

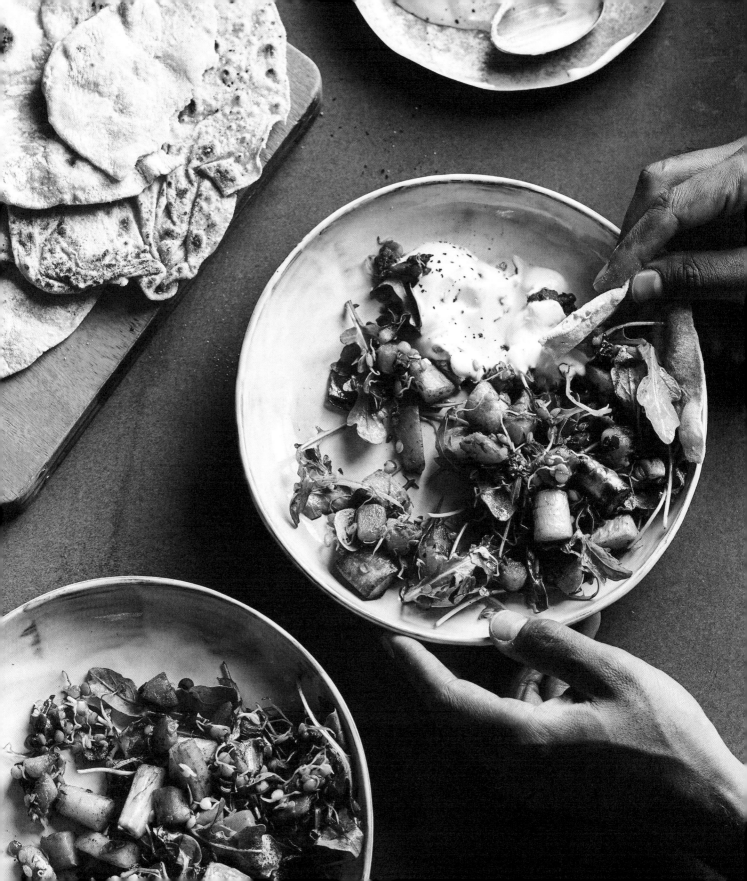

Umami Mushroom Tacos

My number one meal for sharing has to be tacos. I absolutely adore Mexican flavors, and the vibrant colors and sweet Cajun spice packed into these mushrooms is hard to beat. Adding lots of black beans increases the fiber content, and the fresh avocado salsa cools the dish while adding nutrients from the tomatoes and quality fats from the avocado. I like to use corn tacos as they're another source of whole grains, which adds more fiber to the meal. This will become a firm family favorite.

Preheat the oven to 425°F.

Scatter the mushrooms and onion wedges in an oven dish, and bake for 15 minutes to dry them out.

Meanwhile, mix the marinade ingredients together in a bowl.

After 15 minutes, remove the dish from the oven, and reduce the temperature to 400°F. Add the beans to the mushrooms and onion, drizzle on the Cajun marinade and mix thoroughly, then return to the oven for a further 15 minutes.

Dry-cook the corn in a large frying pan over medium-high heat for 3–4 minutes until slightly browned. Slice the kernels off into a bowl, then add a drizzle of olive oil plus the lime zest and chili flakes and some salt to taste.

Combine the avocado salsa ingredients in a bowl with the oil and the juice from the zested lime, and season with salt and pepper.

Warm the tacos in the oven, and serve everything for assembling at the table. Pile the mushroom bean filling on the warm tacos, followed by the toasted corn, then the avocado salsa.

Serves 4

10½ oz shiitake mushrooms, ripped into shreds or pulled apart using forks

1 red onion, halved and cut into thin wedges

14 oz canned black beans, drained and rinsed (or try pinto beans or black-eyed peas)

2 ears sweet corn

½ tbsp olive oil

grated zest of 1 lime

½ tsp dried chili flakes

sea salt and freshly ground black pepper

For the Cajun marinade

3 tbsp extra-virgin olive oil

2 tsp Cajun spice blend

1 tbsp maple syrup

1 tbsp soy sauce

1 tsp black pepper

For the avocado salsa

2 ripe avocados, stoned, peeled, and cut into ½-inch cubes

1 shallot, finely diced

3½ oz cherry tomatoes, finely diced

1 tbsp extra-virgin olive oil

juice of a zested lime

To serve

8 corn tacos (or whole-wheat flour tacos)

Poke Bowl

Serves 2

5½ oz Camargue or brown rice, soaked in water for at least 20 minutes, then drained

4 tsp tamari (or soy sauce)

½ oz peeled gingerroot, grated

1 tsp coconut sugar (or brown sugar)

5 tsp toasted or plain sesame oil

juice of 1 lime

¼ tsp cayenne pepper

½ tsp ground black pepper

3 spring onions, trimmed and thinly sliced at an angle

3½ oz edamame beans

¼ oz coriander (a small handful), leaves picked

2 tsp sesame seeds

Topping options:

Fish

7 oz sashimi-grade tuna, cut into ¾-inch cubes

Veg

7 oz peeled butternut squash, cut into ¾-inch cubes

3½ oz yellow or red beet, cut into ¾-inch cubes

1 tbsp coconut oil

When I lived in Sydney, I would regularly visit the fish markets and make fresh dishes just like this Hawaiian poke bowl. It makes a fantastic starter, or you can turn it into the main event by adding a few extra ingredients. The flavors in this dish are beautiful, and the sweet marinade with a sharp lime hint makes a fantastic contrast. You can make this vegetarian or with fish, but do try it with all the ingredients below; they work really well together and make a substantial meal.

Preheat the oven to 425°F if you're serving the rice with roasted vegetables.

Bring a pan of water to a boil, add the rice, and cook for 20–25 minutes, then drain and set aside to cool to room temperature.

If you're serving vegetables with the rice instead of tuna, toss them with the coconut oil in a tray, and roast for 25 minutes. Allow the vegetables to cool.

Put the tamari, ginger, sugar, sesame oil, lime juice, and spices in a bowl, and mix. Add the spring onions and edamame beans along with the tuna or cooled roasted vegetables (or both), and mix well. Add more sesame oil and lime juice if needed.

Divide the rice between two bowls, and top with the marinated tuna or roasted vegetables. Top with coriander and sesame seeds, and serve immediately.

VARIATION

+ Try other vegetables using the same poke marinade, such as cherry tomatoes, cucumber, or even roasted carrots. You could add diced mango for an exotic summery twist, too.

TIP

+ Togarashi powder is a fantastic seasoning. If you can find it, use 2 teaspoons of this instead of the cayenne and black pepper.

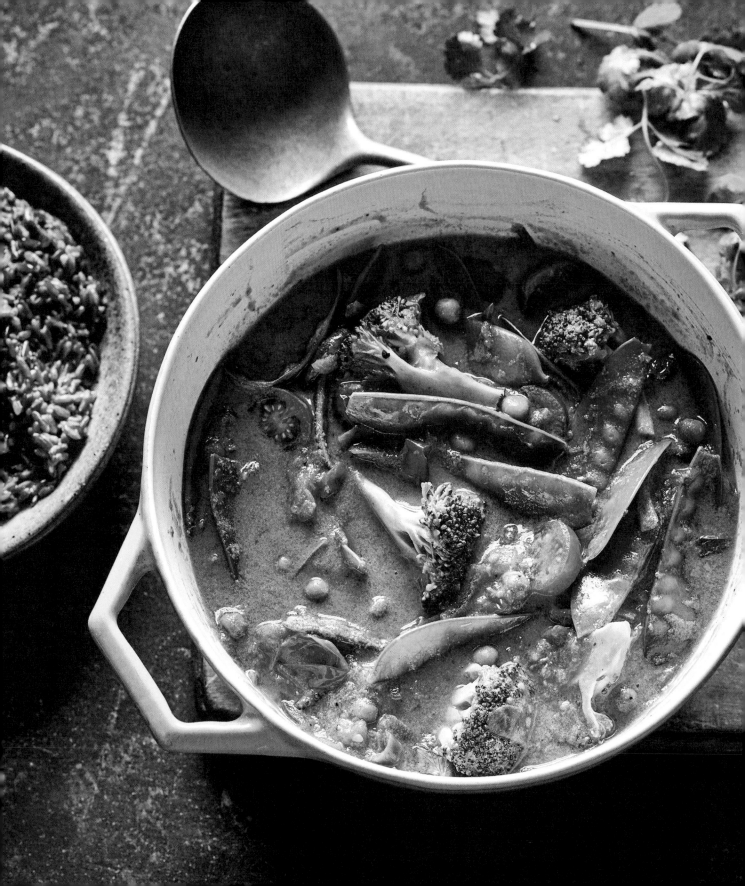

Ethiopian Berbere Curry

Serves 4

2 tbsp coconut oil

2 red onions, thinly sliced into half-moons

3 tsp berbere spice blend

3½ oz cherry tomatoes, halved

3½ oz peas (fresh or thawed)

7 oz snow peas

5½ oz broccoli, florets broken into 1¼-inch pieces

14 oz canned chopped tomatoes

14 oz canned coconut milk

9 oz red Camargue rice, soaked in water for at least 20 minutes, then drained

1½ cups vegetable stock

1 tbsp peanut butter (smooth or crunchy)

1 oz fresh coriander, finely chopped

This delicious curry is inspired by Ethiopian cuisine and uses a spice blend called berbere. I would describe it as a spicy masala—it has a fantastic heat to it. It tastes phenomenal with the snow peas and greens, but you could use any vegetables you have at hand. I learned the trick of adding nut butter to rice from a young Zimbabwean chef who told me it was a staple in their cuisine. It adds protein to the whole-grain rice and tastes wonderful with this curry.

Melt the oil in a large saucepan over medium heat, then add the onions with the spice blend, and cook for 2 minutes, stirring. Add the cherry tomatoes, and cook for a further minute. Toss in the peas, snow peas, and broccoli florets, stirring to coat them in the spices, then add the chopped tomatoes and coconut milk. Bring to a simmer, and cook for 10 minutes while you cook the rice.

Tip the rice into a dry saucepan over medium heat. Cook the grains for 1–2 minutes until they are dry and smell toasted, then add the vegetable stock and peanut butter, stir, cover, and simmer for 15 minutes until the rice has absorbed the water and the grains are cooked.

Fold most of the coriander into the curry, and scatter the rest on top of the rice as a garnish, then serve.

TIP

+ You can find berbere spice blend in most supermarkets, but Jamaican jerk spice can work well as a substitute.

Asian-Style Lettuce Wraps with Mint and Thai Basil

Using fresh herbs is the easiest way to get anti-inflammatory ingredients onto your plate, and they are the star of this crowd-pleasing dish, which uses widely available ingredients and involves minimal prep. I sometimes serve this light meal with a simple Asian-style omelette made with a little cinnamon, so I have included the recipe here.

Serves 2

2 tbsp sesame oil, plus extra for greasing

7 oz firm tofu, cut into ½-inch dice

1 tbsp soy sauce

3½ oz celery stalks, finely diced

2 oz spring onions, trimmed and finely diced

1 red pepper, halved, deseeded, and cut into thin strips

5½ oz bean sprouts

1 red chili, deseeded and thinly sliced

For the omelettes

3 eggs

4 tsp milk

1 tbsp soy sauce

small pinch of ground cinnamon

To serve

¾ oz mint leaves

¾ oz Thai basil leaves

8 baby gem lettuce leaves

Heat the sesame oil in a large non-stick frying pan over medium-high heat, add the diced tofu, and sauté for 8–10 minutes until lightly golden. Add the soy sauce and stir, then add the celery, spring onions, pepper strips, bean sprouts, and chili, and cook for another 3 minutes until softened. Transfer to a plate and set aside.

Put the mint and basil leaves and lettuce cups on a large platter.

To make the Asian-style omelettes, whisk the eggs in a bowl with the rest of the omelette ingredients. Grease the frying pan you cooked the tofu in with a little sesame oil, and place it over medium-high heat. Pour in half the omelette mixture, and swirl it around to coat the pan. Cook for 2–3 minutes, transfer to the platter, and repeat the process for the rest of the omelette mixture.

Serve the fried tofu and vegetables in an omelette next to the fresh herbs and lettuce cups on the platter.

VARIATIONS

+ Add fermented veggies, kimchi, or slaw to the platter alongside the lettuce cups and herbs.
+ Leave out the omelette to make this a completely plant-based dish.
+ Try serving a nuoc cham dipping sauce with the omelette-wrapped vegetables.

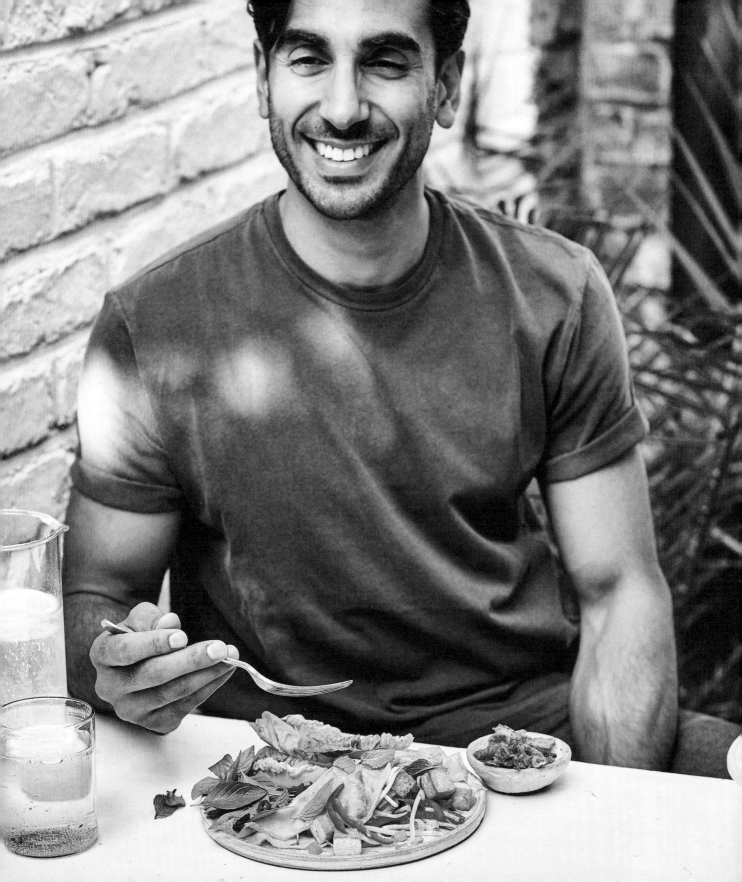

Roast Squash Curry with Cashew Sauce

Serves 4

18 oz unpeeled acorn or butternut squash, sliced into 1¼-inch-thick wedges, seeds removed

5½ oz unsalted cashews

1 tbsp coconut oil

½ large white onion, diced

4 garlic cloves, grated

½ oz gingerroot, peeled and grated

2 tsp garam masala

1 green chili, halved and deseeded

9 oz cherry tomatoes, diced, or 14 oz canned chopped tomatoes

2 tsp tomato puree

2 oz spinach, finely chopped

sea salt and freshly ground black pepper

½ oz fresh coriander leaves, finely chopped, to serve

For the cashew sauce

2 tsp smooth cashew butter

1 tsp ground cumin

juice of ½ lemon

¼ cup hot water

For the masala marinade

2 tbsp coconut oil, melted

1 tsp garam masala

1 tsp maple syrup

1 tsp ground turmeric

Curry dishes can be the healthiest and most comforting dishes to make. Ginger, garlic, and onion, the typical base ingredients for a curry, are a powerful trio that have all been shown to have anti-inflammatory properties and may have a role in improving the resilience of our immune system. The wealth of spices used in curries gives them so much flavor, and this is one of the quickest dishes to make. Serve with whole-wheat chapatis, brown rice, or simply on its own.

Preheat the oven to 400°F.

Mix the marinade ingredients together in a small bowl. Spread the squash pieces over a baking tray with the cashews, and coat with the masala marinade and some salt and pepper. Bake for 20–25 minutes, stirring occasionally so the cashews don't burn, until the slices are cooked through and the cashews are lightly browned.

Meanwhile, heat the coconut oil in a large frying pan over low–medium heat. Add the onion, garlic, and ginger, and cook for 2 minutes, then add the garam masala, green chili, tomatoes, and tomato puree. Season with salt and pepper, and cook for 6–8 minutes, allowing the tomatoes to break down. Add the roasted squash, cashews, and spinach to the mixture, and stir for 2–3 minutes to coat them in the sauce.

Whisk the cashew sauce ingredients in a bowl to make a light, creamy sauce. Dress the curry with the sauce, and finish by topping with the chopped coriander.

Herbes de Provence Chicken Skewers

Serves 2

14 oz skinless chicken breasts, cut into 1½-inch chunks

2 oz cherry tomatoes, halved

2 oz sun-dried tomatoes, roughly chopped

3½ oz watercress, roughly chopped

sea salt and freshly ground black pepper

½ oz lightly toasted pine nuts, to serve

For the marinade

2 tbsp extra-virgin olive oil

3 tsp herbes de Provence

grated zest and juice of 1 lemon

2 garlic cloves, finely chopped

For the basil dressing

¾ oz fresh basil leaves

¾ oz sunflower seeds

1 garlic clove

3 tbsp extra-virgin olive oil

Herbes de Provence is one of my go-to dry herb blends, and you'll find it in most supermarkets. Oregano and thyme are an absolutely splendid combination, and this is a firm favorite summer dish that will work on the barbecue, too. Combining both fresh and sun-dried tomatoes delivers an assortment of sweet and sharp flavors and pairs well with the citrus notes of the marinated chicken. The basil dressing is super quick to make, but you could use a store-bought pesto to save time.

Combine the marinade ingredients with some salt and pepper in a bowl. Add the chicken chunks, stir to coat in the marinade, and leave for at least 10 minutes (or overnight).

Push the marinated chicken onto 6 skewers (if using bamboo or wood skewers, soak them in water first for 20 minutes, to prevent them burning). Heat a dry griddle pan over medium heat, add the skewers, and cook for 7–8 minutes, turning them frequently until the chicken is cooked through with a lovely golden crust.

Meanwhile, make the basil dressing. Put the basil, sunflower seeds, garlic, and oil in a mini food processor with some salt and pepper, and blitz to create a thick dressing (or bash everything together with a pestle and mortar).

Combine the fresh and sun-dried tomatoes and the watercress in a bowl, and drop spoonfuls of the basil dressing onto them. Serve the grilled skewers on top of the salad, and garnish with the pine nuts.

TIP

+ Add more olive oil and some lemon juice to the basil dressing if you prefer it a little thinner.

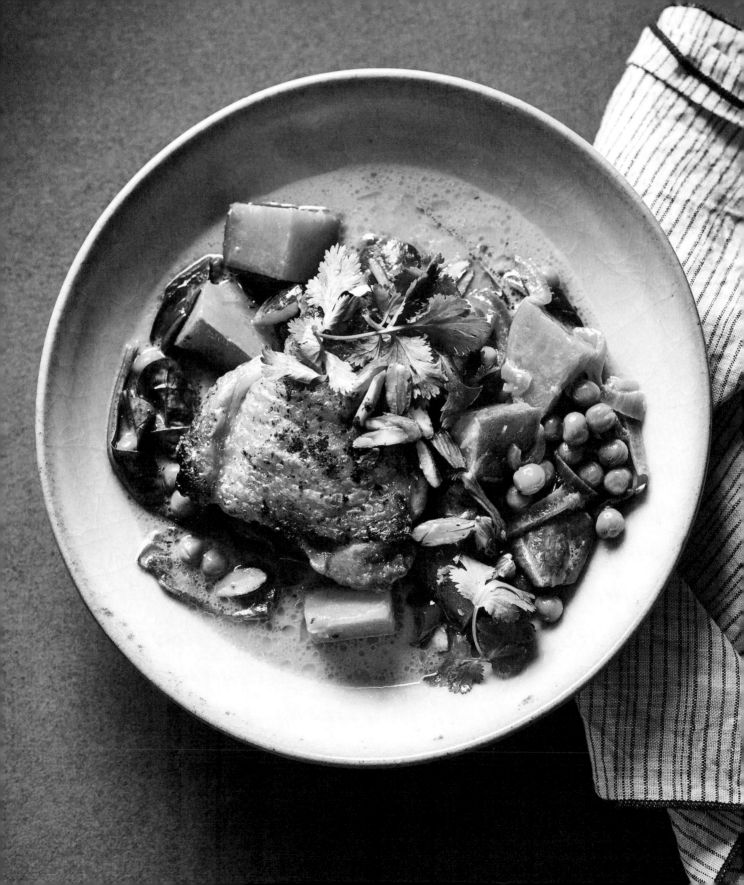

Coconut Chicken with Spicy Peas and Potato

Serves 4

2 tbsp coconut oil

½ red onion, thinly sliced

3 garlic cloves, roughly chopped

1 red chili, deseeded and roughly chopped

2 tsp yellow mustard seeds

2-inch piece of gingerroot, peeled and grated

1 tsp ground turmeric

1¼-inch cinnamon stick (or ½ tsp ground cinnamon)

4 bone-in, skin-on chicken thighs

¾ cup coconut milk

¾ cup vegetable stock (use a stock cube dissolved in water if needed)

7 oz peas (fresh or thawed)

18 oz peeled sweet potato, cut into 1¼-inch cubes

3½ oz spinach, roughly chopped

sea salt and freshly ground black pepper

½ oz fresh coriander, leaves and stalks finely chopped, to serve

I love making this one-pan dish on autumn evenings. The turmeric and mustard seeds deliver delicious earthy notes, while the onion and chili bring heat, resulting in a well-balanced, complex flavor. The peas and potatoes are the stars of this meal, as they provide nutrient density and fiber. I like to serve this dish with a simple green side salad; it also makes a great lunch the next day.

Preheat the oven to 400°F.

Melt the coconut oil in a large ovenproof saucepan or casserole dish over medium heat.

Add the onion, garlic, chili, mustard seeds, and ginger with some salt and pepper, and sauté for 3–4 minutes, then stir the turmeric and cinnamon into the oil, and cook for a minute before adding the chicken, skin side down. Fry the chicken gently for 5–6 minutes, stirring every now and again to ensure the onions don't burn, until the skin lightly browns.

Flip the chicken thighs over, and pour in the coconut milk and stock. Add the peas, sweet potato cubes, and spinach, making sure they are all covered in the coconut sauce. Cover with a lid, and transfer the dish to the oven. Bake for 30 minutes until the chicken is cooked through (the juices run clear when you pierce the thighs with a sharp knife) and the sweet potato is soft.

Remove from the oven, and serve garnished with the coriander.

VARIATION

+ Try swapping the chicken for fish, or even cooked chickpeas for a vegetarian version.

TIP

+ Garnish the dish with toasted coconut flakes or toasted almonds for added crunch and texture.

Mussels in Parsley and Lemon Dressing with Rye Croutons

Serves 2

18 oz live mussels, rinsed under cold running water and scrubbed

3 tbsp white wine or water

3½ oz rye bread, cut into chunky 1¼-inch cubes

1 tbsp olive oil

3¼ oz watercress, roughly chopped

5½ oz heirloom tomatoes (or other tomatoes), roughly quartered

½ oz Parmesan cheese, grated

½ oz sunflower seeds

For the parsley and lemon dressing

¼ cup extra-virgin olive oil

½ oz fresh flat-leaf parsley leaves, finely chopped

juice of 2 lemons

1 red chili, finely chopped (deseeded if you like)

1 tsp fennel seeds, finely ground

2 anchovy fillets from a can, finely chopped (optional)

½ tsp freshly ground black pepper

2 tsp capers, rinsed and finely chopped

1 garlic clove, finely chopped

I absolutely love the depth of flavor and freshness in this dish. The dressing, made with good-quality olive oil, parsley, and sharp lemon, combines wholesome fats and plant chemicals to deliver an anti-inflammatory boost to the mussels. Watercress is a phenomenal ingredient that contains phytochemicals such as lutein, which is good for eye health, and rye croutons deliver great texture and additional fiber.

Debeard the mussels, discarding any mussels with open shells that don't close when tapped.

Heat a large saucepan over high heat, add the mussels and wine or water, cover, and cook for 2–3 minutes until all the shells are open and the mussels are cooked through (discard any that remain closed). Remove the mussels from the pan, and allow to cool before picking the meat out of the shells and placing it in a bowl (discard the shells).

Mix all the dressing ingredients together in a medium bowl. Toss in the cooked mussels, and set to one side for them to soak in all the flavors of the dressing.

Toast the cubes of rye bread in a dry frying pan over medium heat for a few minutes until slightly colored, then add the olive oil and continue to toast, moving them gently around the pan until they are evenly golden.

Bring all the elements together on a large platter: arrange the watercress and tomatoes on the platter, scatter over the warm croutons, then add the mussels, drizzling with the dressing they've been sitting in. Garnish with the grated Parmesan and sunflower seeds, and serve.

VARIATION

+ To make this dish plant-based, replace the anchovies with 1 teaspoon of red miso paste, and the mussels with canned white beans, drained, rinsed, and warmed in a pan.

TIP

+ Use the dressing on vegetarian staples too, such as cannellini beans, puy lentils, or even the humble chickpea.

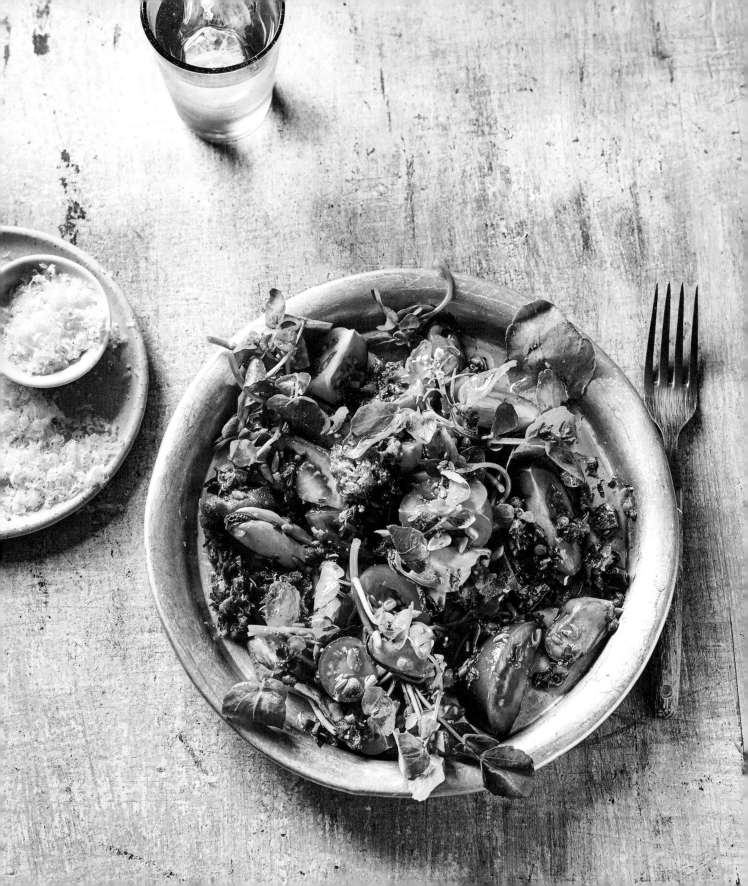

Spinach and Vegetable Lasagne

When I have a lot of people coming over and I want a no-fuss comfort meal, this classic family-style dish hits the spot every time. I like to make a simple green salad to go with it—you can add vegetables to the salad, too. The creamy white sauce made with nut milk works great and can be made completely plant-based by substituting oil for the butter. It's also a fantastic way of introducing more vegetables into children's diets as well as your own.

Preheat the oven to 400°F.

Heat the olive oil in a large saucepan over medium heat, add the onion, and cook, stirring, for 2 minutes before adding the garlic. Cook for another minute, then toss in the mushrooms, eggplant, and zucchini with the oregano, and sauté for 4–5 minutes until softened. Add the basil, vinegar, and chopped tomatoes, and simmer for 10 minutes.

While the vegetables are simmering, make the white sauce. Melt the butter in a small saucepan over medium heat, then gradually whisk in the flour until thickened. Cook the flour and butter mixture for a minute, then whisk in the cashew milk a little at a time until you achieve a béchamel sauce consistency (you may need more or less milk), then add the nutritional yeast flakes (or cheese) and nutmeg. Remove from the heat.

Build your lasagne by layering half the vegetables on the bottom of a lasagne dish (about 8 x 10 x 3 inches), then placing 2 or 3 lasagne sheets on top. Smother the pesto on top of the sheets, then add a layer of spinach, with some white sauce on top. Repeat the layers of vegetables, lasagne sheets, spinach and white sauce until you run out of mixture: the top layer should be the white sauce, which will crisp up nicely in the oven. Bake for 35–40 minutes and allow to cool a little on the work surface for 5 minutes before serving with arugula leaves or a simple side salad.

Serves 6

2 tbsp extra-virgin olive oil

1 red onion, sliced

6 garlic cloves, finely chopped

7 oz mushrooms, roughly diced

5½ oz eggplant, cut into 1¼-inch cubes

5½ oz zucchini, cut into 1¼-inch cubes

2 tsp dried (or fresh) oregano

½ oz fresh basil leaves, roughly torn

2 tsp balsamic vinegar

14 oz canned chopped tomatoes

arugula or simple salad leaves, to serve

For the white sauce

2 tbsp butter

1 oz all-purpose flour

1 cup cashew milk

3 tbsp nutritional yeast flakes (or grated Parmesan)

½ tsp freshly grated or ground nutmeg

3½ oz fresh green pesto (store-bought or homemade)

6 spinach or whole-grain pasta lasagne sheets (about 3¼ x 8 inches) (buy bean pasta sheets if you want a gluten-free version)

3½ oz spinach

Split Green Pea and Pearl Barley Pan

Serves 4

2 tbsp extra-virgin olive oil

4 garlic cloves, finely chopped

1 red onion, finely diced

2 oz cooked chestnuts, roughly sliced

½ oz rosemary needles, roughly chopped

1 tsp cayenne pepper

5½ oz pearl barley flakes, soaked in water for 30 minutes, then drained (or whole-grain oats)

3½ oz split green peas (or split yellow peas), soaked in water for 30 minutes, then drained

2½ cups hot vegetable stock

3½ oz cherry tomatoes, halved

2½ oz spinach, roughly chopped

¼ oz fresh flat-leaf parsley leaves, finely chopped

sea salt and freshly ground black pepper

This comforting autumnal dish provides a wealth of flavor and nutrition. The pearl barley flakes are wonderfully nutty, and the split peas are an excellent fiber-rich protein source. I've heightened the nutrient density of this meal-in-a-pan by using a variety of herbs and spices and including two different sources of fiber. It's a fantastic, easy meal to make, and you can easily use different pulses or beans instead of the peas.

Heat the oil in a large saucepan over medium heat. Add the garlic, onion, chestnuts, and rosemary, and sauté for 2–3 minutes, then scatter in the cayenne, drained pearl barley, and split peas, along with a pinch each of salt and pepper, and stir for a couple of minutes.

Pour in 2 cups of the vegetable stock, and add the halved tomatoes. Reduce the heat to medium-low, cover, and simmer for 35–40 minutes until the split peas are cooked through. Top up with the remaining stock if the ingredients at the bottom of the pan are sticking slightly during cooking.

Remove from the heat, stir in the spinach, and cover for another 2 minutes to allow the leaves to wilt. Stir, and serve in bowls, scattered with the chopped parsley.

VARIATION

+ Use different spices to suit your taste. Two teaspoons of my Creole Spice Blend (see page 245) would work really well in this meal.

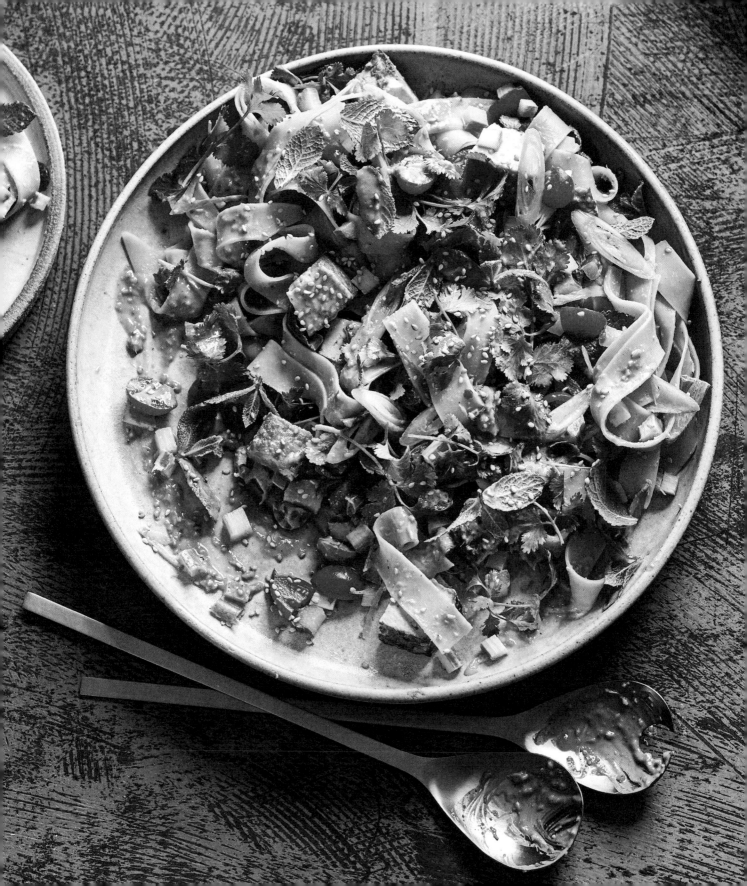

Vibrant Malay Salad

This has got to be one of the most flavorful dishes in this book. Bursting with incredible colors inspired by Malaysian cuisine, it is a celebration of how the healthiest way of eating can be vibrant and exciting. Don't be put off by the long list of ingredients: it's actually very quick to make, and you can find all the components in most supermarkets. The large quantity of fresh herbs represents the concentrated sources of polyphenols known to fight inflammation; they're a perfect balance for the heat and citrus in this delicious recipe.

Serves 2

For the dressing

1 red chili, deseeded and finely chopped

1 tbsp peanut butter (smooth or crunchy)

2-inch piece of gingerroot, peeled and grated

3 garlic cloves, grated

2-inch piece of lemongrass (tender base only), very finely chopped

2 tsp palm sugar (or honey/maple syrup)

1 tsp fish sauce (or tamari if vegan)

2 tsp soy sauce

2 tsp sesame oil

For the salad

2 oz cherry tomatoes, diced

grated zest and juice of 1 lime

½ oz Thai basil leaves (or regular basil), roughly chopped

½ oz fresh mint leaves, finely chopped

½ oz fresh coriander leaves, finely chopped

4-inch piece of rhubarb, finely diced

3 spring onions, trimmed and finely chopped

3½ oz brown rice noodles

1 tbsp sesame oil

10½ oz smoked tofu

1 oz sesame seeds

Mix the dressing ingredients together in a large bowl, or blitz them in a small food processor if you want the dressing to be smooth.

Toss the cherry tomatoes, lime zest, and juice into the bowl of dressing. Once combined, add the herbs, rhubarb, and spring onions.

Put the rice noodles in a saucepan of boiling water (off the heat), and cover for 5 minutes (or cook according to the packet instructions), then drain, cool, and toss through the salad.

Heat the sesame oil in a small frying pan over low-medium heat, add the tofu, and brown it on both sides until crisp on the outside and soft within. Remove from the pan and slice into 1¼-inch cubes.

Toast the sesame seeds in a dry pan for 30 seconds, scatter them over the salad with the fried tofu, and serve.

TIP

+ If rhubarb isn't in season, just leave it out.

Thai-Style Salmon Burgers

These beautiful aromatic Omega-3-rich salmon burgers are an absolute favorite of mine. The punchy herbs and lemongrass give them incredible depth of flavor and add nutritional value, too. I sometimes use pumpernickel bread or rye bread instead of whole-grain bread, for extra fiber. These burgers are delicious on their own, as part of a platter, or with this quick salad dressed with spiced coconut cream.

Put the bread in a food processor, and blitz into coarse breadcrumbs, then add the herbs, spring onions, ginger, chili, lemongrass, and soy sauce, and blend to form a paste. Add the salmon, and blitz to create a rough burger mixture. Transfer the mixture to a bowl, then shape it into four small patties with wet hands.

Melt the coconut oil in a frying pan over medium heat, add the patties, and fry for 5–6 minutes on each side until cooked through.

Warm the coconut cream in a saucepan over medium heat with the curry paste for a few minutes until combined and hot through. Divide the cream among four shallow bowls, and top with the pea shoots and watercress.

Serve the burgers on top of the salad, garnish with the lime zest and peanuts, and squeeze the lime juice over the top.

TIP

+ If you prefer, you can also bake the salmon burgers on a parchment-lined baking tray in an oven preheated to 400°F for about 12 minutes.

Serves 4

2 slices (2½ oz) of whole-grain bread (or gluten-free equivalent)

½ oz Thai basil leaves, roughly chopped

½ oz fresh coriander, leaves and stalks roughly chopped

2 spring onions, trimmed and roughly chopped

¾ oz gingerroot, peeled and roughly chopped

1 red chili, roughly chopped

4-inch stick of lemongrass (tender base only), roughly chopped

2 tsp soy sauce (or tamari if you're making the meal gluten free)

9 oz skinless salmon fillet, cut into thick chunks

1 tbsp coconut oil

For the salad

3½ oz coconut cream

2 tsp red curry paste

3½ oz pea shoots, roughly chopped

3½ oz watercress, roughly chopped

To serve

grated zest and juice of 1 lime

½ oz unsalted peanuts, toasted and roughly chopped

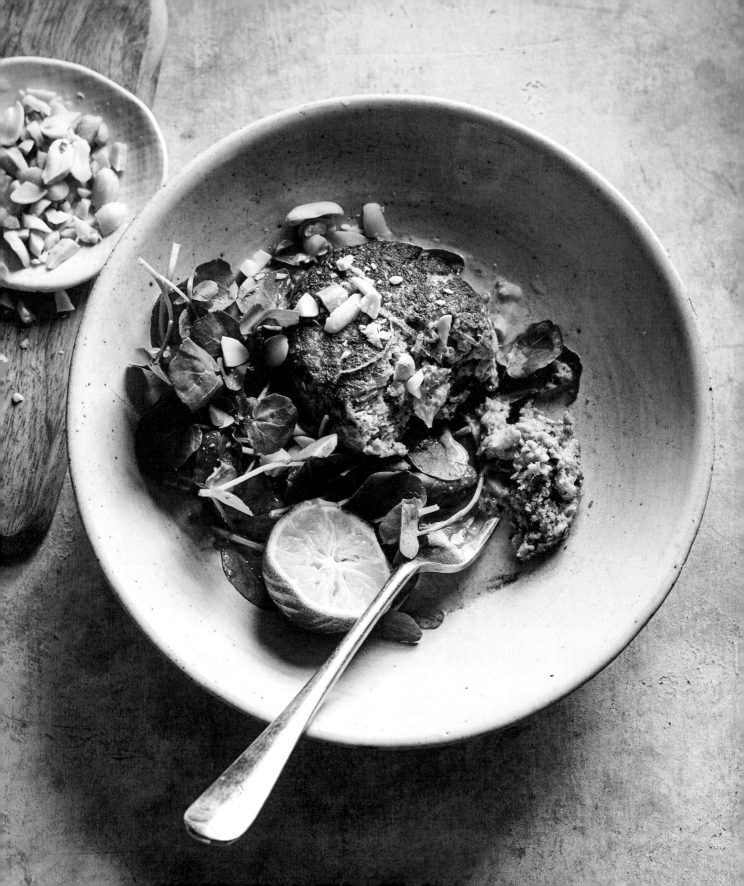

228

6 servings

7 oz red rice (or brown basmati), soaked in water for at least 20 minutes, then drained

1¼ cups water

1 bay leaf

28 oz boneless, skinless cod, cut into 4 fillets

For the spice paste

1 tsp cumin seeds

2 tsp black (or yellow) mustard seeds

1 tsp coconut oil

4 garlic cloves

¼ oz fresh turmeric root (or 1 tsp ground)

½ white onion, roughly chopped

sea salt and freshly ground black pepper

For the salad

5½ oz cucumber, finely diced

3½ oz cherry tomatoes, finely diced

1 oz fresh coriander, finely chopped

grated zest and juice of 1 lime

½ tsp dried chili flakes (optional)

Bengali-Style Cod

Making a spice paste from scratch is such a pleasure, and it doesn't take much effort at all. Once you start making your own, you'll realize how vibrant and fresh the ingredients taste, plus the spices have distinguished health properties. Garlic is a well-recognized anti-inflammatory ingredient that also contains a special type of fiber that benefits the gut microbe population. The dish's prominent mustard flavor is a familiar characteristic of Bengali cuisines, and it gives the cod an earthy, deep flavor.

Preheat the oven to 425°F.

To make the paste, toast the cumin and mustard seeds in a dry frying pan over medium heat for 1 minute, then grind with a pestle and mortar.

Put the pan back over medium heat, and add the coconut oil. When it has melted, add the whole garlic cloves, turmeric, and onion, and cook for 5 minutes until softened. Transfer the dry ground spices and the contents of the pan to a small food processor, add some salt and pepper, and blitz to form a paste.

Tip the rice into a dry pan, and toast it for 1 minute while you boil the 1¼ cups water. Add the boiling water, seasoning, and bay leaf to the rice, and simmer for 15 minutes until the rice is cooked and the water has been absorbed.

While the rice is cooking, coat the fish fillets all over with the spice paste, and cover individually with baking parchment. Place on a baking tray, and bake in the oven for 10 minutes, or until the fish is cooked through.

Put the cucumber, tomatoes, and coriander in a bowl, and stir in the lime zest and juice. Sprinkle with the chili flakes (if using).

Plate up the rice, flake the baked fish on top of the rice, and serve with the salad.

VARIATION

+ You can use any sustainable white fish if you don't like cod: try haddock, pollock, or hake.

TIP

+ To make a quick version of this dish, use any good-quality curry paste instead of making one from scratch. I suggest a madras curry paste.

Celeriac and Broad Bean Rendang Curry

Serves 4

2 tbsp coconut oil

10½ oz celeriac, peeled and cut into 1¼-inch cubes

1 red onion, thinly sliced

4 tsp Rendang Curry Paste (see page 246) or store-bought paste

5½ oz podded broad beans (or frozen edamame beans)

7 oz coconut cream

1¾ cups vegetable stock

1 tbsp soy sauce

5½ oz green beans

1 oz fresh coriander, leaves and stalks finely chopped

sesame oil, for frying (optional)

3–4 kaffir lime leaves (optional)

grated zest and juice of 1 lime

½ oz unsalted cashews, toasted and crushed

3 tbsp coconut flakes, lightly toasted

I love making big curries with different types of vegetables. Combining celeriac with rendang curry paste gives this subtle-flavored vegetable a fiery boost. This curry is an easy way to increase your vegetable intake, and it's endlessly adaptable, suiting all manner of vegetables and spice blends. Topping the finished dish with kaffir lime leaves gives this particular curry an authentic finish and looks incredible. Serve with whole-grain rice for a complete meal.

Melt the oil in a large saucepan over medium heat. Add the celeriac and cook for 10 minutes, stirring frequently, then add the onion and cook for a further 5 minutes until both the celeriac and onion are lightly colored. Add the curry paste and broad beans and stir for a minute, then add the coconut cream and continue stirring for another minute. Add the stock and soy sauce, bring to a simmer, and cook uncovered for 10 minutes, or until the celeriac is tender.

Once the celeriac is tender, add the green beans, cover, and cook for a final 2–3 minutes.

Remove from the heat, mix in the coriander, and divide among wide bowls.

Heat a little sesame oil in a frying pan, add the kaffir lime leaves, and fry for 4 minutes (if using), then scatter them over the curry.

Squeeze over the lime juice, scatter over the cashews and the coconut flakes, and garnish with the lime zest. Serve with whole-grain rice.

VARIATION

+ Try making this curry with different cubed veggies, such as eggplant, rutabaga, or parsnip.

TIP

+ Add a teaspoon of honey, maple syrup, palm sugar, or coconut sugar for added sweetness.

I usually eat fruit, nuts, and good-quality dark chocolate during the week as a sweet treat after meals, but when you're feeling a little more indulgent, try these delicious dishes. Also, don't try to kid yourself that there is such a thing as a "guilt-free" or "healthy" sweet dish; sugar is still sugar, whether it's from natural sources or refined, so indulge in these as you would any other dessert recipe.

Desserts

Coconut Bananas with Maple Cream

Serves 2

¾ oz shelled, unsalted pistachios

1 tbsp coconut oil

2 medium firm bananas, peeled and sliced in half lengthways

3½ oz thick coconut cream

1 tbsp maple syrup

½ tsp ground cinnamon

2 oz pomegranate seeds

½ oz dark chocolate (minimum 75% cocoa solids), grated

This recipe makes use of some delicious wholesome ingredients like pomegranate, pistachio, and banana. I could talk about the benefits of pomegranate extract in preventing cancer cells from growing, demonstrated in the POMI-T trials, or perhaps the fantastic fatty acids found in pistachios, but it's worth pointing out that this delightful dessert is sweet and indulgent, so please only enjoy occasionally. A firm, almost ripe banana works better in this recipe that an overly ripe one. You'll love making this!

Toast the pistachios in a large dry frying pan over medium heat for 3–4 minutes until lightly browned and fragrant. Remove from the pan, and roughly chop.

Add the coconut oil to the pan, and warm it over medium heat. Add the banana halves to the pan, cut side down, and let them sizzle in the oil for 4–5 minutes, until the slices begin to caramelize. Flip them over and fry on the other side for 1–2 minutes until softened.

Combine the coconut cream in a bowl with the maple syrup and cinnamon to create an indulgent sauce. Spread the cream onto two dessert plates, and place the fried bananas on top.

Scatter the pomegranate seeds, chopped pistachios, and chocolate on top to serve.

TIP

+ Use honey as a sweetener instead of maple syrup, if you wish.

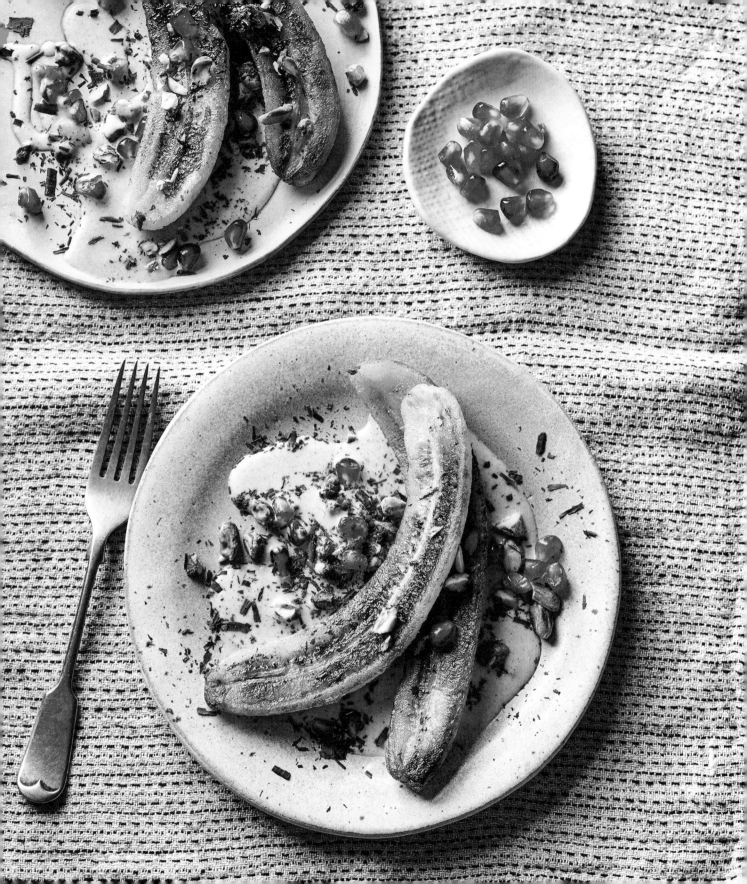

Candied Almonds with Spiced Strawberries

Serves 2

1 oz raw almonds, roughly chopped

1 tbsp maple syrup

7 oz strawberries, hulled and halved

1 tsp coconut sugar or demerara sugar

½ oz mint leaves, finely chopped

seeds from 3–4 green cardamom pods, freshly ground

2½ oz unsweetened dairy-free coconut yogurt

Almonds, cardamom, and strawberries are a wonderful combination commonly found in Middle Eastern desserts. The strawberries are wonderfully nutritious—they contain a plethora of plant chemicals including anthocyanins and phenolic acids that promote health and prevent disease. The cardamom really enhances the sweet flavors in the dish, and a dusting of sugar helps draw moisture out of the fruit to create a light syrup.

Toast the almonds in a small dry frying pan over medium heat for about 3 minutes until fragrant and lightly golden, then add the maple syrup and continue to cook for 1–2 minutes until the nuts are coated in the syrup and have caramelized. Set aside on a piece of baking parchment to cool.

Toss the strawberries in a bowl with the sugar, chopped mint, and cardamom.

Pile the berries into two bowls, spoon over the coconut yogurt, and top with the candied almonds.

TIPS

+ Use plain full-fat Greek yogurt if you can't find coconut yogurt.
+ If you prefer to keep the sugar content as low as possible, leave out the maple syrup or coconut sugar so the nuts will be toasted but not candied.

Roasted Apricots with Cardamom and Lime

Serves 2

pared peel and juice of 1 lime,
  plus extra grated zest to serve
pared peel and juice of ½ orange
3 cardamom pods, lightly crushed
4 apricots, stoned and quartered
2 tsp coconut sugar (or demerara
  sugar or maple syrup)
1 oz shelled, unsalted pistachios
  (or flaked almonds or chopped
  walnuts)
coconut ice cream, to serve

This dessert makes fantastic use of the natural sweetness found in stone fruit, with just a touch of sugar to encourage caramelization. The sweetness of the apricot and coconut sugar is balanced by the bitter notes in the citrus fruit. I love using different types of nuts for added texture, and they make this a more satiating sweet dish, too.

Preheat the oven to 400°F.

Pour the citrus juices into a small baking tray with the orange and lime peels and the cardamom pods. Toss the quartered apricots in the liquid, and dust them with the sugar. Bake in the oven for 15–20 minutes until the liquid has caramelized.

Gently toast the pistachios in a dry pan over medium heat for a few minutes, then roughly chop them.

Serve the warm apricots with coconut ice cream, the toasted nuts, and some lime zest scattered over.

VARIATION

+ Try swapping the apricots for other stone fruits, such as nectarines, plums, or peaches, and use the same roasting method.

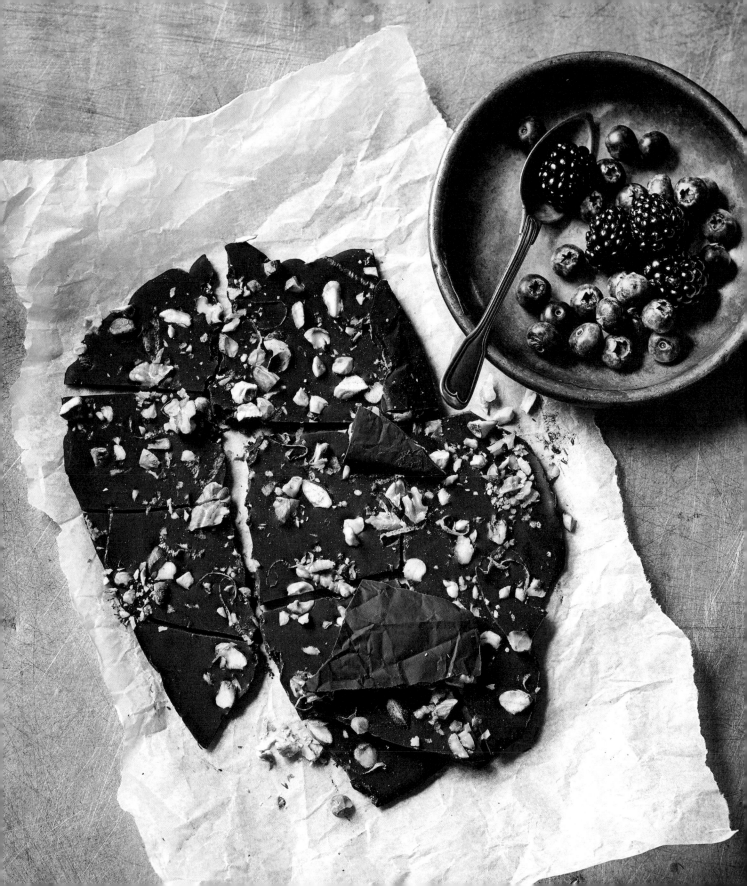

Orange-Zest Chocolate Bark with Berries

Makes one large piece of bark (serves 4–6)

7 oz dark chocolate (minimum 70% cocoa solids), broken into small pieces

½ oz shelled, unsalted pistachios, roughly chopped

½ oz walnuts, roughly chopped

grated zest of ½ small orange

small pinch of ground cinnamon

5½ oz blackberries or a selection of seasonal fruits such as nectarines, pears, apples, or raspberries

Chocolate has been promoted as a healthy ingredient for a variety of reasons, including its flavonol content, which can have a positive effect on heart health. However, simply adding your favorite chocolate bar to your regular diet and expecting it to benefit your health is misguided. Chocolate may have been found to have some marginal benefits, but it's your overall lifestyle that determines health outcomes. That being said, I eat a small amount of good-quality dark chocolate as a treat. The bitter notes of chocolate with 75 percent (or higher) cocoa content can be overwhelming for those used to the average commercial chocolate bar, so I've introduced other sweet notes into this bark recipe, which will help ease you into appreciating the deep flavors of dark chocolate.

Set a heatproof bowl over a pan of simmering water, making sure the bowl doesn't touch the water. Place the chocolate into the bowl and let it melt, stirring it occasionally. Meanwhile, line a small baking tray or chopping board with baking parchment.

Spread the melted chocolate over the tray to a thickness of about 1¼ inches. Scatter all the remaining ingredients (apart from the fresh fruit) evenly over the melted chocolate, and place in the freezer for 20–25 minutes to harden.

Snap and enjoy with seasonal fruits.

Serves 2

2 medium bananas, peeled,
   cut into chunks, and frozen
   (7 oz peeled weight)

7 oz frozen mixed berries

3½ oz coconut cream

¾ oz pecans, roughly chopped,
   plus extra to serve

1 oz dark chocolate, grated

Banana Berry Scoops

This is one of the easiest desserts to make, and I always have a batch of it, or the ingredients, in my freezer. Frozen mixed berries are widely available and super cheap. They maintain their nutritional value even when frozen and are a great source of polyphenols, which have been shown to protect our brain cells from oxidative stress. This dessert is a great way to introduce berries into our diet regularly, and the chocolate shavings deliver some bitter notes to complement the sweetness from the bananas.

Put the frozen bananas, berries, and coconut cream into a food processor or blender, and blitz until combined and smooth. Add the chopped pecans, and combine using a spoon.

Divide between two bowls, and scatter with the grated dark chocolate and a few extra pecans. Enjoy immediately.

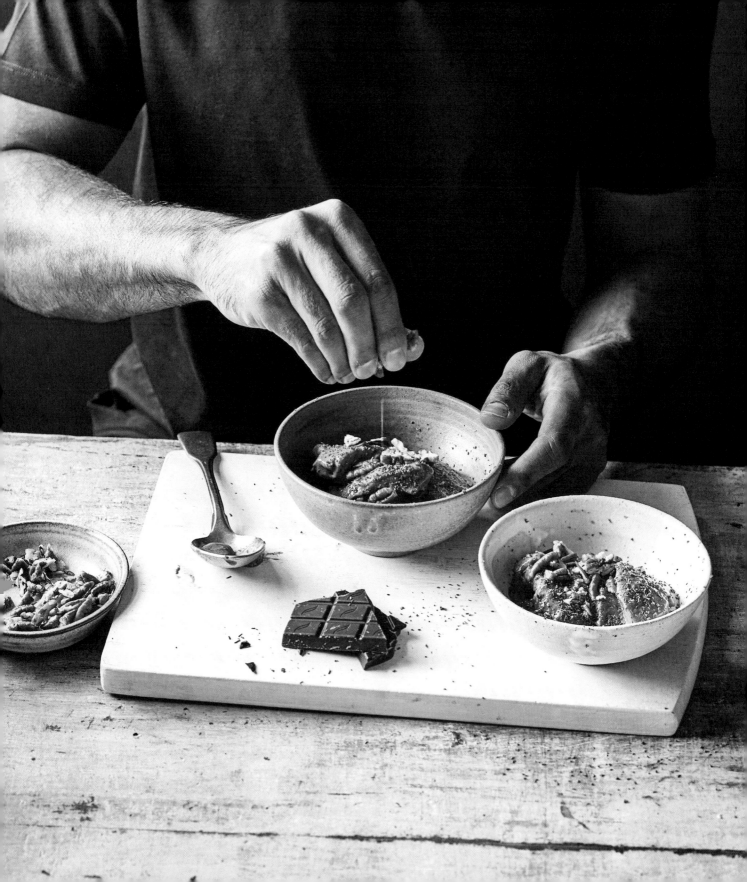

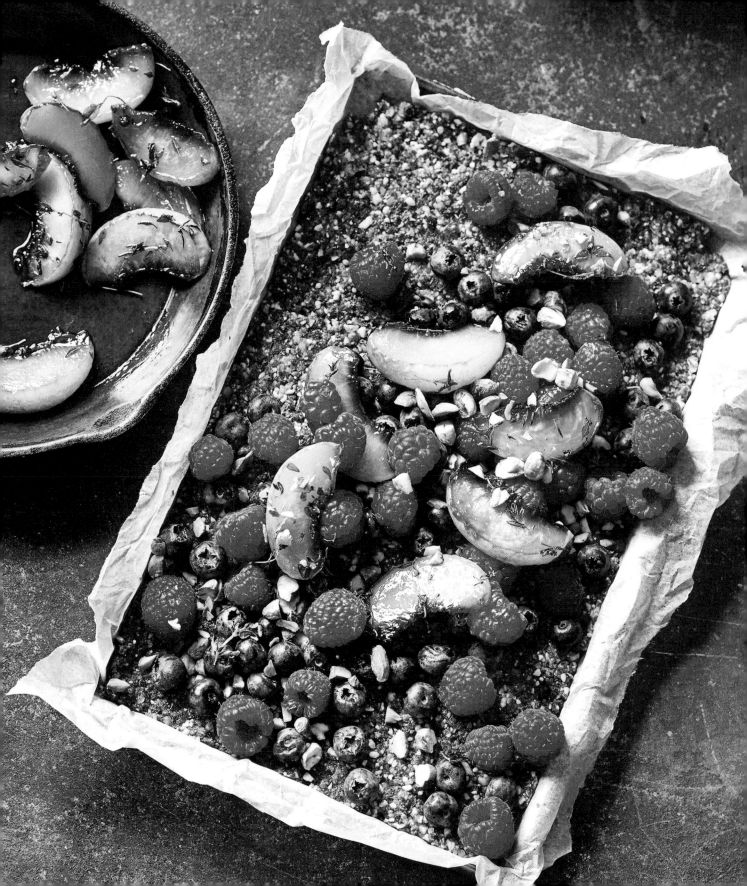

Glazed Peaches with Thyme

Since learning more about the impact of berries on brain health and how they generally reduce inflammation, I try to sneak them into recipes wherever I can. The sharp taste of the berries in this recipe contrasts with the sweet stone fruit, and the delicious base has plenty of fiber from the nuts and more flavor than a traditional biscuit base.

Serves 4

7 oz pitted dates

pinch of salt

10½ oz raw hazelnuts, soaked in warm water for 10 minutes, then drained

1½ tbsp coconut oil

7 oz ripe peaches, stoned and cut into ¾-inch-thick slices

2 tsp honey or maple syrup (optional)

¼ oz fresh thyme leaves, chopped

3½ oz fresh berries (blueberries and raspberries work well)

½ oz shelled, unsalted pistachios, toasted and crushed

Put the dates, salt, and drained hazelnuts in a blender, and blitz until you get a coarse mixture that sticks together when pressed.

Line a small 12 x 16-inch flat baking tray, and grease it with ½ tablespoon of the coconut oil. Press the date crust into the tray to make an even ½-inch-thick layer, and place in the fridge or freezer to set.

Melt the remaining tablespoon of coconut oil in a pan over medium heat,w and toss in the sliced peaches. Sauté for 4–5 minutes until lightly colored, then drizzle over the honey or maple syrup (if using), and scatter with the thyme before taking it off the heat.

Allow to cool slightly, then scatter the fruit on top of the chilled nutty crust, along with the fresh berries and pistachios, and slice.

These simple blends will inspire you to be more creative in the kitchen and introduce you to a world of flavors that will lift any simple ingredients to new heights. Try making one from scratch and comparing the flavor with a store-bought version. The differences in flavor are incomparable.

Pastes, spices, and teas

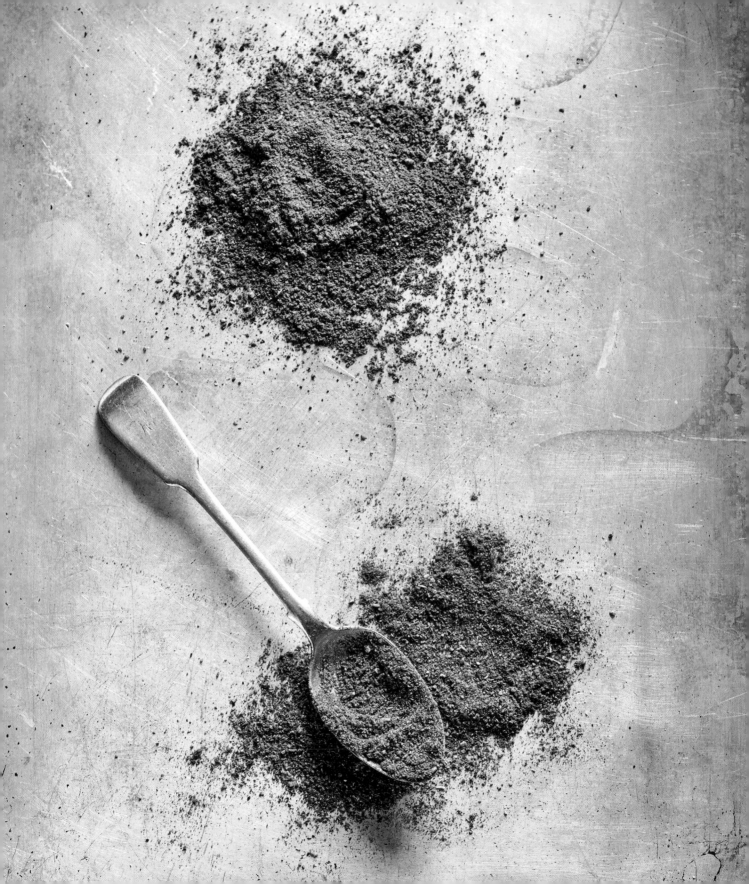

Creole Spice Blend

Ever since I tasted my first authentic Louisianan Creole dish while visiting New Orleans during my childhood, I've been obsessed with Creole spice blends. As diverse as the region itself, the spice combinations reflect a mix of European, African, and Caribbean heritage. I use this blend on everything from scrambled eggs and mixed roast vegetables to my vegetarian Jambalaya (see page 204).

Makes about 2 oz

4 tsp black peppercorns
2 tsp fennel seeds
4 tsp dried oregano
4 tsp dried thyme
4 tsp sweet paprika
2 tsp garlic powder
2 tsp onion powder
2 tsp cayenne pepper

Heat a dry frying pan over medium heat. Add the black peppercorns and fennel seeds, and toast them for 2–3 minutes until aromatic. Remove from the heat and allow to cool, then pound using a pestle and mortar or blitz in a coffee grinder until finely ground.

Mix the rest of the ingredients with the ground black peppercorns and fennel seeds. The spice blend will keep in an airtight jar for up to 6–8 weeks.

TIP

+ Use pre-ground pepper and fennel for ease, if you prefer.

Rupy's Ras El Hanout

This spice blend translates as "head of the shop," which is taken to mean the best that a spice seller has to offer. It's essentially the garam masala of Northern Africa—it uses similar spices but has a distinct fragrance. The blend contains some of the most potent culinary spices, known to have strong antioxidant properties, which can reduce oxidative stress. Mixed with garlic and oil, ras el hanout makes a delicious paste that works well in curries or simply smothered over white fish and baked. Use the spices as a simple seasoning for roasted vegetables such as fennel, cauliflower, or red onion, and it will transform your cooking.

Makes about 1½ oz

1 tbsp cumin seeds
2 tbsp coriander seeds
1 tsp black peppercorns
1½ tbsp ground cinnamon or 1 cinnamon stick
½ tsp cardamom seeds (from about 5 green cardamom pods)
1 tsp sweet paprika
2 tsp ground ginger
½ tsp ground turmeric

Heat a dry frying pan over low-medium heat, add the cumin, coriander, black peppercorns, cinnamon stick (if using), and cardamom seeds, and toast for 3–4 minutes until aromatic (be careful not to burn them). Remove from the heat and allow to cool, then pound using a pestle and mortar or blitz in a coffee grinder until finely ground.

Mix with the ground cinnamon (if using), paprika, ginger and turmeric, and store in an airtight jar for 6–8 weeks.

Malaysian Laksa Paste

This is simple to prepare and totally worth the extra effort—you'll notice a massive difference between store-bought paste and this homemade version. It gives dishes an indulgent flavor while delivering fantastic nutritional value by way of anti-inflammatory chemicals found in the lemongrass and ginger. I use it in my Carrot and Zucchini Laksa on page 158—give it a try!

Makes about 5½ oz

5 garlic cloves, roughly chopped
2-inch piece of lemongrass (tender base only), bruised and roughly chopped
¾ oz gingerroot, peeled and roughly chopped
1 red chili, halved
1 shallot or 2 oz trimmed spring onions, roughly chopped
1 tsp fish sauce
1 tbsp soy sauce
1 tbsp smooth cashew butter (or any smooth nut butter)
½ oz fresh coriander, leaves and stalks
1 tsp ground turmeric
1 tbsp palm sugar (or coconut sugar, honey, or maple syrup)
juice of 2 limes

Heat a dry frying pan over medium heat, add the garlic, lemongrass, ginger, chili and shallot or spring onions, and toast, gently stirring, for about 4 minutes.

Place the spices in a blender or small food processor along with the remaining ingredients, and blitz to form a smooth paste. Store in an airtight jar in the fridge for up to 4 weeks.

Rendang Curry Paste

This spice paste, popular in Indonesia and Malaysia, is usually combined with red meats like beef, but the incredible flavor works perfectly with vegetables and in stir-fries. I tend to make a big batch and keep it in my fridge, so it's ready to go when I want to make my Rendang Stir-Fry on page 162.

Makes 7 oz

1 tsp cumin seeds
2-inch piece of cinnamon stick
seeds from 5 green cardamom pods
1 star anise
2 cloves
2-inch piece of lemongrass (tender base only), roughly chopped
1 shallot, roughly chopped (or ½ red onion)
5 garlic cloves, smashed
¾ oz gingerroot, peeled and roughly chopped
1 red chili, deseeded and roughly chopped
¼ oz fresh turmeric root, peeled (or use 1 tsp ground turmeric)
½ oz desiccated coconut
2 tsp tamarind paste (or grated zest and juice of 1 lime)

Heat a dry frying pan over low-medium heat, add the cumin seeds, cinnamon, cardamom seeds, star anise, and cloves, and toast them for a few minutes until aromatic (be careful not to burn them).

Remove from the heat and allow to cool, then pound using a pestle and mortar or blitz in a coffee grinder until finely ground.

Put the pan over medium heat. Add the lemongrass, shallot, garlic, ginger, chili, and turmeric, and toast for 2–3 minutes, stirring gently, until they release their flavors and start to color, then add the coconut, and toast for a further minute, being careful not to let it burn.

Blitz the wet and dry spices in a blender or small food processor with the tamarind paste, adding a little water or oil to help the ingredients come together and scraping the mixture down from the side of the blender to make sure everything is well incorporated. Store in an airtight jar in the fridge for up to 4 weeks.

TIPS

+ When you are making a curry with the paste, add a bit of sweetness—e.g., 1 teaspoon of honey, maple syrup, palm sugar, or coconut sugar.
+ Combine 3 teaspoons of paste with a 14-ounce can of coconut milk for an amazing curry sauce.

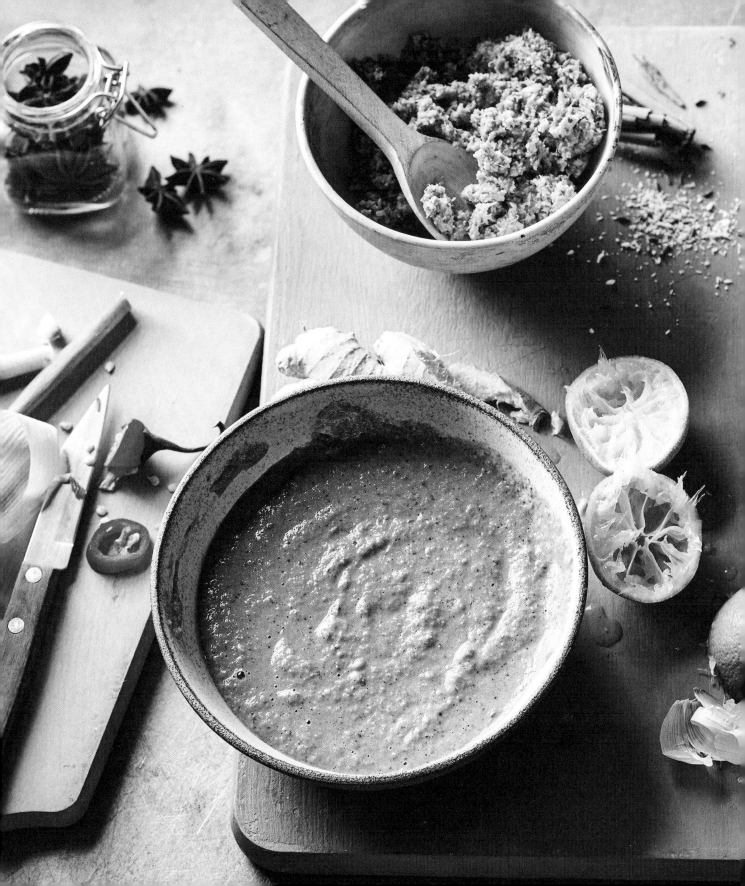

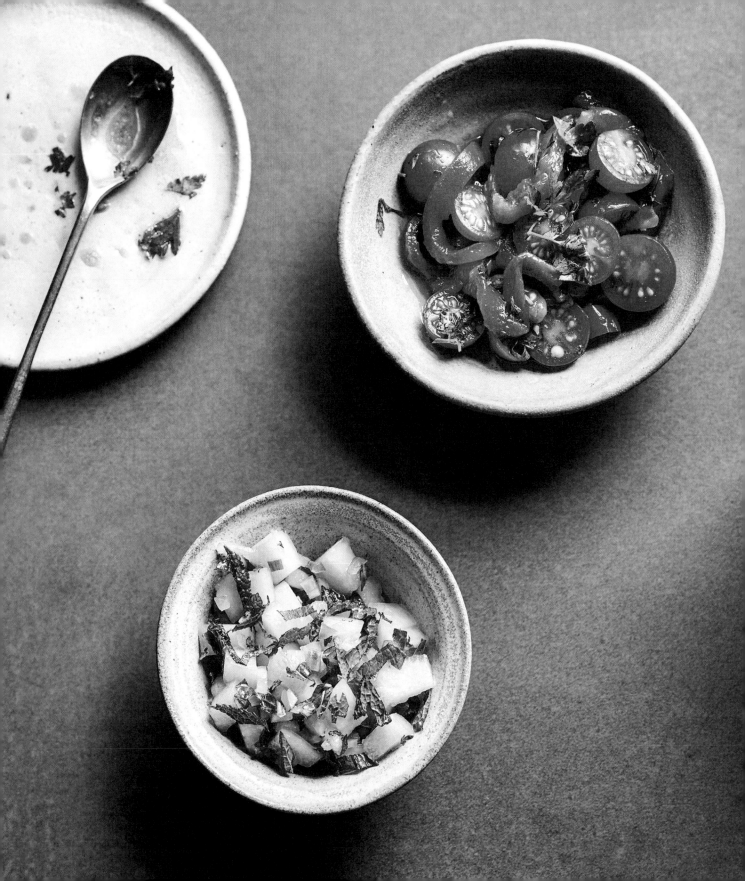

Chili Melon Relish

It's quite common to find savory and sweet flavors blended in Indian and Southeast Asian cuisine. I think the combination of summer fruits and hot spice works really well, plus it's an ingenious way of introducing more fruit and color into your diet. The antioxidant value of having more fruits on your plate could positively impact your skin and eye health, so the more colors we add to our plates and the more inventive we can be with our food, the better. Relishes like this one will ignite much more excitement and enjoyment in your food, and they are perfect for pairing with high protein foods such as beans, lentils, or even simple poached chicken.

Serves 2

5½ oz cantaloupe, skin removed and cut into
 1¼-inch cubes (diced weight)
¼ oz fresh mint leaves, finely chopped
1 green chili, deseeded and finely diced
½ shallot, finely diced
1 tbsp apple cider vinegar
2 tbsp extra-virgin olive oil
sea salt and freshly ground black pepper

Combine all the ingredients in a bowl, and add a little salt and pepper to taste. Let the flavors infuse for 10 minutes before serving.

Roasted Red Pepper Salsa

One of my favorite antipasto ingredients has to be roasted red peppers. They're a bit of a fuss to make yourself, so I often use the delicious jarred ones you can find in most supermarkets. They pair beautifully with a side of simple greens or traditional Spanish white beans and paprika. They're usually sweet and salty enough and don't require seasoning, so be wary of this before adding salt. This salsa is a sure-fire way to lift any meal. Try it on top of a tuna steak or muddled with cannellini beans and oregano.

Serves 2

5½ oz cherry tomatoes, halved
3½ oz roasted red peppers from a jar, thinly sliced
½ oz fresh flat-leaf parsley leaves, roughly chopped
1 tbsp red wine vinegar
2 tbsp extra-virgin olive oil
¼–½ tsp dried chili flakes (to taste)
sea salt and freshly ground black pepper

Combine all the ingredients in a bowl, and add salt and pepper to taste.

VARIATION

+ Try adding sweet shallots, fresh red peppers, or even sweet cooked beet to the salsa.

Aromatic Citrus-ade

Serves 6

1¼ cups water

½ oz fresh turmeric root, scrubbed and chopped

½ oz gingerroot, scrubbed and chopped

1 star anise

½ tsp freshly ground black pepper

½ oz fresh mint

½ oz fresh rosemary

2 lemons

2 red or pink grapefruits

2 oranges

2 cups spring water or carbonated water

Social media opened up a host of new connections for me. One of my earliest followers when I was still living in Sydney was Kellie from "Food to Glow" in Scotland, a health educator and nutrition adviser with Maggie's Cancer Center. I instantly resonated with her beautiful recipes and writing. We actually had the chance to meet and collaborate with a charity called Trekstock, which provides information and support to young people with cancer. This recipe is a twist on one of her delicious drinks. I tend to make a big batch of this to keep in the fridge for a few days, but it's best drunk on the day it's made to make the most of the vitamin C content from the fruit. I like to drink a small glass of it with dark greens or dishes with pulses, as citrus-based drinks are shown to aid the absorption of iron and minerals from food.

Pour the water into a saucepan, and add the turmeric, ginger, star anise and black pepper. Bring to a boil, then remove from the heat, add the mint and rosemary, and allow to cool for 20 minutes.

Meanwhile, juice the citrus fruits through a sieve directly into a large jug. Discard the seeds.

Pass the cooled, aromatic water through a sieve into the jug, along with the spring or carbonated water, and cool in the fridge. Serve chilled.

TIP

+ If the drink is too tart for your liking, add ½ teaspoon of maple syrup per serving for sweetness.

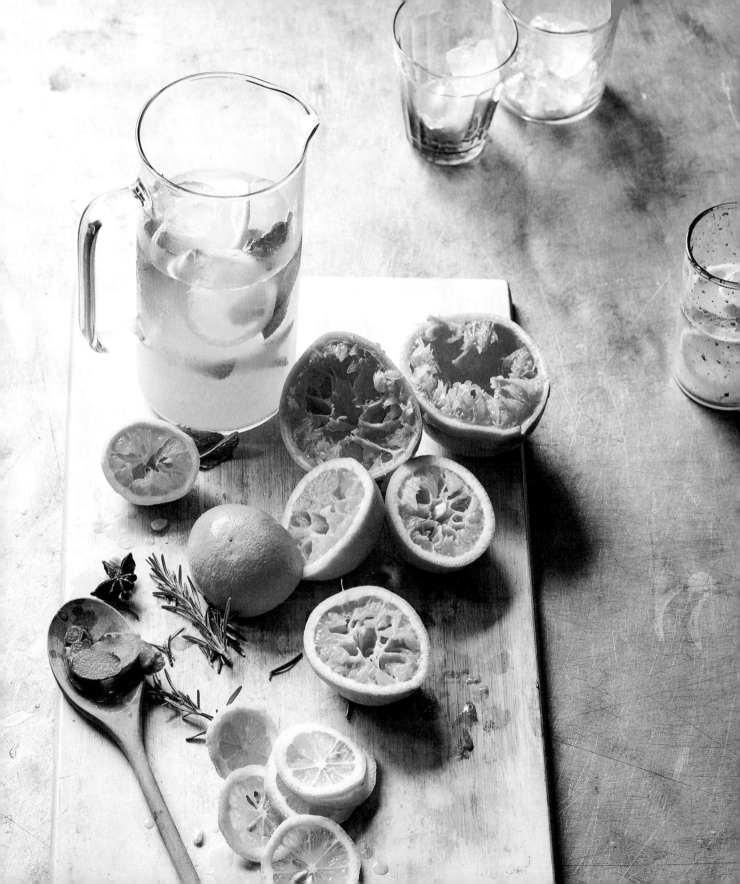

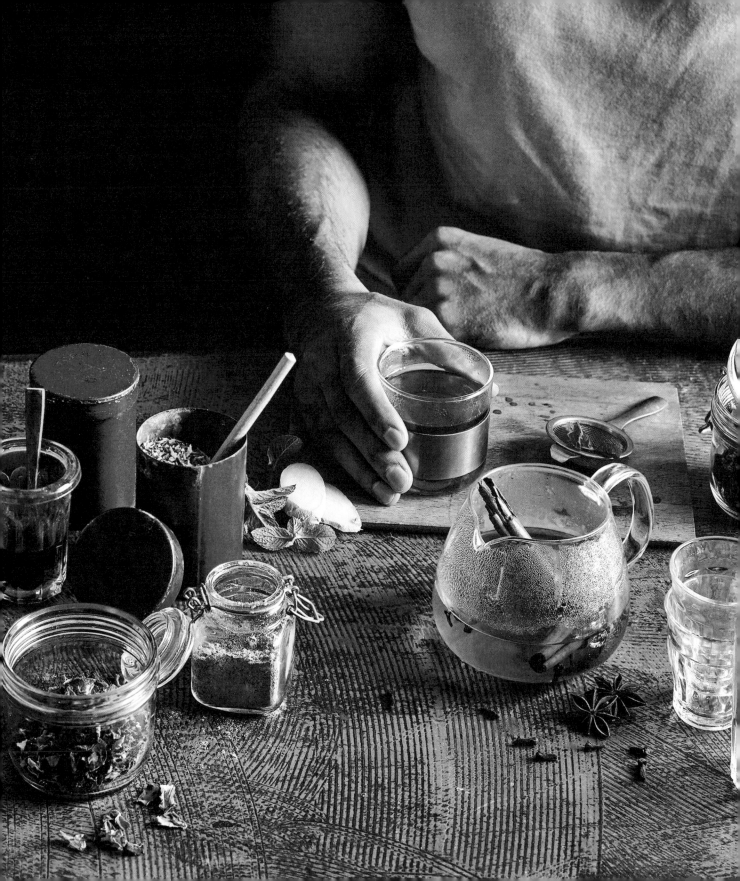

Fresh Tea Blends

I love experimenting with different tea blends. Combining fresh aromatic ingredients, like lemon rind and ginger, creates a wonderfully intense, crisp taste that blends beautifully with tea leaves and heightens the flavor of the tea. Little research into the health benefits of tea blends has been conducted, but there are some studies that suggest drinking green tea regularly helps protect us from cancer by lowering inflammation levels. Either way, these blends are comforting, delicious, and a great way to experiment with different flavors.

Each blend serves 4

Citrus Chamomile Tea

1 chamomile tea bag (or 2 tsp loose leaf)
4–5 strips of unwaxed orange peel
1 tsp fennel seeds
2 tsp honey (optional)

Black Aromatic Tea

1 black tea bag (English breakfast)
 (or 2 tsp loose leaf)
1 star anise
2 cloves
1¼–1½-inch piece of cinnamon stick
2 tsp honey (optional)

Citrus Mint and Maple Tea

½ oz mint leaves
4–5 strips of unwaxed lime peel
1 tsp maple syrup
1 black tea bag (English Breakfast) (or 2 tsp loose leaf)
 (fresh mint also pairs well with fruit teas: instead of black tea, try using berry, apricot, apple, or even cherry tea bags)

Lemon and Ginger Matcha Tea

1 tsp ceremonial-grade matcha powder
 (or 1 tea bag of green tea)
4–5 strips of unwaxed lemon peel
5 thin slices of peeled gingerroot
2 tsp maple syrup (optional)

Rose Cinnamon Tea

1 rooibos tea bag
1¼-inch piece of cinnamon stick
½ tsp dried rose petals
1 tsp coconut sugar or sweetener of choice (optional)

TIP

+ Be aware of the caffeine content in tea. I tend to have only black teas early in the day and opt for the decaffeinated ones like chamomile, valerian root, and rooibos in the evening.

NOTES

1 Fineberg NA, Haddad PM, Carpenter L, et al. The size, burden and cost of disorders of the brain in the UK. *J Psychopharmacol*. 2013. doi:10.1177/0269881113495118.

2 NHS England. Neurological conditions. https://www.england.nhs.uk/ourwork/ltc-op-eolc/ltc-eolc/our-work-on-long-term-conditions/si-areas/neurological/. Accessed 4 July 2018.

3 Gómez-Pinilla F. Brain foods: the effects of nutrients on brain function. *Nat Rev Neurosci*. 2008. doi:10.1038/nrn2421.

4 Korczyn AD. Is dementia preventable? *Dialogues Clin Neurosci*. 2009. PMC3181911.

5 Barnett JH, Hachinski V, Blackwell AD. Cognitive health begins at conception: addressing dementia as a lifelong and preventable condition. *BMC Med*. 2013. doi:10.1186/1741-7015-11-246.

6 Ramscar M, Hendrix P, Shaoul C, Milin P, Baayen H. The myth of cognitive decline: non-linear dynamics of lifelong learning. *Top Cogn Sci*. 2014. doi:10.1111/tops.12078.

7 Phillips C. Lifestyle modulators of neuroplasticity: how physical activity, mental engagement, and diet promote cognitive health during aging. *Neural Plast*. 2017. doi:10.1155/2017/3589271.

8 Fuchs E, Flügge G. Adult neuroplasticity: more than 40 years of research. *Neural Plast*. 2014. doi:10.1155/2014/541870.

9 Cramer SC, Sur M, Dobkin BH, et al. Harnessing neuroplasticity for clinical applications. *Brain*. 2011. doi:10.1093/brain/awr039.

10 Hsu TM, Kanoski SE. Blood-brain barrier disruption: mechanistic links between western diet consumption and dementia. *Front Aging Neurosci*. 2014. doi:10.3389/fnagi.2014.00088.

11 Jacka FN, Cherbuin N, Anstey KJ, Sachdev P, Butterworth P. Western diet is associated with a smaller hippocampus: a longitudinal investigation. *BMC Med*. 2015. doi:10.1186/s12916-015-0461-x.

12 Figueira I, Garcia G, Pimpão RC, et al. Polyphenols journey through blood-brain barrier towards neuronal protection. *Sci Rep*. 2017. doi:10.1038/s41598-017-11512-6.

13 Medina-Remón A, Casas R, Tressserra-Rimbau A, et al. Polyphenol intake from a Mediterranean diet decreases inflammatory biomarkers related to atherosclerosis: a substudy of the PREDIMED trial. *Br J Clin Pharmacol*. 2017. doi:10.1111/bcp.12986.

14 Macpherson H, Formica M, Harris E, Daly RM. Brain functional alterations in Type 2 diabetes: a systematic review of fMRI studies. *Front Neuroendocrinol*. 2017. doi:10.1016/j.yfrne.2017.07.001.

15 Valls-Pedret C, Lamuela-Raventós RM, Medina-Remón A, et al. Polyphenol-rich foods in the Mediterranean diet are associated with better cognitive function in elderly subjects at high cardiovascular risk. *J Alzheimer's Dis*. 2012. doi:10.3233/JAD-2012-111799.

16 Vauzour D. Dietary polyphenols as modulators of brain functions: biological actions and molecular mechanisms underpinning their beneficial effects. *Oxid Med Cell Longev*. 2012. doi:10.1155/2012/914273.

17 Morris MC, Tangney CC, Wang Y, Sacks FM, Bennett DA, Aggarwal NT. MIND diet associated with reduced incidence of Alzheimer's disease. *Alzheimer's Dement*. 2015. doi:10.1016/j.jalz.2014.11.009.

18 Morris MC, Wang Y, Barnes LL, Bennett DA, Dawson-Hughes B, Booth SL. Nutrients and bioactives in green leafy vegetables and cognitive decline. *Neurology*. 2018. doi:10.1212/WNL.0000000000004815.

19 Warren KN, Beason-Held LL, Carlson O, et al. Elevated markers of inflammation are associated with longitudinal changes in brain function in older adults. *Journals Gerontol Ser A*. 2018. doi:10.1093/gerona/glx199.

20 Ozdal T, Sela DA, Xiao J, Boyacioglu D, Chen F, Capanoglu E. The reciprocal interactions between polyphenols and gut microbiota and effects on bioaccessibility. *Nutrients*. 2016. doi:10.3390/nu8020078.

21 Su HM. Mechanisms of n-3 fatty acid-mediated development and maintenance of learning memory performance. *J Nutr Biochem*. 2010. doi:10.1016/j.jnutbio.2009.11.003.

22 Lieberman, HR. The role of protein and amino acids in sustaining and enhancing performance. http://www.nap.edu/catalog/9620.html. Accessed 5 July 2018.

256

23 Subash S, Essa MM, Al-Adawi S, Memon MA, Manivasagam T, Akbar M. Neuroprotective effects of berry fruits on neurodegenerative diseases. *Neural Regen Res.* 2014. doi:10.4103/1673-5374.139483.

24 Beilharz JE, Maniam J, Morris MJ. Diet-induced cognitive deficits: the role of fat and sugar, potential mechanisms and nutritional interventions. *Nutrients.* 2015. doi:10.3390/nu7085307.

25 Maniam J, Antoniadis CP, Youngson NA, Sinha JK, Morris MJ. Sugar consumption produces effects similar to early life stress exposure on hippocampal markers of neurogenesis and stress response. *Front Mol Neurosci.* 2016. doi:10.3389/fnmol.2015.00086.

26 Riebl SK, Davy BM. The hydration equation: update on water balance and cognitive performance. *ACSMs Health Fit J.* 2013. doi:10.1249/FIT.0b013e3182a9570f.

27 Libro R, Giacoppo S, Rajan TS, Bramanti P, Mazzon E. Natural phytochemicals in the treatment and prevention of dementia: an overview. *Molecules.* 2016. doi:10.3390/molecules21040518.

28 Park DC, Bischof GN. The aging mind: neuroplasticity in response to cognitive training. *Dialogues Clin Neurosci.* 2013. doi:10.1007/s11065-009-9119-9.

29 Hölzel BK, Carmody J, Vangel M, et al. Mindfulness practice leads to increases in regional brain gray matter density. *Psychiatry Res.* 2011. doi:10.1016/j.pscychresns.2010.08.006.

30 Menard C, Pfau ML, Hodes GE, et al. Social stress induces neurovascular pathology promoting depression. *Nat Neurosci.* 2017. doi:10.1038/s41593-017-0010-3.

31 Shansky RM, Lipps J. Stress-induced cognitive dysfunction: hormone–neurotransmitter interactions in the prefrontal cortex. *Front Hum Neurosci.* 2013. doi:10.3389/fnhum.2013.00123.

32 Sasmita AO, Kuruvilla J, Ling APK. Harnessing neuroplasticity: modern approaches and clinical future. *Int J Neurosci.* 2018. doi:10.1080/00207454.2018.1466781.

33 Baek S-S. Role of exercise on the brain. *J Exerc Rehabil.* 2016. doi:10.12965/jer.1632808.404.

34 Jessen NA, Munk ASF, Lundgaard I, Nedergaard M. The glymphatic system: a beginner's guide. *Neurochem Res.* 2015. doi:10.1007/s11064-015-1581-6.

35 McGill HC, McMahan CA, Herderick EE, Malcom GT, Tracy RE, Jack P. Origin of atherosclerosis in childhood and adolescence. *Am J Clin Nutr.* 2000. doi:10.1093/ajcn/72.5.1307s.

36 Ornish D, Scherwitz LW, Billings JH, et al. Intensive lifestyle changes for reversal of coronary heart disease. *JAMA.* doi:10.1097/00008483-199905000-00016.

37 Tuso P. A plant-based diet, atherogenesis, and coronary artery disease prevention. *Perm J.* 2015. doi:10.7812/TPP/14-036.

38 Esselstyn CB. A plant-based diet and coronary artery disease: a mandate for effective therapy. *J Geriatr Cardiol.* 2017. doi:10.11909/j.issn.1671-5411.2017.05.004.

39 Razavi M, Fournier S, Shepard DS, Ritter G, Strickler GK, Stason WB. Effects of lifestyle modification programs on cardiac risk factors. *PLoS One.* 2014. doi:10.1371/journal.pone.0114772.

40 Aldana SG, Greenlaw R, Salberg A, Merrill RM, Hager R, Jorgensen RB. The effects of an intensive lifestyle modification program on carotid artery intima-media thickness: a randomized trial. *Am J Health Promot.* 2007. doi:10.4278/0890-1171-21.6.510.

41 Widmer RJ, Flammer AJ, Lerman LO, Lerman A. The Mediterranean diet, its components, and cardiovascular disease. *Am J Med.* 2015. doi:10.1016/j.amjmed.2014.10.014.

42 Dinu M, Pagliai G, Casini A, Sofi F. Mediterranean diet and multiple health outcomes: an umbrella review of meta-analyses of observational studies and randomized trials. *Eur J Clin Nutr.* 2018. doi:10.1038/ejcn.2017.58.

43 Blekkenhorst LC, Sim M, Bondonno CP, et al. Cardiovascular health benefits of specific vegetable types: a narrative review. *Nutrients.* 2018. doi:10.3390/nu10050595.

44 Pollock RL. The effect of green leafy and cruciferous vegetable intake on the incidence of cardiovascular disease: a meta-analysis. *JRSM Cardiovasc Dis.* 2016. doi:10.1177/2048004016661435.

45 Madmani ME, Yusuf Solaiman A, Tamr Agha K, et al. Coenzyme Q10 for heart failure. *Cochrane Database Syst Rev.* 2014. doi:10.1002/14651858.CD008684.pub2.

46 Tangney CC, Rasmussen HE. Polyphenols, inflammation, and cardiovascular disease. *Curr Atheroscler Rep.* 2013. doi:10.1007/s11883-013-0324-x.

47 British Heart Foundation. *BHF CVD Statistics Factsheet – UK.* 2016. doi:10.1017/CBO9781107415324.004.

48 Khera AV, Emdin CA, Drake I, et al. Genetic risk, adherence to a healthy lifestyle, and coronary disease. *N Engl J Med.* 2016. doi:10.1056/NEJMoa1605086.

49 Garaulet M. The Mediterranean diet and obesity from a nutrigenetic and epigenetics perspective. In *The Mediterranean Diet: An Evidence-Based Approach.* Elsevier. 2014. doi:10.1016/B978-0-12-407849-9.00022-1.

50 Corella D, Ordovas JM. Nutrigenomics in cardiovascular medicine. *Circ Cardiovasc Genet.* 2009. doi:10.1161/CIRCGENETICS.109.891366.

51 Yang X, Li Y, Li Y, et al. Oxidative stress-mediated atherosclerosis: mechanisms and therapies. *Front Physiol.* 2017. doi:10.3389/fphys.2017.00600.

52 Hegab Z, Gibbons S, Neyses L, Mamas MA. Role of advanced glycation end products in cardiovascular disease. *World J Cardiol.* 2012. doi:10.4330/wjc.v4.i4.90.

53 DiNicolantonio JJ, O'Keefe JH, Wilson W. Subclinical magnesium deficiency: a principal driver of cardiovascular disease and a public health crisis. *Open Heart.* 2018. doi:10.1136/openhrt-2017-000668.

54 Bai Y, Wang X, Zhao S, Ma C, Cui J, Zheng Y. Sulforaphane protects against cardiovascular disease via Nrf2 activation. *Oxid Med Cell Longev.* 2015. doi:10.1155/2015/407580.

55 Ros E. Health benefits of nut consumption. *Nutrients.* 2010. doi:10.3390/nu2070652.

56 Mohamed S. Functional foods against metabolic syndrome (obesity, diabetes, hypertension and dyslipidemia) and cardiovascular disease. *Trends Food Sci Technol.* 2014. doi:10.1016/j.tifs.2013.11.001.

57 Simopoulos A. The importance of the Omega-6/Omega-3 fatty acid ratio in cardiovascular disease and other chronic diseases. *Exp Biol Med.* 2008. doi:10.3181/0711-MR-311.

58 Simopoulos AP. Evolutionary aspects of diet, essential fatty acids and cardiovascular disease. *Eur Heart J Suppl.* 2001. doi:10.1016/s1520-765x(01)90113-0.

59 Billingsley HE, Carbone S. The antioxidant potential of the Mediterranean diet in patients at high cardiovascular risk: an in-depth review of the PREDIMED. *Nutr Diabetes.* 2018. doi:10.1038/s41387-018-0025-1.

60 Vendrame S, Del Bo' C, Ciappellano S, Riso P, Klimis-Zacas

D. Berry fruit consumption and metabolic syndrome. *Antioxidants*. 2016. doi:10.3390/antiox5040034.

61 Basu A, Rhone M, Lyons TJ. Berries: emerging impact on cardiovascular health. *Nutr Rev*. 2010. doi:10.1111/j.1753-4887.2010.00273.x.

62 Erlund I, Koli R, Alfthan G, et al. Favorable effects of berry consumption on platelet function, blood pressure, and HDL cholesterol. *Am J Clin Nutr*. 2008. doi:87/2/323.

63 Slingerland AE, Schwabkey Z, Wiesnoski DH, Jenq RR. Clinical evidence for the microbiome in inflammatory diseases. *Front Immunol*. 2017. doi:10.3389/fimmu.2017.00400.

64 Bakker GCM, Van Erk MJ, Pellis L, et al. An antiinflammatory dietary mix modulates inflammation and oxidative and metabolic stress in overweight men: a nutrigenomics approach. *Am J Clin Nutr*. 2010. doi:10.3945/ajcn.2009.28822.

65 Mullington JM, Haack M, Toth M, Serrador JM, Meier-Ewert HK. Cardiovascular, inflammatory, and metabolic consequences of sleep deprivation. *Prog Cardiovasc Dis*. 2009. doi:10.1016/j.pcad.2008.10.003.

66 Greer SM, Goldstein AN, Walker MP. The impact of sleep deprivation on food desire in the human brain. *Nat Commun*. 2013. doi:10.1038/ncomms3259.

67 Heidt T, Sager HB, Courties G, et al. Chronic variable stress activates hematopoietic stem cells. *Nat Med*. 2014. doi:10.1038/nm.3589.

68 Dimsdale JE. Psychological stress and cardiovascular disease. *J Am Coll Cardiol*. 2008. doi:10.1016/j.jacc.2007.12.024.

69 Garaulet M, Madrid JA. Chronobiology, genetics and metabolic syndrome. *Curr Opin Lipidol*. 2009. doi:10.1097/MOL.0b013e3283292399.

70 Longo VD, Panda S. Fasting, circadian rhythms, and time-restricted feeding in healthy lifespan. *Cell Metab*. 2016. doi:10.1016/j.cmet.2016.06.001.

71 Chaix A, Zarrinpar A, Miu P, Panda S. Time-restricted feeding is a preventative and therapeutic intervention against diverse nutritional challenges. *Cell Metab*. 2014. doi:10.1016/j.cmet.2014.11.001.

72 Manoogian ENC, Panda S. Circadian rhythms, time-restricted feeding, and healthy aging. *Ageing Res Rev*. 2017. doi:10.1016/j.arr.2016.12.006.

73 Hatori M, Vollmers C, Zarrinpar A, et al. Time-restricted feeding without reducing caloric intake prevents metabolic diseases in mice fed a high-fat diet. *Cell Metab*. 2012. doi:10.1016/j.cmet.2012.04.019.

74 Hotamisligil GS. Inflammation and metabolic disorders. *Nature*. 2006. doi:10.1038/nature05485.

75 Minihane AM, Vinoy S, Russell WR, et al. Low-grade inflammation, diet composition and health: current research evidence and its translation. *Br J Nutr*. 2015. doi:10.1017/S0007114515002093.

76 Rubio-Ruiz ME, Peredo-Escárcega AE, Cano-Martínez A, Guarner-Lans V. An evolutionary perspective of nutrition and inflammation as mechanisms of cardiovascular disease. *Int J Evol Biol*. 2015. doi:10.1155/2015/179791.

77 Hotamisligil GS. Inflammation, metaflammation and immunometabolic disorders. *Nature*. 2017. doi:10.1038/nature21363.

78 Miller AH, Raison CL. The role of inflammation in depression: from evolutionary imperative to modern treatment target. *Nat Rev Immunol*. 2016. doi:10.1038/nri.2015.5.

79 Hunter P. The inflammation theory of disease. the growing realization that chronic inflammation is crucial in many diseases opens new avenues for treatment. *EMBO Rep*. 2012. doi:10.1038/embor.2012.142.

80 Lopez-Candales A, Hernández Burgos PM, Hernandez-Suarez DF, Harris D. Linking chronic inflammation with cardiovascular disease: from normal aging to the metabolic syndrome. *J Nat Sci*. 2017.

81 Fernández-Sánchez A, Madrigal-Santillán E, Bautista M, et al. Inflammation, oxidative stress, and obesity. *Int J Mol Sci*. 2011. doi:10.3390/ijms12053117.

82 Hotamisligil GS. Inflammation and metabolic disorders. *Nature*. 2006. doi:10.1038/nature05485.

83 Ortega-Gómez A, Perretti M, Soehnlein O. Resolution of inflammation: an integrated view. *EMBO Mol Med*. 2013. doi:10.1002/emmm.201202382.

84 Manzel A, Muller DN, Hafler DA, Erdman SE, Linker RA, Kleinewietfeld M. Role of "western diet" in inflammatory autoimmune diseases. *Curr Allergy Asthma Rep*. 2014. doi:10.1007/s11882-013-0404-6.

85 Galland L. Diet and inflammation. *Nutr Clin Pract*. 2010. doi:10.1177/0884533610385703.

86 Chrysohoou C, Panagiotakos DB, Pitsavos C, Das UN, Stefanadis C. Adherence to the Mediterranean diet attenuates inflammation and coagulation process in healthy adults: the ATTICA study. *J Am Coll Cardiol*. 2004. doi:10.1016/j.jacc.2004.03.039.

87 Genné-Bacon EA. Thinking evolutionarily about obesity. *Yale J Biol Med*. 2014.

88 Coelho M, Oliveira T, Fernandes R. Biochemistry of adipose tissue: an endocrine organ. *Arch Med Sci*. 2013. doi:10.5114/aoms.2013.33181.

89 Moschen AR, Molnar C, Geiger S, et al. Anti-inflammatory effects of excessive weight loss: potent suppression of adipose interleukin 6 and tumour necrosis factor alpha expression. *Gut*. 2010. doi:10.1136/gut.2010.214577.

90 Sears B, Ricordi C. Anti-inflammatory nutrition as a pharmacological approach to treat obesity. *J Obes*. 2011. doi:10.1155/2011/431985.

91 Schirmer M, Smeekens SP, Vlamakis H, et al. Linking the human gut microbiome to inflammatory cytokine production capacity. *Cell*. 2016. doi:10.1016/j.cell.2016.10.020.

92 Ma D, Forsythe P, Bienenstock J. Live Lactobacillus reuteri is essential for the inhibitory effect on tumor necrosis factor alpha-induced interleukin-8 expression. *Infect Immun*. 2004. doi:10.1128/IAI.72.9.5308-5314.2004.

93 Zhang L, Li N, Caicedo R, Neu J. Alive and dead Lactobacillus rhamnosus GG decrease tumor necrosis factor-alpha-induced interleukin-8 production in Caco-2 cells. *J Nutr*. 2005. doi:135/7/1752 [pii].

94 O'Hara AM, O'Regan P, Fanning Á, et al. Functional modulation of human intestinal epithelial cell responses by Bifidobacterium infantis and Lactobacillus salivarius. *Immunology*. 2006. doi:10.1111/j.1365-2567.2006.02358.x.

95 Kelly D, Campbell JI, King TP, et al. Commensal anaerobic gut bacteria attenuate inflammation by regulating nuclear-cytoplasmic shuttling of PPAR-gamma and RelA. *Nat Immunol*. 2004. doi:10.1038/ni1018.

96 Flint HJ, Scott KP, Louis P, Duncan SH. The role of the gut microbiota in nutrition and health. *Nat Rev Gastroenterol Hepatol*. 2012. doi:10.1038/nrgastro.2012.156.

97 Allen AP, Hutch W, Borre YE, et al. Bifidobacterium longum 1714 as a translational psychobiotic: modulation of stress,

258

electrophysiology and neurocognition in healthy volunteers. *Transl Psychiatry*. 2016. doi:10.1038/tp.2016.191.

98 Calder PC. Long chain fatty acids and gene expression in inflammation and immunity. *Curr Opin Clin Nutr Metab Care*. 2013. doi:10.1097/MCO.0b013e3283620616.

99 Wall R, Ross RP, Fitzgerald GF, Stanton C. Fatty acids from fish: the anti-inflammatory potential of long-chain omega-3 fatty acids. *Nutr Rev*. 2010. doi:10.1111/j.1753-4887.2010 .00287.x.

100 Yubero-Serrano EM, Gonzalez-Guardia L, Rangel-Zuñiga O, et al. Mediterranean diet supplemented with coenzyme Q10 modifies the expression of proinflammatory and endoplasmic reticulum stress–related genes in elderly men and women. *Journals Gerontol*. 2012. doi:10.1093/gerona/glr167.

101 Konstantinidou V, Khymenets O, Fito M, et al. Characterization of human gene expression changes after olive oil ingestion: an exploratory approach. *Folia Biol (Praha)*. 2009.

102 Santangelo C, Varì R, Scazzocchio B, Di Benedetto R, Filesi C, Masella R. Polyphenols, intracellular signalling and inflammation. *Ann Ist Super Sanita*. 2007.

103 González R, Ballester I, López-Posadas R, et al. Effects of flavonoids and other polyphenols on inflammation. *Crit Rev Food Sci Nutr*. 2011. doi:10.1080/10408390903584094.

104 Yoon J-H, Baek SJ. Molecular targets of dietary polyphenols with anti-inflammatory properties. *Yonsei Med J*. 2005. doi:10.3349/ymj.2005.46.5.585.

105 Sears B. Anti-inflammatory diets. *J Am Coll Nutr*. 2015. doi:10.1080/07315724.2015.1080105.

106 Ricker MA, Haas WC. Anti-inflammatory diet in clinical practice: a review. *Nutr Clin Pract*. 2017. doi:10.1177 /0884533617700353.

107 Guerrero-Beltrán CE, Calderón-Oliver M, Pedraza-Chaverri J, Chirino YI. Protective effect of sulforaphane against oxidative stress: recent advances. *Exp Toxicol Pathol*. 2012. doi:10.1016/j.etp.2010.11.005.

108 Tarozzi A, Angeloni C, Malaguti M, Morroni F, Hrelia S, Hrelia P. Sulforaphane as a potential protective phytochemical against neurodegenerative diseases. *Oxid Med Cell Longev*. 2013. doi:10.1155/2013/415078.

109 Khoo HE, Azlan A, Tang ST, Lim SM. Anthocyanidins and anthocyanins: colored pigments as food, pharmaceutical ingredients, and the potential health benefits. *Food Nutr Res*. 2017. doi:10.1080/16546628.2017.1361779.

110 Giugliano D, Ceriello A, Esposito K. The effects of diet on inflammation: emphasis on the metabolic syndrome. *J Am Coll Cardiol*. 2006. doi:10.1016/j.jacc.2006.03.052.

111 Esposito K, Nappo F, Marfella R, et al. Inflammatory cytokine concentrations are acutely increased by hyperglycemia in humans: role of oxidative stress. *Circulation*. 2002. doi:10.1161/01.CIR.0000034509.14906.AE.

112 North CJ, Venter CS, Jerling JC. The effects of dietary fiber on C-reactive protein, an inflammation marker predicting cardiovascular disease. *Eur J Clin Nutr*. 2009. doi:10.1038 /ejcn.2009.8.

113 Chin KY. The spice for joint inflammation: anti-inflammatory role of curcumin in treating osteoarthritis. *Drug Des Devel Ther*. 2016. doi:10.2147/DDDT.S117432.

114 Kunnumakkara AB, Sailo BL, Banik K, et al. Chronic diseases, inflammation, and spices: how are they linked? *J Transl Med*. 2018. doi:10.1186/s12967-018-1381-2.

115 Khanna S, Jaiswal KS, Gupta B. Managing rheumatoid arthritis with dietary interventions. *Front Nutr*. 2017. doi:10.3389/fnut.2017.00052.

116 Jungbauer A, Medjakovic S. Anti-inflammatory properties of culinary herbs and spices that ameliorate the effects of metabolic syndrome. *Maturitas*. 2012. doi:10.1016/j .maturitas.2011.12.009.

117 Agarwal AK. Spice up your life: adipose tissue and inflammation. *J Lipids*. 2014. doi:10.1155/2014/182575.

118 Daubenmier J, Kristeller J, Hecht FM, et al. Mindfulness intervention for stress eating to reduce cortisol and abdominal fat among overweight and obese women: an exploratory randomized controlled study. *J Obes*. 2011. doi:10.1155/2011 /651936.

119 Creswell JD, Irwin MR, Burklund LJ, et al. Mindfulness-based stress reduction training reduces loneliness and pro-inflammatory gene expression in older adults: a small randomized controlled trial. *Brain Behav Immun*. 2012. doi:10.1016/j.bbi.2012.07.006.

120 Buric I, Farias M, Jong J, Mee C, Brazil IA. What is the molecular signature of mind-body interventions? A systematic review of gene expression changes induced by meditation and related practices. *Front Immunol*. 2017. doi:10.3389 /fimmu.2017.00670.

121 Bower JE, Irwin MR. Mind–body therapies and control of inflammatory biology: a descriptive review. *Brain Behav Immun*. 2016. doi:10.1016/j.bbi.2015.06.012.

122 Hansen MM, Jones R, Tocchini K. Shinrin-yoku (forest bathing) and nature therapy: a state-of-the-art review. *Int J Environ Res Public Health*. 2017. doi:10.3390/ ijerph14080851.

123 Song C, Ikei H, Miyazaki Y. Physiological effects of nature therapy: a review of the research in Japan. *Int J Environ Res Public Health*. 2016. doi:10.3390/ijerph13080781.

124 Mullington JM, Simpson NS, Meier-Ewert HK, Haack M. Sleep loss and inflammation. *Best Pract Res Clin Endocrinol Metab*. 2010. doi:10.1016/j.beem.2010.08.014.

125 Miller M, Cappuccio F. Inflammation, sleep, obesity and cardiovascular disease. *Curr Vasc Pharmacol*. 2007. doi:10.2174/157016107780368280.

126 Alberts B, Johnson A, Lewis J, Raff M, Roberts K, Walter P. *Molecular Biology of the Cell*. 4th ed. Garland Science. 2008. doi:10.1002/1521-3773(20010316)40:6<9823::AID -ANIE9823>3.3.CO;2-C.

127 Chandel NS. *Navigating Metabolism*. CSHL Press. 2015. doi:10.1016/B978-0-08-025486-9.50014-1.

128 Clemente JC, Manasson J, Scher JU. The role of the gut microbiome in systemic inflammatory disease. *BMJ*. 2018. doi:10.1136/bmj.j5145.

129 Vighi G, Marcucci F, Sensi L, Di Cara G, Frati F. Allergy and the gastrointestinal system. *Clin Exp Immunol*. 2008. doi:10.1111/j.1365-2249.2008.03713.x.

130 Belkaid Y, Hand TW. Role of the microbiota in immunity and inflammation. *Cell*. 2014. doi:10.1016/j.cell.2014.03.011.

131 Kumar V, Abbas AK, Fausto N, Aster JC. *Robbins & Cotran Pathologic Basis of Disease*. Elsevier. 2010.

132 Li B, Selmi C, Tang R, Gershwin ME, Ma X. The microbiome and autoimmunity: a paradigm from the gut–liver axis. *Cell Mol Immunol*. 2018. doi:10.1038/cmi.2018.7.

133 Yurkovetskiy LA, Pickard JM, Chervonsky AV. Microbiota and autoimmunity: exploring new avenues. *Cell Host Microbe*. 2015. doi:10.1016/j.chom.2015.04.010.

134 Fujimura KE, Lynch SV. Microbiota in allergy and asthma and the emerging relationship with the gut microbiome. *Cell Host Microbe*. 2015. doi:10.1016/j.chom.2015.04.007.

135 Mu Q, Kirby J, Reilly CM, Luo XM. Leaky gut as a danger

signal for autoimmune diseases. *Front Immunol.* 2017. doi:10.3389/fimmu.2017.00598.

136 Konijeti GG, Kim N, Lewis JD, et al. Efficacy of the autoimmune protocol diet for inflammatory bowel disease. *Inflamm Bowel Dis.* 2017. doi:10.1097/MIB .0000000000001221.

137 Fasano A. Leaky gut and autoimmune diseases. *Clin Rev Allergy Immunol.* 2012. doi:10.1007/s12016-011-8291-x.

138 West AP, Shadel GS, Ghosh S. Mitochondria in innate immune responses. *Nat Rev Immunol.* 2011. doi:10.1038 /nri2975.

139 Weinberg SE, Sena LA, Chandel NS. Mitochondria in the regulation of innate and adaptive immunity. *Immunity.* 2015. doi:10.1016/j.immuni.2015.02.002.

140 De Felice FG, Ferreira ST. Inflammation, defective insulin signaling, and mitochondrial dysfunction as common molecular denominators connecting type 2 diabetes to Alzheimer's disease. *Diabetes.* 2014. doi:10.2337/db13-1954.

141 Willis JCD, Lord GM. Immune biomarkers: the promises and pitfalls of personalized medicine. *Nat Rev Immunol.* 2015. doi:10.1038/nri3820.

142 Mora JR, Iwata M, Von Andrian UH. Vitamin effects on the immune system: vitamins A and D take centre stage. *Nat Rev Immunol.* 2008. doi:10.1038/nri2378.

143 Wintergerst ES, Maggini S, Hornig DH. Immune-enhancing role of vitamin C and zinc and effect on clinical conditions. *Ann Nutr Metab.* 2006. doi:10.1159/000090495.

144 Nieman DC, Henson DA, McAnulty SR, et al. Influence of vitamin C supplementation on oxidative and immune changes after an ultramarathon. *J Appl Physiol.* 2002. doi:10.1152 /japplphysiol.00961.2001.

145 Heuser G, Vojdani A. Enhancement of natural killer cell activity and T and B cell function by buffered vitamin C in patients exposed to toxic chemicals: the role of protein kinase-C. *Immunopharmacol Immunotoxicol.* 1997. doi:10.3109/08923979709046977.

146 Hoffmann PR, Berry MJ. The influence of selenium on immune responses. *Mol Nutr Food Res.* 2008. doi:10.1002 /mnfr.200700330.

147 Prasad AS. Zinc in human health: effect of zinc on immune cells. *Mol Med.* 2008. doi:10.2119/2008-00033.Prasad.

148 Pekmezci D. Vitamin E and immunity. *Vitam Horm.* 2011. doi:10.1016/B978-0-12-386960-9.00008-3.

149 Meijer K, De Vos P, Priebe MG. Butyrate and other short-chain fatty acids as modulators of immunity: what relevance for health? *Curr Opin Clin Nutr Metab Care.* 2010. doi:10.1097/MCO.0b013e32833eebe5.

150 Triantafyllidi A, Xanthos T, Papalois A, Triantafillidis JK. Herbal and plant therapy in patients with inflammatory bowel disease. *Ann Gastroenterol.* 2015. PMC4367210.

151 Haddad PS, Azar GA, Groom S, Boivin M. Natural health products, modulation of immune function and prevention of chronic diseases. *Evid Based Complement Alternat Med.* 2005. doi:10.1093/ecam/neh125.

152 Simpson RJ, Kunz H, Agha N, Graff R. Exercise and the regulation of immune functions. In *Progress in Molecular Biology and Translational Science.* 2015. doi:10.1016/bs .pmbts.2015.08.001.

153 Eluamai A, Brooks K. Effect of aerobic exercise on mitochondrial DNA and aging. *J Exerc Sci Fit.* 2013. doi:10.1016/j.jesf.2013.03.003.

154 Robinson MM, Dasari S, Konopka AR, et al. Enhanced protein translation underlies improved metabolic and physical adaptations to different exercise training modes in young and old humans. *Cell Metab.* 2017. doi:10.1016/j .cmet.2017.02.009.

155 Gunzer W, Konrad M, Pail E. Exercise-induced immuno-depression in endurance athletes and nutritional intervention with carbohydrate, protein and fat: what is possible, what is not? *Nutrients.* 2012. doi:10.3390/nu4091187.

156 Qu S, Olafsrud SM, Meza-Zepeda LA, Saatcioglu F. Rapid gene expression changes in peripheral blood lymphocytes upon practice of a comprehensive yoga program. *PLoS One.* 2013. doi:10.1371/journal.pone.0061910.

157 Bauer ME. Stress, glucocorticoids and ageing of the immune system. *Stress.* 2005. doi:10.1080/10253890500100240.

158 Li Q, Kobayashi M, Wakayama Y, et al. Effect of phytoncide from trees on human natural killer cell function. *Int J Immunopathol Pharmacol.* 2009. doi:10.1177/039463200 902200410.

159 Prietl B, Treiber G, Pieber TR, Amrein K. Vitamin D and immune function. *Nutrients.* 2013. doi:10.3390/nu5072502.

160 Hewison M. Vitamin D and immune function: an overview. *Proc Nutr Soc.* 2012. doi:10.1017/S0029665111001650.

161 Besedovsky L, Lange T, Born J. Sleep and immune function. *Pflugers Arch Eur J Physiol.* 2012. doi:10.1007/s00424-011 -1044-0.

162 Myles IA. Fast food fever: reviewing the impacts of the Western diet on immunity. *Nutr J.* 2014. doi:10.1186/1475 -2891-13-61.

163 Steward WP, Brown K. Cancer chemoprevention: a rapidly evolving field. *Br J Cancer.* 2013. doi:10.1038/bjc.2013.280.

164 Sofi F, Cesari F, Abbate R, Gensini GF, Casini A. Adherence to Mediterranean diet and health status: meta-analysis. *BMJ.* 2008. doi:10.1136/bmj.a1344.

165 Boffetta P, Couto E, Wichmann J, et al. Fruit and vegetable intake and overall cancer risk in the European prospective investigation into cancer and nutrition (EPIC). *J Natl Cancer Inst.* 2010. doi:10.1093/jnci/djq072.

166 Sofi F, Macchi C, Abbate R, Gensini GF, Casini A. Mediterranean diet and health status: an updated meta-analysis and a proposal for a literature-based adherence score. *Public Health Nutr.* 2013. doi:10.1017/S13689800 13003169.

167 Theodoratou E, Tzoulaki I, Zgaga L, Ioannidis JPA. Vitamin D and multiple health outcomes: umbrella review of systematic reviews and meta-analyses of observational studies and randomized trials. *BMJ.* 2014. doi:10.1136 /bmj.g2035.

168 Borek C. Dietary antioxidants and human cancer. *Integr Cancer Ther.* 2004. doi:10.1177/1534735404270578.

169 Bidlack WR, Brown RC, Mohan C. Nutritional parameters that alter hepatic drug metabolism, conjugation, and toxicity. *Fed Proc.* 1986.

170 Hodges RE, Minich DM. Modulation of metabolic detoxification pathways using foods and food-derived components: a scientific review with clinical application. *J Nutr Metab.* 2015. doi:10.1155/2015/760689.

171 Pecorino L. *Molecular Biology of Cancer: Mechanisms, Targets, and Therapeutics.* OUP. 2008. doi:10.1038 /nchembio840.

172 Kurutas EB. The importance of antioxidants which play the role in cellular response against oxidative/nitrosative stress: current state. *Nutr J.* 2016. doi:10.1186/s12937-016-0186-5.

173 Elsamanoudy AZ, Neamat-Allah MAM, Mohammad FAH, Hassanien M, Nada HA. The role of nutrition related genes and

nutrigenetics in understanding the pathogenesis of cancer. *J Microsc Ultrastruct*. 2016. doi:10.1016/j.jmau.2016.02.002.

174　Riboli E, Hunt KJ, Slimani N, et al. European prospective investigation into cancer and nutrition (EPIC): study populations and data collection. *Public Health Nutr*. 2002. doi:10.1079/PHN2002394.

175　Donohoe CL, Doyle SL, Reynolds JV. Visceral adiposity, insulin resistance and cancer risk. *Diabetol Metab Syndr*. 2011. doi:10.1186/1758-5996-3-12.

176　Brody JG, Rudel RA. Environmental pollutants and breast cancer. *Environ Health Perspect*. 2003. doi:10.1289/ehp.6310.

177　Goodman B, Gardner H. The microbiome and cancer. *J Pathol*. 2018. doi:10.1002/path.5047.

178　Gopalakrishnan V, Helmink BA, Spencer CN, Reuben A, Wargo JA. The influence of the gut microbiome on cancer, immunity, and cancer immunotherapy. *Cancer Cell*. 2018. doi:10.1016/j.ccell.2018.03.015.

179　Surh YJ. Cancer chemoprevention with dietary phytochemicals. *Nat Rev Cancer*. 2003. doi:10.1038/nrc1189.

180　Rafter JJ. Scientific basis of biomarkers and benefits of functional foods for reduction of disease risk: cancer. *Br J Nutr*. 2002. doi:10.1079/BJN2002686.

181　Trejo-Solis C, Pedraza-Chaverri J, Torres-Ramos M, et al. Multiple molecular and cellular mechanisms of action of lycopene in cancer inhibition. *Evid Based Complement Alternat Med*. 2013. doi:10.1155/2013/705121.

182　Holzapfel NP, Holzapfel BM, Champ S, Feldthusen J, Clements J, Hutmacher DW. The potential role of lycopene for the prevention and therapy of prostate cancer: from molecular mechanisms to clinical evidence. *Int J Mol Sci*. 2013. doi:10.3390/ijms140714620.

183　Roy S, Khanna S, Alessio HM, et al. Anti-angiogenic property of edible berries. *Free Radic Res*. 2002. doi:10.1080/1071576021000006662.

184　Bagchi D, Sen CK, Bagchi M, Atalay M. Anti-angiogenic, antioxidant, and anti-carcinogenic properties of a novel anthocyanin-rich berry extract formula. *Biochemistry (Mosc)*. 2004. doi:10.1023/B:BIRY.0000016355.19999.93.

185　Manson MM. Cancer prevention: the potential for diet to modulate molecular signalling. *Trends Mol Med*. 2003. doi:10.1016/S1471-4914(02)00002-3.

186　Kristo A, Klimis-Zacas D, Sikalidis A. Protective role of dietary berries in cancer. *Antioxidants*. 2016. doi:10.3390/antiox5040037.

187　Seeram NP, Adams LS, Zhang Y, et al. Blackberry, black raspberry, blueberry, cranberry, red raspberry, and strawberry extracts inhibit growth and stimulate apoptosis of human cancer cells in vitro. *J Agric Food Chem*. 2006. doi:10.1021/jf061750g.

188　Van Breda SGJ, Wilms LC, Gaj S, et al. Can transcriptomics provide insight into the chemopreventive mechanisms of complex mixtures of phytochemicals in humans? *Antioxid Redox Signal*. 2014. doi:10.1089/ars.2013.5528.

189　Yoshida K, Ushida Y, Ishijima T, et al. Broccoli sprout extract induces detoxification-related gene expression and attenuates acute liver injury. *World J Gastroenterol*. 2015. doi:10.3748/wjg.v21.i35.10091.

190　Melchini A, Traka MH. Biological profile of erucin: a new promising anticancer agent from cruciferous vegetables. *Toxins (Basel)*. 2010. doi:10.3390/toxins2040593.

191　Egner PA, Chen JG, Zarth AT, et al. Rapid and sustainable detoxication of airborne pollutants by broccoli sprout beverage: Results of a randomized clinical trial in China. *Cancer Prev Res*. 2014. doi:10.1158/1940-6207.CAPR-14-0103.

192　Surh YJ. Molecular mechanisms of chemopreventive effects of selected dietary and medicinal phenolic substances. In *Mutation Research—Fundamental and Molecular Mechanisms of Mutagenesis*. 1999. doi:10.1016/S1383-5742(99)00057-5.

193　David LA, Maurice CF, Carmody RN, et al. Diet rapidly and reproducibly alters the human gut microbiome. *Nature*. 2014. doi:10.1038/nature12820.

194　West NJ, Clark SK, Phillips RKS, et al. Eicosapentaenoic acid reduces rectal polyp number and size in familial adenomatous polyposis. *Gut*. 2010. doi:10.1136/gut.2009.200642.

195　Stephenson JA, Al-Taan O, Arshad A, Morgan B, Metcalfe MS, Dennison AR. The multifaceted effects of omega-3 polyunsaturated fatty acids on the hallmarks of cancer. *J Lipids*. 2013. doi:10.1155/2013/261247.

196　Park JM, Kwon SH, Han YM, Hahm KB, Kim EH. Omega-3 polyunsaturated fatty acids as potential chemopreventive agent for gastrointestinal cancer. *J Cancer Prev*. 2013. doi:10.15430/JCP.2013.18.3.201.

197　White MP, Pahl S, Ashbullby KJ, Burton F, Depledge MH. The effects of exercising in different natural environments on psycho-physiological outcomes in post-menopausal women: a simulation study. *Int J Environ Res Public Health*. 2015. doi:10.3390/ijerph120911929.

198　Gladwell VF, Brown DK, Wood C, Sandercock GR, Barton JL. The great outdoors: how a green exercise environment can benefit all. *Extrem Physiol Med*. 2013. doi:10.1186/2046-7648-2-3.

199　Woods JA, Wilund KR, Martin SA, Kistler BM. Exercise, inflammation and aging. *Aging Dis*. 2012. PMC3320801.

200　Friedenreich CM, Shaw E, Neilson HK, Brenner DR. Epidemiology and biology of physical activity and cancer recurrence. *J Mol Med*. 2017. doi:10.1007/s00109-017-1558-9.

201　Garland CF, Garland FC, Gorham ED, et al. The role of vitamin D in cancer prevention. *Am J Public Health*. 2006. doi:10.2105/AJPH.2004.045260.

202　Révész D, Milaneschi Y, Verhoeven JE, Penninx BW. Telomere length as a marker of cellular aging is associated with prevalence and progression of metabolic syndrome. *J Clin Endocrinol Metab*. 2014. doi:10.1210/jc.2014-1851.

203　Jacobs TL, Epel ES, Lin J, et al. Intensive meditation training, immune cell telomerase activity, and psychological mediators. *Psychoneuroendocrinology*. 2011. doi:10.1016/j.psyneuen.2010.09.010.

204　Epel E, Daubenmier J, Moskowitz JT, Folkman S, Blackburn E. Can meditation slow rate of cellular aging? Cognitive stress, mindfulness, and telomeres. *Ann N Y Acad Sci*. 2009. doi:10.1111/j.1749-6632.2009.04414.x.

205　Moreno-Smith M, Lutgendorf SK, Sood AK. Impact of stress on cancer metastasis. *Future Oncol*. 2011. doi:10.2217/fon.10.142.

206　Ornish D, Magbanua MJM, Weidner G, et al. Changes in prostate gene expression in men undergoing an intensive nutrition and lifestyle intervention. *Proc Natl Acad Sci*. 2008. doi:10.1073/pnas.0803080105.

207　Hidaka BH. Depression as a disease of modernity: explanations for increasing prevalence. *J Affect Disord*. 2012. doi:10.1016/j.jad.2011.12.036.

208 Sarris J, Logan AC, Akbaraly TN, et al. Nutritional medicine as mainstream in psychiatry. *The Lancet Psychiatry*. 2015. doi:10.1016/S2215-0366(14)00051-0.

209 Moylan S, Berk M, Dean O, et al. Oxidative and nitrosative stress in depression: why so much stress? *Neurosci Biobehav Rev*. 2014. doi:10.1016/j.neubiorev.2014.05.007.

210 Louveau A, Smirnov I, Keyes TJ, et al. Structural and functional features of central nervous system lymphatic vessels. *Nature*. 2015. doi:10.1038/nature14432.

211 Schiepers OJG, Wichers MC, Maes M. Cytokines and major depression. *Prog Neuro-Psychopharmacology Biol Psychiatry*. 2005. doi:10.1016/j.pnpbp.2004.11.003.

212 Galea I, Bechmann I, Perry VH. What is immune privilege (not)? *Trends Immunol*. 2007. doi:10.1016/j.it.2006.11.004.

213 Lucas M, Chocano-Bedoya P, Shulze MB, et al. Inflammatory dietary pattern and risk of depression among women. *Brain Behav Immun*. 2014. doi:10.1016/j.bbi.2013.09.014.

214 Parletta N, Zarnowiecki D, Cho J, et al. A Mediterranean-style dietary intervention supplemented with fish oil improves diet quality and mental health in people with depression: a randomized controlled trial (HELFIMED). *Nutritional Neuroscience*. 2017.

215 Jacka FN, O'Neil A, Opie R, et al. A randomized controlled trial of dietary improvement for adults with major depression (the "SMILES" trial). *BMC Med*. 2017. doi:10.1186/s12916-017-0791-y.

216 Sánchez-Villegas A, Henríquez P, Bes-Rastrollo M, Doreste J. Mediterranean diet and depression. *Public Health Nutr*. 2006. doi:10.1017/S1368980007668578.

217 Lynch SV, Pedersen O. The human intestinal microbiome in health and disease. *N Engl J Med*. 2016. doi:10.1056/NEJMra1600266.

218 Clapp M, Aurora N, Herrera L, Bhatia M, Wilen E, Wakefield S. Gut microbiota's effect on mental health: the gut-brain axis. *Clin Pract*. 2017. doi:10.4081/cp.2017.987.

219 Sarkar A, Lehto SM, Harty S, Dinan TG, Cryan JF, Burnet PWJ. Psychobiotics and the manipulation of bacteria–gut–brain signals. *Trends Neurosci*. 2016. doi:10.1016/j.tins.2016.09.002.

220 Bravo JA, Forsythe P, Chew MV, et al. Ingestion of Lactobacillus strain regulates emotional behavior and central GABA receptor expression in a mouse via the vagus nerve. *Proc Natl Acad Sci*. 2011. doi:10.1073/pnas.1102999108.

221 Tillisch K, Labus J, Kilpatrick L, et al. Consumption of fermented milk product with probiotic modulates brain activity. *Gastroenterology*. 2013. doi:10.1053/j.gastro.2013.02.043.

222 Rieder R, Wisniewski PJ, Alderman BL, Campbell SC. Microbes and mental health: a review. *Brain Behav Immun*. 2017. doi:10.1016/j.bbi.2017.01.016.

223 Molteni R, Barnard RJ, Ying Z, Roberts CK, Gómez-Pinilla F. A high-fat, refined sugar diet reduces hippocampal brain-derived neurotrophic factor, neuronal plasticity, and learning. *Neuroscience*. 2002. doi:10.1016/S0306-4522(02)00123-9.

224 Knüppel A, Shipley MJ, Llewellyn CH, Brunner EJ. Sugar intake from sweet food and beverages, common mental disorder and depression: prospective findings from the Whitehall II study. *Sci Rep*. 2017. doi:10.1038/s41598-017-05649-7.

225 Riediger ND, Othman RA, Suh M, Moghadasian MH. A systemic review of the roles of n-3 fatty acids in health and disease. *J Am Diet Assoc*. 2009. doi:10.1016/j.jada.2008.12.022.

226 Grosso G, Pajak A, Marventano S, et al. Role of omega-3 fatty acids in the treatment of depressive disorders: a comprehensive meta-analysis of randomized clinical trials. *PLoS One*. 2014. doi:10.1371/journal.pone.0096905.

227 Sublette ME, Ellis SP, Geant AL, Mann JJ. Meta-analysis: effects of eicosapentaenoic acid in clinical trials in depression. *J Clin Psychiatry*. 2011. doi:10.4088/JCP.10m06634.

228 Jacka FN. Nutritional psychiatry: where to next? *EBioMedicine*. 2017. doi:10.1016/j.ebiom.2017.02.020.

229 Bodnar LM, Wisner KL. Nutrition and depression: implications for improving mental health among childbearing-aged women. *Biol Psychiatry*. 2005. doi:10.1016/j.biopsych.2005.05.009.

230 Mikkelsen K, Stojanovska L, Polenakovic M, Bosevski M, Apostolopoulos V. Exercise and mental health. *Maturitas*. 2017. doi:10.1016/j.maturitas.2017.09.003.

231 Dunn AL, Trivedi MH, Kampert JB, Clark CG, Chambliss HO. Exercise treatment for depression: efficacy and dose response. *Am J Prev Med*. 2005. doi:10.1016/j.amepre.2004.09.003.

232 Teychenne M, Ball K, Salmon J. Sedentary behavior and depression among adults: a review. *Int J Behav Med*. 2010. doi:10.1007/s12529-010-9075-z.

233 Deslandes A, Moraes H, Ferreira C, et al. Exercise and mental health: many reasons to move. *Neuropsychobiology*. 2009. doi:10.1159/000223730.

234 Reddy AB, O'Neill JS. Healthy clocks, healthy body, healthy mind. *Trends Cell Biol*. 2010. doi:10.1016/j.tcb.2009.10.005.

235 Knutsson A. Health disorders of shift workers. *Occup Med*. 2003. doi:10.1093/occmed/kqg048.

236 Anderson KN, Bradley AJ. Sleep disturbance in mental health problems and neurodegenerative disease. *Nat Sci Sleep*. 2013. doi:10.2147/NSS.S34842.

237 Koopman FA, Chavan SS, Miljko S, et al. Vagus nerve stimulation inhibits cytokine production and attenuates disease severity in rheumatoid arthritis. *Proc Natl Acad Sci*. 2016. doi:10.1073/pnas.1605635113.

238 Tracey KJ. The inflammatory reflex. *Nature*. 2002. doi:10.1038/nature01321.

239 Ma X, Yue ZQ, Gong ZQ, et al. The effect of diaphragmatic breathing on attention, negative affect and stress in healthy adults. *Front Psychol*. 2017. doi:10.3389/fpsyg.2017.00874.

240 Evans JA, Johnson EJ. The role of phytonutrients in skin health. *Nutrients*. 2010. doi:10.3390/nu2080903.

241 D'Orazio J, Jarrett S, Amaro-Ortiz A, Scott T. UV radiation and the skin. *Int J Mol Sci*. 2013. doi:10.3390/ijms140612222.

242 Grether-Beck S, Marini A, Jaenicke T, Stahl W, Krutmann J. Molecular evidence that oral supplementation with lycopene or lutein protects human skin against ultraviolet radiation: results from a double-blinded, placebo-controlled, crossover study. *Br J Dermatol*. 2017. doi:10.1111/bjd.15080.

243 Aust O, Stahl W, Sies H, Tronnier H, Heinrich U. Supplementation with tomato-based products increases lycopene, phytofluene, and phytoene levels in human serum and protects against UV-light-induced erythema. *Int J Vitam Nutr Res*. 2005. doi:10.1024/0300-9831.75.1.54.

244 Matsumura Y, Ananthaswamy HN. Toxic effects of ultraviolet radiation on the skin. *Toxicol Appl Pharmacol*. 2004. doi:10.1016/j.taap.2003.08.019.

245 Stahl W, Sies H. Carotenoids and flavonoids contribute to nutritional protection against skin damage from sunlight. *Mol Biotechnol*. 2007. doi:10.1007/s12033-007-0051-z.

246 Gollnick HPM, Hopfenmüller W, Hemmes C, et al. Systemic beta carotene plus topical UV-sunscreen are an optimal protection against harmful effects of natural UV-sunlight: results of the Berlin-Eilath study. *Eur J Dermatology*. 1996. doi:10.1556/AAlim.2015.0002.

247 Nicolaou A. Eicosanoids in skin inflammation. *Prostaglandins Leukot Essent Fat Acids*. 2013. doi:10.1016/j.plefa.2012.03.009.

248 Calder PC. Omega-3 fatty acids and inflammatory processes. *Nutrients*. 2010. doi:10.3390/nu2030355.

249 Cordain L, Lindeberg S, Hurtado M, Hill K, Eaton SB, Brand-Miller J. Acne vulgaris: a disease of Western civilization. *Arch Dermatol*. 2002. doi:10.1001/archderm.138.12.1584.

250 Danby FW. Nutrition and acne. *Clin Dermatol*. 2010. doi:10.1016/j.clindermatol.2010.03.017.

251 Thappa D, Kaimal S. Diet in dermatology: revisited. *Indian J Dermatology, Venereol Leprol*. 2010. doi:10.4103/0378-6323.60540.

252 Skroza N, Tolino E, Proietti I, et al. Mediterranean diet and familial dysmetabolism as factors influencing the development of acne. *Scand J Public Health*. 2012. doi:10.1177/1403494812454235.

253 Sies H, Stahl W. Nutritional protection against skin damage from sunlight. *Annu Rev Nutr*. 2004. doi:10.1146/annurev.nutr.24.012003.132320.

254 Souyoul SA, Saussy KP, Lupo MP. Nutraceuticals: a review. *Dermatol Ther (Heidelb)*. 2018. doi:10.1007/s13555-018-0221-x.

255 Stratton SP, Liebler DC. Determination of singlet oxygen-specific versus radical-mediated lipid peroxidation in photosensitized oxidation of lipid bilayers: effect of -carotene and -tocopherol. *Biochemistry*. 1997. doi:10.1021/bi9708646.

256 Fiedor J, Burda K. Potential role of carotenoids as antioxidants in human health and disease. *Nutrients*. 2014. doi:10.3390/nu6020466.

257 Philips N, Auler S, Hugo R, Gonzalez S. Beneficial regulation of matrix metalloproteinases for skin health. *Enzyme Res*. 2011. doi:10.4061/2011/427285.

258 Pickart L. The human tri-peptide GHK and tissue remodeling. *J Biomater Sci Polym Ed*. 2008. doi:10.1163/156856208784909435.

259 Pinnell SR. Cutaneous photodamage, oxidative stress, and topical antioxidant protection. *J Am Acad Dermatol*. 2003. doi:10.1067/mjd.2003.16.

260 Boelsma E, Hendriks HF, Roza L. Nutritional skin care: health effects of micronutrients and fatty acids. *Am J Clin Nutr*. 2001. doi:10.1093/ajcn/73.5.853.

261 Yan D, Issa N, Afifi L, Jeon C, Chang H-W, Liao W. The role of the skin and gut microbiome in psoriatic disease. *Curr Dermatol Rep*. 2017. doi:10.1007/s13671-017-0178-5.

262 Zeeuwen PLJM, Kleerebezem M, Timmerman HM, Schalkwijk J. Microbiome and skin diseases. *Curr Opin Allergy Clin Immunol*. 2013. doi:10.1097/ACI.0b013e328364ebeb.

263 Hall JMF, Cruser D, Podawiltz A, Mummert DI, Jones H, Mummert ME. Psychological stress and the cutaneous immune response: roles of the HPA Axis and the sympathetic nervous system in atopic dermatitis and psoriasis. *Dermatol Res Pract*. 2012. doi:10.1155/2012/403908.

264 Suárez AL, Feramisco JD, Koo J, Steinhoff M. Psychoneuro-immunology of psychological stress and atopic dermatitis: pathophysiologic and therapeutic updates. *Acta Derm Venereol*. 2012. doi:10.2340/00015555-1188.

265 Langan SM, Williams HC. What causes worsening of eczema? A systematic review. *Br J Dermatol*. 2006. doi:10.1111/j.1365-2133.2006.07381.x.

266 Altemus M, Rao B, Dhabhar FS, Ding W, Granstein RD. Stress-induced changes in skin barrier function in healthy women. *J Invest Dermatol*. 2001. doi:10.1046/j.1523-1747.2001.01373.x.

267 Christen WG, Glynn RJ, Ajani UA, et al. Smoking cessation and risk of age-related cataract in men. *JAMA*. 2000. doi:10.1001/jama.284.6.713.

268 Finkel T, Holbrook NJ. Oxidants, oxidative stress and the biology of ageing. *Nature*. 2000. doi:10.1038/35041687.

269 Thiagarajan R, Manikandan R. Antioxidants and cataract. *Free Radic Res*. 2013. doi:10.3109/10715762.2013.777155.

270 Mathew MC, Ervin A-M, Tao J, Davis RM. Antioxidant vitamin supplementation for preventing and slowing the progression of age-related cataract. *Cochrane Database Syst Rev*. 2012. doi:10.1002/14651858.CD004567.pub2.

271 Gritz DC, Srinivasan M, Smith SD, et al. The Antioxidants in Prevention of Cataracts Study: effects of antioxidant supplements on cataract progression in South India. *Br J Ophthalmol*. 2006. doi:10.1136/bjo.2005.088104.

272 Rautiainen S, Lindblad BE, Morgenstern R, Wolk A. Total antioxidant capacity of the diet and risk of age-related cataract: A population-based prospective cohort of women. *JAMA Ophthalmol*. 2014;132(3):247-252. doi:10.1001/jamaophthalmol.2013.6241.

273 Kaur A, Gupta V, Christopher AF, Malik MA, Bansal P. Nutraceuticals in prevention of cataract: an evidence based approach. *Saudi J Ophthalmol*. 2017. doi:10.1016/j.sjopt.2016.12.001.

274 Reidy A, Minassian DC, Vafidis G, et al. Prevalence of serious eye disease and visual impairment in a north London population: population based, cross sectional study. *BMJ*. 1998. doi:10.1136/bmj.316.7145.1643.

275 Simkiss P, Dennison C, Edwards E, et al. *The State of the Nation Eye Health 2016*. RNIB. 2016.

276 Eye TA, Study D. Lutein + zeaxanthin and omega-3 fatty acids for age-related macular degeneration. *JAMA*. 2013. https://jamanetwork.com/journals/jama/fullarticle/1684847.

277 AREDS Research Group. A randomized, placebo-controlled, clinical trial of high-dose supplementation with vitamins C and E, beta carotene, and zinc for age-related macular degeneration and vision loss: AREDS report no. 8. *Arch Ophthalmol*. 1960/2001. doi:10.1016/j.bbi.2008.05.010.

278 Mozaffarieh M, Sacu S, Wedrich A. The role of the carote-noids, lutein and zeaxanthin, in protecting against age-related macular degeneration: a review based on controversial evidence. *Nutr J*. 2003. doi:10.1186/1475-2891-2-20.

279 Klein BEK, Klein R. Lifestyle exposures and eye diseases in adults. *Am J Ophthalmol*. 2007. doi:10.1016/j.ajo.2007.08.016.

280 Hogg R, Chakravarthy U. AMD and micronutrient antioxidants. *Curr Eye Res*. 2004. doi:10.1080/02713680490517890.

281 Krinsky NI, Landrum JT, Bone RA. Biologic mechanisms of the protective role of lutein and zeaxanthin in the eye. *Annu Rev Nutr*. 2003. doi:10.1146/annurev.nutr.23.011702.073307.

282 Wu PC, Huang HM, Yu HJ, Fang PC, Chen CT. Epidemiology of myopia. *Asia-Pacific J Ophthalmol*. 2016. doi:10.1097/APO.0000000000000236.

283 Williams KM, Bertelsen G, Cumberland P, et al. Increasing prevalence of myopia in europe and the impact of education. *Ophthalmology*. 2015. doi:10.1016/j.ophtha.2015.03.018.

284 Pan CW, Ramamurthy D, Saw SM. Worldwide prevalence and risk factors for myopia. *Ophthalmic Physiol Opt*. 2012. doi:10.1111/j.1475-1313.2011.00884.x.

285 Cordain L, Eaton SB, Brand Miller J, Lindeberg S, Jensen C. An evolutionary analysis of the aetiology and pathogenesis of juvenile-onset myopia. *Acta Ophthalmol Scand*. 2002. doi:10.1034/j.1600-0420.2002.800203.x.

286 Goldschmidt E, Jacobsen N. Genetic and environmental effects on myopia development and progression. *Eye (Lond)*. 2014. doi:10.1038/eye.2013.254.

287 Rasmussen HM, Johnson EJ. Nutrients for the aging eye. *Clin Interv Aging*. 2013. doi:10.2147/CIA.S45399.

288 Kalt W, Hanneken A, Milbury P, Tremblay F. Recent research on polyphenolics in vision and eye health. *J Agric Food Chem*. 2010. doi:10.1021/jf903038r.

289 Eisenhauer B, Natoli S, Liew G, Flood VM. Lutein and zeaxanthin: food sources, bioavailability and dietary variety in age-related macular degeneration protection. *Nutrients*. 2017. doi:10.3390/nu9020120.

290 Ganea E, Harding JJ. Glutathione-related enzymes and the eye. *Curr Eye Res*. 2006. doi:10.1080/02713680500477347.

291 Ghavami A, Coward WA, Bluck LJC. The effect of food preparation on the bioavailability of carotenoids from carrots using intrinsic labelling. *Br J Nutr*. 2012. doi:10.1017/S0007 11451100451X.

292 Pärssinen O. The increased prevalence of myopia in Finland. *Acta Ophthalmol*. 2012. doi:10.1111/j.1755-3768.2011 .02210.x.

293 Rose KA, Morgan IG, Ip J, et al. Outdoor activity reduces the prevalence of myopia in children. *Ophthalmology*. 2008. doi:10.1016/j.ophtha.2007.12.019.

294 Charman WN. Myopia, posture and the visual environment. *Ophthalmic Physiol Opt*. 2011. doi:10.1111/j.1475-1313.2011 .00825.x.

295 Sherwin JC, Reacher MH, Keogh RH, Khawaja AP, Mackey DA, Foster PJ. The association between time spent outdoors and myopia in children and adolescents: a systematic review and meta-analysis. *Ophthalmology*. 2012. doi:10.1016/j .ophtha.2012.04.020.

INDEX

acne 90–1, 93
adaptogens 18, 78–9
adipose tissue *see* body fat
advanced glycemic end products
    (AGEs) 26
aerobic exercise 57
aging: cataracts 99
    immune system 57
    skin 87–8
    telomeres 70
alcohol 78, 81–2, 99, 100
algae oil 26
almonds 28, 55, 93
    almond and hazelnut lentils 147
    candied almonds with spiced
        strawberries 234
amino acids 17, 79–80
anthocyanins 27, 42, 67, 104
antioxidants: and brain 14, 17, 18
    and cancer prevention 64–6, 67
    and eyes 99–101, 103–4
    gut microbes and 40
    and heart 26, 27
    and inflammation 42
    and skin 88, 93
anxiety *see* mood disorders
apoptosis 67
apples 41, 42, 68
    chicken thighs with red onion, apple,
        and chestnuts 190
apricots: baked rainbow chard with apricot
        and walnuts 151
    roasted apricots with cardamom and
        lime 235
AREDS formulation 100–1
arteries 23, 25
arthritis 41, 45
artichokes 42, 94

one-pan Greek breakfast 119
    see also Jerusalem artichokes
arugula 16, 41, 68
ashwaganda 18, 78–9
Asian-style lettuce wraps 214
asparagus: spring asparagus and pea
        scallops 133
asthma 53
atherosclerosis 23
autoimmune conditions 53–4, 59, 75, 94
avocado oil 28
avocados 78
    avocado salsa 210
    mint and red cabbage salad 181
    one-pan Cajun scramble 119

bacteria: in gut 16, 27, 40, 50–3, 67, 76,
        79, 94
    and immune system 49
    and inflammation 35
    and mood disorders 76
    probiotics 40, 79
balsamic croutons 148
bananas: banana berry scoops 238
    coconut bananas with maple cream 232
barley 17
    split green pea and pearl barley pan 223
basil 18
    basil dressing 217
    red pesto 186
beans 27, 42, 54, 68, 79, 93, 103
    see also butter beans, flageolet
        beans, etc.
bean sprouts: Asian-style lettuce
        wraps 214
    citrus and pineapple Asian salad 142
    5-spice sticky eggplant bake 175
    spicy peanut and lime stir-fry 172

beets 27, 33, 64, 78, 93
    poke bowl 211
    spinach and sorrel borscht 161
Bengali-style cod 228
berbere curry 213
berries 17, 27, 42, 67, 104
    banana berry scoops 238
    glazed peaches with thyme 241
    see also blackberries, strawberries, etc.
beta-carotene 88, 93, 103–4
betalains 27
black beans 42
    black bean goulash 167
    Cajun corn bites 141
    one-pan Cajun scramble 119
    umami mushroom tacos 210
blackberries 67, 104
    orange-zest chocolate bark with
        berries 237
Blackburn, Dr. Elizabeth 70
blindness 100, 104
blood-brain barrier 14, 75
blood pressure *see* high blood pressure
blood sugar levels 30, 40, 66, 76, 91,
        99, 103
blood vessels 23, 25, 26, 30
blueberries 67, 104
body fat: excess 38–40
    exercise and 70
body mass index (BMI) 38, 70
bok choy 41
bone marrow 50
borlotti beans: one-pan spicy bean and
        mushroom breakfast 120
borscht, spinach and sorrel 161
box breathing 81
brain 12–21
    dementia 13

inflammation 14, 16
lifestyle 18–19
lymphatic system 19, 75–6
mental training and stimulation 18
mood disorders 74–85
neuroplasticity 13
stroke 13, 14, 23
brain-derived neurotrophic factor
(BDNF) 17
brassicas 41, 68, 104
Brazil nuts 55, 91, 93
bread 42, 78, 90, 110
balsamic croutons 148
flatbreads 208
rye croutons 220
breathing exercises 19, 30, 44, 57, 71,
81, 112
broad beans: celeriac and broad bean
rendang curry 229
crispy mushroom bowl 194
seasonal soup with red pesto 186
broccoli 26, 41, 55, 66, 68, 78, 93, 104
Ethiopian berbere curry 213
harissa beans and greens 164
pea orecchiette with purple sprouting
broccoli and hazelnuts 169
rendang stir-fry 162
sage eggplant and broccoli 134
Brussels sprouts 16, 26, 41, 55, 68, 104
buckwheat uttapam 200
burgers, Thai-style salmon 226
butter beans: butter beans, butternut
squash, and spicy couscous 165
Greek-style giant beans 154
harissa beans and greens 164
my best breakfast bowl 127
oats and butter bean breakfast 125
butternut squash see squash
butyrate 56

cabbage 68, 93, 104
chicken thighs with red onion, apple,
and chestnuts 190
rendang stir-fry 162
see also red cabbage
Cajun corn bites 141
Cajun marinade 210
Cajun scramble 119
Cajun sweet potato hash 116
cakes 42, 78, 110
calcium 23, 24, 27
cancer 62–73
antioxidants and 64–6
enzyme processes and 66
fiber and 66–9
genetic expression 66
and immune system 49
lifestyle and 69–71
and sleep 45, 59
candied almonds with spiced
strawberries 234
cannellini beans: Creole couscous with
white beans and parsley 166

carbohydrates 17
and acne 90
excess of sugar 78
and inflammation 14, 38, 42
cardiovascular disease 19, 23–4, 45,
50, 99
carotenoids 55, 93, 104, 105
carrots 42, 93, 104
black bean goulash 167
carrot and zucchini laksa 158
fennel and carrots with star anise 146
glazed Asian vegetable rice bowls 193
lemon, thyme, and hazelnut roast
vegetables 138
seasonal soup with red pesto 186
spicy peanut and lime stir-fry 172
thyme and ginger comfort soup 207
cashews 55
herby walnut and cashew roast 195
roast squash curry 216
Sri Lankan cashew curry 203
cataracts 99–100
catechins 69
cauliflower 66, 68
herby cauliflower steaks 145
cavolo nero 16, 27, 93
polenta and greens 153
celeriac and broad bean rendang curry 229
cells: brain cells 13
cancer cells 67, 68
and immune system 49
inflammation 35
mitochondria 54–5, 57, 80–1
nerve cells 17
telomeres 70
cereals 26, 42
chamomile tea 253
chard: baked rainbow chard with apricot
and walnuts 151
Creole couscous with white beans and
parsley 166
Greek-style giant beans 154
cherries 67
chestnuts: chicken thighs with red onion,
apple, and chestnuts 190
wild mushroom and herb frittata 124
chia seeds 69, 79
chicken: aromatic Vietnamese pho 199
chicken thighs with red onion, apple,
and chestnuts 190
coconut chicken with spicy peas and
potato 219
herbes de Provence chicken
skewers 217
chickpeas 27, 79, 91
crispy mushroom bowl 194
Spanish chickpea stew with roasted
peppers 170
Sri Lankan cashew curry 203
chicory 27, 56, 68, 79, 94
roast walnut and squash medley with
persillade 188
chilies: chili and lime fish skewers with

mint and red cabbage 181
chili melon relish 249
chocolate: banana berry scoops 238
orange-zest chocolate bark with
berries 237
cholesterol 28
chromosomes 70
chronic stress 18–19
chutney, coconut, and mint 200
cinnamon: rose cinnamon tea 253
circadian rhythm 30
citrus-ade, aromatic 250
citrus and pineapple Asian salad 142
citrus chamomile tea 253
citrus fruit 55, 104
see also grapefruit, lemons, limes, oranges
citrus mint and maple tea 253
cloves 42, 78
co-enzyme Q10 24, 66
coconut and mint chutney 200
coconut cream: banana berry
scoops 238
coconut bananas with maple
cream 232
coconut milk: coconut chicken with spicy
peas and potato 219
Ethiopian berbere curry 213
Sri Lankan cashew curry 203
cod: Bengali-style cod 228
cod bites with lemon and seaweed 176
coffee 94
collagen 93, 94
collard greens: jambalaya 204
color, rainbow diet 27, 33, 41–2, 55, 67,
78, 93, 103–4, 110
computers, screen breaks 105
cookies 27, 42, 78, 90
cooking techniques 109–10
copper 93
corn 17, 26
cortisol 44
couscous: butter beans, butternut squash
and spicy couscous 165
Creole couscous with white beans
and parsley 166
cravings 28
crayfish: watercress, walnut and
crayfish 121
Creole couscous with white beans and
parsley 166
Creole spice blend 245
croutons: balsamic croutons 148
rye croutons 220
cruciferous vegetables 67
cucumber: glazed Asian vegetable rice
bowls 193
speedy gazpacho 137
tzatziki 130
curcumin 18, 68
curry: celeriac and broad bean rendang
curry 229
Ethiopian berbere curry 213
okra and lentil curry 200

266

curry (continued)
 rendang curry paste 246
 rendang stir-fry 162
 roast squash curry 216
 Sri Lankan cashew curry 203
cycling 57

dairy products 90
dates: glazed peaches with thyme 241
dehydration 17–18, 23, 94
dementia 13
depression see mood disorders
dermatitis 88, 94
diabetes: and eyes 99, 103
 immune system and 50
 and inflammation 36
 Mediterranean diet and 14
 and mood disorders 75, 78
 and sleep 45, 59
digestive system: fiber and 67
 gut microbes 16, 27, 40, 50–3, 67, 76, 79, 94
 and immune system 50–3
 and mood disorders 76
 shift workers 30
DNA 24–5, 64, 66, 88, 93
Dr. Ornish Program for Reversing Heart Disease 30
dopamine 105
drinks: alcohol 78, 81–2, 99, 100
 aromatic citrus-ade 250
 fresh tea blends 253
 water 17–18, 94
dry skin 88

eating slowly 44
echinacea 56
eczema 53, 94
edamame beans: glazed Asian vegetable rice bowls 193
 poke bowl 211
eggplant: eggplant and walnut ragu 197
 5-spice sticky eggplant bake 175
 sage eggplant and broccoli 134
 spinach and vegetable lasagne 222
eggs 80
 Asian-style lettuce wraps 214
 Cajun sweet potato hash 116
 and eyes 104–5
 my best breakfast bowl 127
 one-pan Greek breakfast 119
 wild mushroom and herb frittata 124
elderberry 56
elimination diets 53–4
endive 56
endurance exercise 19, 57
energy: mitochondria 54, 80–1
 storage in body fat 38
enzyme processes 66
Epel, Dr. Elissa 70
epigallocatechin gallate 66
epigenetics 24
Ethiopian berbere curry 213

exercise 112
 and brain 19
 and cancer prevention 69–70
 and immune system 57
 and inflammation 44–5
 and mood disorders 80–1
eyes 98–107
 cataracts 99–100
 lifestyle 105
 myopia 103, 105
 retinal health 100–1

fat tissue see body fat
fats 110–11
 and eyes 104–5
 and heart health 23, 26–7, 28
 and inflammation 38, 41
 and mood disorders 78
 and skin 88
fatty acids see Omega-3 fats, Omega-6 fats
fennel 56
 black bean goulash 167
 fennel and carrots with star anise 146
 fennel, cumin, and mackerel salad 152
 fennel sardines with pine nuts 180
 radicchio, peach, and fennel salad 148
 seasonal soup with red pesto 186
fiber 111
 and cancer prevention 66–9
 and eyes 103
 in grains 17
 green vegetables 16
 and heart health 27
 and immune system 56
 and inflammation 42
 and mood disorders 79
 and skin 91, 94
"fight or flight" system 28
fish see monkfish, oily fish, salmon, etc.
5-spice sticky eggplant bake 175
flageolet beans: spring asparagus and pea scallops 133
flatbreads 208
flavonoids 42, 104
flavonols 55, 69, 104–5
flaxseeds 55, 69, 104–5
folate 79
food synergy 18
forest bathing 45, 112
free radicals 93, 94, 95, 100–1
French beans: celeriac and broad bean rendang curry 229
fried foods 27, 78
frittata, wild mushroom and herb 124
fruit: and cancer prevention 64
 colored fruit 27
 and eyes 100
 and heart 23
 polyphenols 14
 and skin 88
 see also apples, berries, strawberries, etc.

garlic 27, 56, 67, 68, 79, 104

gazpacho, speedy 137
genetics 24–5, 44, 57, 66, 70, 71
ginger 56, 67, 68
 lemon and ginger matcha tea 253
 thyme and ginger comfort soup 207
gingerols 68
gingko 18
glucose, and brain 17
glucosinolates 68
glutathione 104
gluten 54
glycemic index (GI) foods 42
goulash, black bean 167
grains 17, 42, 66, 80, 93
grapefruit 104
 aromatic citrus-ade 250
grapes 27
Greek skewers with tzatziki 130
Greek-style giant beans 154
green tea 66, 69
green vegetables: and brain 16
 and cancer prevention 68
 and eyes 104
 and heart health 24, 26, 27
 heirloom tomatoes, horta, and mackerel 182
 and immune system 55
 and inflammation 41
 and skin 93
 see also chard, spinach, etc.
"grey matter" 18
grounding techniques 81
guava 67
gut see digestive system

harissa beans and greens 164
hazelnuts: almond and hazelnut lentils 147
 glazed peaches with thyme 241
heart 14, 22–33
 heart attack 23
 lifestyle and 28–31
 and mood disorders 75
 muscles 23, 24
 and sleep 59
heirloom tomatoes, horta, and mackerel 182
herbes de Provence chicken skewers 217
herbs: and brain 18
 and cancer prevention 68
 and immune system 56
 and mood disorders 78–9
 see also mint, parsley, etc.
high blood pressure: and eyes 99, 100
 and inflammation 36
 Mediterranean diet and 23, 26
 oxidative stress and 25, 26
 sleep deprivation and 28
high-intensity interval training (HIIT) 19, 57, 80–1
hormones: and acne 90
 exercise and 70, 80

and mood disorders 76
and sleep 45
stress hormones 28, 30, 44, 57
horta 182
hydration 17–18, 94

immune system 48–61
autoimmune conditions 53–4, 59, 75, 94
and digestive system 50–3
inflammation 35
lifestyle 56–9
mitochondria 54–5
and stress 30
immunosenescence 57
indole-3-carbinol 26, 41, 66
inflammation 34–47
and brain 14, 16
and cancer 64
and heart disease 25–6, 27
lifestyle 44–5
and mood disorders 75–6
Omega-6 fats and 26
skin 88
and sleep 45, 59
triggers 36–8
inflammatory bowel disease 94
insulin 66, 90, 103
insulin resistance 36

jambalaya 204
Jerusalem artichokes 56, 79

kale 41, 55, 93, 104
Cajun sweet potato hash 116
kimchi 79

laksa: carrot and zucchini laksa 158
Malaysian laksa paste 246
large intestine 50
lasagne, spinach and vegetable 222
lectins 54
leeks 27, 68, 94
black bean goulash 167
jambalaya 204
legumes 27, 68, 91
lemons 104
aromatic citrus-ade 250
lemon and ginger matcha tea 253
lemon, thyme, and hazelnut roast
vegetables 138
parsley and lemon dressing 220
lentils 24, 27, 42, 79, 103
almond and hazelnut lentils 147
eggplant and walnut ragu 197
jambalaya 204
okra and lentil curry 200
lettuce wraps, Asian-style 214
lifestyle 111–13
brain 18–19
cancer 69–71
eyes 105
heart 28–31
immune system 56–9

inflammation 44–5
mood disorders 80–2
skin 94–5
light see sunlight
limes: citrus mint and maple tea 253
liver: micronutrients 66
shift workers 30
stress hormones and 30
vitamin A content 55
lutein 93, 100, 101, 104
lycopene 67, 93
lymph nodes 50
lymphatic system, in brain 19, 75–6
Lyon Heart Study 24

maca root 78–9
macadamia nuts 41
mackerel 79
fennel, cumin, and mackerel
salad 152
heirloom tomatoes, horta, and
mackerel 182
macular degeneration 100–1, 104
magnesium 23, 24, 26, 55, 66
Malaysian laksa paste 246
mangoes 93
maple syrup: coconut bananas with
maple cream 232
masala marinade 216
matcha tea, lemon and ginger 253
mealtimes 30–1, 111
meditation 112
and the brain 18, 19
and cancer risk 71
and heart health 30
and immune system 57
and inflammation 44
and mood disorders 81
Mediterranean diet: and brain 14
and cancer prevention 64, 66
and heart health 23–4, 25
and inflammation 38
and oxidative stress 26
melatonin 45
melon: chili melon relish 249
memory 13
mental health see mood disorders
mental training 18
meta-inflammation 35–6
microbes, in gut 16, 27, 40, 50–3, 67,
76, 79, 94
micronutrients: and cancer prevention 66
and eyes 100
for heart health 23, 24, 26
and inflammation 42
and mood disorders 79
and skin 91, 93
milk 90
millet 17
mind-body interventions, and
inflammation 44
MIND diet 14–21
mindfulness 18, 57, 71, 81, 94–5, 112

minerals see calcium, micronutrients,
potassium, etc.
mint 18, 68
citrus mint and maple tea 253
coconut and mint chutney 200
mint and red cabbage salad 181
miso marinade 193
mitochondria 54–5, 57, 80–1
monkfish: chili and lime fish skewers
with mint and red cabbage 181
mood disorders 74–85
digestive system and 76
fats and 78
inflammation and 36, 75–6
lifestyle 80–2
movement see exercise
muscles, heart 23, 24
mushrooms 56, 66
crispy mushroom bowl 194
Greek skewers with tzatziki 130
my best breakfast bowl 127
oats and butter bean breakfast 125
one-pan spicy bean and mushroom
breakfast 120
roast walnut and squash medley with
persillade 188
spinach and vegetable lasagne 222
sunflower sprouts with caraway and
porcini mushrooms 173
umami mushroom tacos 210
watercress, walnut, and crayfish 121
wild mushroom and herb frittata 124
mussels in parsley and lemon
dressing 220
my best breakfast bowl 127
myopia 103, 105

National Cancer Institute 67
natural light see sunlight
neural synapses 13
neuroplasticity 13
neurotransmitters 17, 76, 79
neurotrophic factors 19
night-shift workers 30
noodles: aromatic Vietnamese pho 199
carrot and zucchini laksa 158
rendang stir-fry 162
vibrant Malay salad 225
nutraceuticals 18
nutrient deficiencies 35
nutrigenetics 24–5
nutrigenomics 24–5, 66
nuts: and brain 16–17
and cancer prevention 66, 68
and heart health 26–7
and immune system 55–6
and inflammation 38, 41
and skin 88, 91, 93
see also almonds, cashews, etc.

oats 17, 79
herby walnut and cashew roast 195
oats and butter bean breakfast 125

268 oats (continued)
    pimenton oats with poached salmon 122
    Sri Lankan–style oats 135
obesity 45, 70, 78, 82
oils 23, 28
    see also olive oil
oily fish: and brain 16–17
    and cancer prevention 69
    and heart health 26, 28
    and inflammation 41
    and mood disorders 79
    and skin 88, 91, 93
    vitamin A 55
okra and lentil curry 200
olive oil: and brain 16
    and cancer prevention 69
    and heart health 26, 27, 28
    and inflammation 41
    and mood disorders 79
olives: one-pan Greek breakfast 119
    tapenade 194
Omega-3 fats: and brain 16–17
    and cancer prevention 69
    and eyes 105
    and heart health 26–7
    and inflammation 35, 41
    and mood disorders 78, 79
    and skin 88, 91
Omega-6 fats 26–7
omelettes: Asian-style lettuce
    wraps 214
one-pan Cajun scramble 119
one-pan Greek breakfast 119
one-pan spicy bean and mushroom
    breakfast 120
onions 27, 42, 67, 68, 104
    chicken thighs with red onion, apple,
    and chestnuts 190
orange foods 55, 93
oranges 104
    aromatic citrus-ade 250
    orange-zest chocolate bark with
    berries 237
oregano 18
organ meats 55
Ornish, Dr. Dean 71
osteoarthritis 42
oxidative stress: and brain 14, 18
    and cancer 64, 67, 69
    and eyes 100–1
    green vegetables and 41
    gut microbes and 40
    and heart disease 25–6, 30
    and skin 93
painkillers 41
pancakes: buckwheat uttapam 200
pancreas 30
papaya 88, 93
parsley 26, 55, 78, 100, 104
    parsley and lemon dressing 220
    persillade 188
parsnips: lemon, thyme, and hazelnut roast
    vegetables 138

parsnip and butternut squash 208
pasta 42, 78, 90, 110
    pea orecchiette with purple sprouting
    broccoli and hazelnuts 169
    spinach and vegetable lasagne 222
peaches 68
    glazed peaches with thyme 241
    radicchio, peach, and fennel salad 148
peanut dressing 172
pearl barley: split green pea and pearl
    barley pan 223
peas 41, 79, 93
    coconut chicken with spicy peas and
    potato 219
    5-spice sticky eggplant bake 175
    pea orecchiette with purple sprouting
    broccoli and hazelnuts 169
    pimenton oats with poached
    salmon 122
    polenta and greens 153
    spring asparagus and pea scallops 133
    sunflower sprouts with caraway and
    porcini mushrooms 173
    watercress, walnut, and crayfish 121
pecans 26
    banana berry scoops 238
Penny Brohn UK, Bristol 71
peppermint 56
peppers 64, 100, 103–4
    Asian-style lettuce wraps 214
    black bean goulash 167
    citrus and pineapple Asian salad 142
    Creole couscous with white beans and
    parsley 166
    5-spice sticky eggplant bake 175
    Greek skewers with tzatziki 130
    jambalaya 204
    red pesto 186
    roast walnut and squash medley with
    persillade 188
    roasted red pepper salsa 249
    Spanish chickpea stew with roasted
    peppers 170
persillade 188
pesto, red 186
pho, aromatic Vietnamese 199
phytochemicals 18, 26, 27, 42, 68, 78, 93
phytonutrients 16, 88
pickle, quick 193
pimenton oats with poached salmon 122
pine nuts, fennel sardines with 180
pineapple: citrus and pineapple Asian
    salad 142
pistachios 28, 104–5
    orange-zest chocolate bark with
    berries 237
plaque formation, and inflammation 26
poke bowl 211
polenta and greens 153
pollution 49, 68
polyphenols 14, 17, 41, 67, 69
polyunsaturated fats 93–4
pomegranate 104

porcini mushrooms, sunflower sprouts
    with caraway and 173
potassium 23, 24, 27
potatoes 42
    cod bites with lemon and seaweed 176
    fennel sardines with pine nuts 180
    spinach and sorrel borscht 161
    thyme and ginger comfort soup 207
prebiotic fibers 56, 79
PREDIMED studies 24
probiotics 40, 56, 79
processed foods 14, 38, 78, 103,
    109–10
prostate cancer 67, 71
protein 17, 38, 79–80
psoriasis 42, 53, 88, 94
psychobiotics 76
psychogenic environment 82
pulses 27, 66, 79, 103
pumpkin 103–4
pumpkin seeds 41, 80, 91
purple sprouting broccoli 78
    pea orecchiette with purple sprouting
    broccoli and hazelnuts 169

qigong 57
quercetin 17, 26, 68
quinoa 17, 80
    sweet Cajun salmon 179

radicchio, peach, and fennel salad 148
radishes 64
    glazed Asian vegetable rice bowls 193
rainbow diet 27, 33, 41–2, 55, 67, 78,
    93, 103–4, 110
rapeseed oil 28
ras el hanout 245
reactive oxidative species (ROS) 88
red cabbage 27, 42
    mint and red cabbage salad 181
red foods 42, 67, 93, 103–4
relaxation techniques 44
relish, chili melon 249
rendang curry paste 246
rendang stir-fry 162
resveratrol 17
retina 99, 100–1, 105
rheumatoid arthritis 42, 53, 75
rice 42, 80
    Bengali-style cod 228
    Ethiopian berbere curry 213
    glazed Asian vegetable rice bowls 193
    jambalaya 204
    poke bowl 211
    red rice 17
    spicy peanut and lime stir-fry 172
root vegetables 93
rose cinnamon tea 253
rosemary 18, 78, 79
Rupy's ras el hanout 245
rutabaga: lemon, thyme, and hazelnut
    roast vegetables 138
rye croutons 220

sage eggplant and broccoli 134
salads: citrus and pineapple Asian
        salad 142
    fennel, cumin, and mackerel salad 152
    mint and red cabbage salad 181
    radicchio, peach, and fennel salad 148
    vibrant Malay salad 225
salmon: pimenton oats with poached
        salmon 122
    sweet Cajun salmon 179
    Thai-style salmon burgers 226
salsas: avocado salsa 210
    roasted red pepper salsa 249
salt 14
sardines: fennel sardines with pine nuts 180
saturated fats 28
sauerkraut 79
scallops: spring asparagus and pea
        scallops 133
screen breaks, eye health 105
seasonal soup with red pesto 186
seaweed, cod bites with lemon and 176
seeds: and brain 16–17
    and cancer prevention 66, 68
    and heart health 26–7, 28
    and immune system 55–6
    and inflammation 38
    and skin 88, 91
    see also flaxseeds, sunflower seeds, etc.
selenium 26, 55, 69, 79, 91, 93
sesame seeds 27
shift workers 30
shinrin yoku 45
shortsightedness 103, 105
sight see eyes
skewers: Greek skewers 130
    herbes de Provence chicken
        skewers 217
skin 86–97
    acne 90–1, 93
    aging 87–8
    inflammation 88
    and lifestyle 94–5
    wrinkles 93
sleep 111
    and brain 19
    and heart health 28–30
    and immune system 59
    and inflammation 45
    and mood disorders 81
    and skin 95
slow eating 44
smoking 25, 99, 100
snacks 27, 31
snow peas: Ethiopian berbere curry 213
    5-spice sticky eggplant bake 175
    spicy peanut and lime stir-fry 172
soft drinks 78
sorrel: spinach and sorrel borscht 161
soups: aromatic Vietnamese pho 199
    carrot and zucchini laksa 158
    seasonal soup with red pesto 186
    speedy gazpacho 137

spinach and sorrel borscht 161
    thyme and ginger comfort soup 207
soy oils 26
Spanish chickpea stew 170
spice blends: Creole spice blend 245
    Malaysian laksa paste 246
    rendang curry paste 246
    Rupy's ras el hanout 245
spices 18, 42–4, 56, 68, 78–9
spinach 16, 66, 78, 104
    coconut chicken with spicy peas
        and potato 219
    fennel sardines with pine nuts 180
    my best breakfast bowl 127
    one-pan Greek breakfast 119
    one-pan spicy bean and mushroom
        breakfast 120
    spicy peanut and lime stir-fry 172
    spinach and sorrel borscht 161
    spinach and vegetable lasagne 222
    Sri Lankan cashew curry 203
    thyme and ginger comfort soup 207
spleen 50
split peas 42
    split green pea and pearl barley
        pan 223
spring asparagus, peas, and scallops 133
spring greens 27, 55, 93, 104
sprouts see Brussels sprouts
square breathing 81
squash 24, 41, 55, 64, 88, 93
    butter beans, butternut squash, and
        spicy couscous 165
    parsnip and butternut squash 208
    poke bowl 211
    roast walnut and squash medley with
        persillade 188
    roast squash curry 216
Sri Lankan cashew curry 203
Sri Lankan–style oats 135
star anise 78
stew, Spanish chickpea 170
stimulation, brain 18
stir-fries: rendang stir-fry 162
    spicy peanut and lime stir-fry 172
strawberries 67
    candied almonds with spiced
        strawberries 234
stress: and cancer prevention 70–1
    chronic stress 18–19
    and heart health 30
    and mitochondria 54
    and skin 94–5
    stress hormones 28, 30, 44, 57
    see also oxidative stress
stroke 13, 14, 23
sugar: and acne 90
    excess of 78
    fiber and 66
    glycemic index (GI) foods 42
    and inflammation 14, 35, 38
    and mitochondria 54
    and myopia 103

and oxidative stress 26
    and whole grains 17
sugar snap peas: harissa beans
        and greens 164
sulforaphane 26, 41, 55, 66, 68
sun protection 87, 88
sunflower seeds 26, 41, 55, 78, 80, 93
    Cajun sweet potato hash 116
sunflower sprouts with caraway and porcini
        mushrooms 173
sunlight 112
    and eyes 105
    skin damage 49, 87–8
    and vitamin D 59
sweet corn: Cajun corn bites 141
    Cajun sweet potato hash 116
    Sri Lankan cashew curry 203
    sweet Cajun salmon 179
    umami mushroom tacos 210
sweet potatoes 55, 104
    Cajun sweet potato hash 116
    coconut chicken with spicy peas and
        potato 219
sweets 90
swimming 57
Swiss chard 27
    see also chard
synapses, neural 13

tacos, umami mushroom 210
tai chi 44, 57
tapenade 194
tea 66
    black aromatic tea 253
    black tea 94
    citrus chamomile tea 253
    citrus mint and maple tea 253
    green tea 69
    lemon and ginger matcha tea 253
    rose cinnamon tea 253
telomeres 70
tempeh: rendang stir-fry 162
Thai-style salmon burgers 226
thyme 68, 79
    thyme and ginger comfort soup 207
timing meals 30–1, 111
tofu 80
    Asian-style lettuce wraps 214
    Greek skewers with tzatziki 130
    one-pan Cajun scramble 119
    vibrant Malay salad 225
tomatoes 24, 67, 93
    almond and hazelnut lentils 147
    black bean goulash 167
    eggplant and walnut ragu 197
    Ethiopian berbere curry 213
    Greek-style giant beans 154
    heirloom tomatoes, horta, and
        mackerel 182
    herbes de Provence chicken skewers 217
    jambalaya 204
    mussels in parsley and lemon
        dressing 220

270   tomatoes (continued)
        okra and lentil curry 200
        one-pan Greek breakfast 119
        red pesto 186
        roasted red pepper salsa 249
        roast squash curry 216
        Spanish chickpea stew 170
        speedy gazpacho 137
        spinach and vegetable lasagne 222
tonsillitis 59
transcendental meditation 57
tuna: poke bowl 211
turmeric 42, 56, 67, 68, 78
turnips: lemon, thyme, and hazelnut
        roast vegetables 138
tzatziki 130

umami mushroom tacos 210
unsaturated fats 28
uttapam, buckwheat 200
UV light 87–8, 100

vegetables: and cancer prevention
        64, 67
        colored vegetables 27, 33, 41–2
        and eyes 100
        and heart 23–4
        polyphenols 14
        and skin 88, 93
        see also peppers, tomatoes, etc.

vegetarian diet 38
vibrant Malay salad 225
viruses 49
visceral fat 40
vision see eyes
vitamin A 55
vitamin B complex 17, 66
vitamin C 26, 55, 64–5, 93, 99, 101, 104
vitamin D 35, 59, 70
vitamin E 26, 55, 64, 69, 91, 99,
        101, 105
Voltaire 109

Walker, Matthew 45
walking 44–5, 57–9, 71
walnuts 26, 28, 41, 69, 78, 79
        baked rainbow chard with apricot
            and walnuts 151
        eggplant and walnut ragu 197
        herby walnut and cashew roast 195
        orange-zest chocolate bark with
            berries 237
        roast walnut and squash medley
            with persillade 188
        watercress, walnut, and crayfish 121
water, drinking 17–18, 94
watercress: herbes de Provence chicken
        skewers 217
        mussels in parsley and lemon
            dressing 220

sweet Cajun salmon 179
        watercress, walnut, and crayfish 121
watermelon 67
weight gain 45, 70, 78, 82
weight loss 38
wheat 26
white beans: Creole couscous with
        white beans and parsley 166
        white bean purée 145
white sauce 222
whole grains 17, 66, 80, 93
winter squash 55
workers, shift 30
wrinkles 93

yellow foods 55, 93, 103–4
yoga 19, 30, 44, 57, 59
yogurt 79
        tzatziki 130

zeaxanthin 100, 101, 104
zinc 55, 79, 91, 93
zucchini: carrot and zucchini
        laksa 158
        Greek skewers with tzatziki 130
        one-pan spicy bean and mushroom
            breakfast 120
        seasonal soup with red pesto 186
        spinach and vegetable lasagne 222

Acknowledgments

To my sister Jasmin, Mum, and Dad who have shaped my perspective on the world and of myself. Your unconditional love and support is what allows me to chase my ambitions. This would not be possible without you all by my side.

To my patients who teach me as much as I am able to help them. I'm humbled and grateful to have the opportunity to care for people in their most vulnerable state.

To my closest friends, whose messages and gestures of support over the last five years have kept me pushing The Doctor's Kitchen inch by inch. Your love and belief in the mission is what keeps me driving forward, and I cannot thank you all enough.

To my baby godsons Otis and Ike. I hope the work I do in my lifetime will positively impact your future environment, and I will always be there to support you.

To my publishing team at HarperCollins—especially Carolyn Thorne, Georgina Atsiaris, Lucy Sykes-Thompson, Isabel Prodger and Orlando Mowbray—and literary agent, Carly Cook, for their incredible support and vision. My work would not have reached the number of people it has thus far without you all, and I see a lot more work to do in the future to complete the mission. Many thanks also to my amazing photographic team—Faith Mason, Marina Filippelli, Kitty Cole, and Sarah Birks.

To Ash, David, and Dharmesh. You always seem to help me think of the bigger picture. Thank you for fueling my ambition; I'm just getting started.

To Nuwan, who graciously lent his time and opinion to the early drafts. I'm grateful to have had your backing and friendship for this many years, despite your appalling dress sense.

To the scientists in the field of nutritional research whose work forms the very backbone of The Doctor's Kitchen and why I can confidently prescribe and talk about food and lifestyle as medicine. You are the unsung heroes of a movement that should have started decades ago.

And finally, to all the health professionals transforming the way they practice and becoming the beacons of a movement that embraces lifestyle as medicine. Together we will revolutionize well-being and healthcare for the better.

About the Author

Dr. Rupy Aujla is a practicing General Practitioner in London. Trained at Imperial College London, he has been featured and appeared in *Men's Health, Huffington Post,* and more, and is a regular contributor to leading nutrition websites, including NutritionFacts.org.